# THE LONG DISTANCE RUNNER'S GUIDE TO INJURY PREVENTION AND TREATMENT

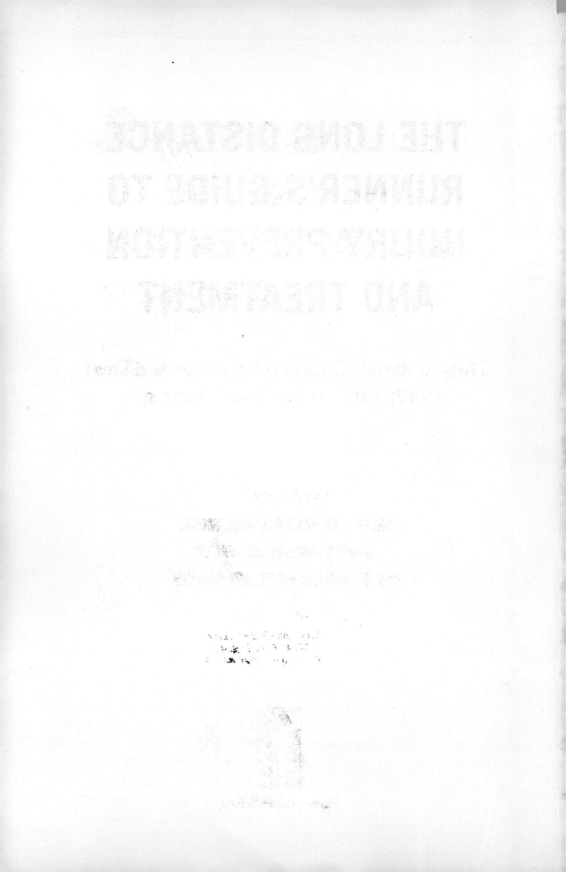

# THE LONG DISTANCE RUNNER'S GUIDE TO INJURY PREVENTION AND TREATMENT

## How to Avoid Common Problems and Deal with Them When They Happen

EDITED BY

BRIAN J. KRABAK, MD, MBA, FACSM

GRANT S. LIPMAN, MD, FACEP

AND BRANDEE L. WAITE, MD, FAAPMR

Skyhorse Publishing

Skyhorse Publishing books may be purchased in bulk at special discounts for sales promotion, corporate gifts, fund-raising, or educational purposes. Special editions can also be created to specifications. For details, contact the Special Sales Department, Skyhorse Publishing, 307 West 36th Street, 11th Floor, New York, NY 10018 or info@skyhorsepublishing.com.

Skyhorse® and Skyhorse Publishing® are registered trademarks of Skyhorse Publishing, Inc.®, a Delaware corporation.

Visit our website at www.skyhorsepublishing.com.

10 9 8 7 6 5 4 3 2 1

Library of Congress Cataloging-in-Publication Data is available on file.

Cover design by Tom Lau
Cover photo credit: XEMPower/Zandy Mangold

Print ISBN: 978-1-5107-1790-9
Ebook ISBN: 978-1-5107-1793-0

Printed in China

# Table of Contents

# FOREWORD

Some might consider me an unlikely candidate to write the foreword for this book. Why? Because in my decades of marathon and ultramarathon running I've never suffered an injury (with the exception of a few lost toenails).

Of course, I am something of an outlier. Nearly three-quarters of all long distance runners will incur some form of an injury during their athletic career. This is the reality most runners face.

In my talks and travels to runners around the globe, one of the most common questions I field is how to treat these various anomalies. The clear-eyed truth is that I'm wholly unqualified to answer such questions. I've never experienced a medical issue from running myself—so I have no practical advice to offer—and I am not a trained medical professional. My typical response is to direct such inquires to the hodgepodge of disparate information available that deals with these topics, often in conflicting and inconsistent ways.

I've long searched for a single unifying resource that I could recommend in such instances, and *The Long Distance Runner's Guide to Injury Prevention and Treatment* is just that. Written by prominent leaders in sports science, as well as accomplished runners in their own right, the book offers guidance on important and diverse themes, like proper nutrition, muscular ailments, skeletal injuries, and medical illnesses caused by racing and proper recovery. This book contains valuable insights, tips, and strategies from more than two dozen medical professionals who specialize in treating endurance athletes, and this information is presented in a way that is understandable and actionable to everyday runners.

While it may be impossible to completely avoid injury, *The Long Distance Runner's Guide to Injury Prevention and Treatment* is an indispensable tool to help those who love to run understand some of the most common causes of injuries, and learn how to best avoid and treat athletic ailments. This book belongs on every runner's shelf and is destined to help all of us run healthier and happier in the miles ahead.

—Dean Karnazes, ultramarathoner and *The New York Times* best-selling author

# INTRODUCTION

Running is one of the most common modes of exercise utilized to promote overall health and well-being. It is not just a workout—running is part of our human fabric. As we evolved, our ancestral survival was predicated on the ability to run long distances. Running has been transformed into a leisure activity, as technological advancements have greatly impacted how and why we run. This is evident by the exponential increase in the number of people participating in running events over the past half-century. It is estimated that in the United States alone, over seventeen million people participated in a running event in 2016, with over five hundred thousand of those completing a marathon. Furthermore, there has been a dramatic increase in the number of endurance running events around the world, with a 10 percent annual increase over the last decade and over ninety thousand participants in ultramarathons last year.

As more athletes participate in long distance running, there is a great opportunity to understand the relationship of running to injury or illness. Studies suggest most runners will eventually sustain some type of injury or illness while training or competing. Hopefully, these injuries or illnesses will have a minimal impact both on time lost from running and the athlete's long-term health, especially considering that a sedentary lifestyle may contribute to significant health-related issues such as cardiovascular disease, obesity, and diabetes. Therefore, prevention, evaluation, and treatment of injuries and illnesses in the long distance runner require a comprehensive understanding of the complete athlete—an assessment that takes into consideration the physical, mental, emotional, and nutritional aspects of the individual athlete.

The aim of *The Long Distance Runner's Guide to Injury Prevention and Treatment* is to discuss the unique aspects of running-related injuries and illnesses potentially encountered by athletes in the unique environments where endurance running takes place, during both training and competition. This book represents a combination of scientific rigor and practical advice written by the leading experts in the fields of sports medicine, emergency medicine, nutrition, and wilderness medicine who provide medical care for these athletes around the world. It aims to educate athletes and health-care practitioners on how to recognize, manage, and treat these injuries and illnesses during long distance running, and how to optimize recovery.

We each have our own reasons to run, whether it's toward something, away from something, to prove something, or simply to do something. We hope that reading this book results in a greater understanding of the human condition for those who love to run, with improved health and education, that will hopefully translate into improved long distance running endeavors and accomplishments around the world. Enjoy the journey.

—Brian J. Krabak, MD, MBA, FACSM, Grant S. Lipman, MD, FACEP, FAWM, and Brandee L. Waite, MD, FAAPMR

# SECTION 1
# The Distance Running Athlete

## CHAPTER 1

# History of Distance Running

## BY DANIEL E. LIEBERMAN

## Key Points

1.  Both comparative and fossil evidence suggest that the first hominins (a species more closely related to today's humans than to chimpanzees) were bipedal but also retained many adaptations to climb trees. Bipedalism was probably initially favored, as it would have improved hominins' ability to walk efficiently, but also made them slower and less steady than their quadrupedal ancestors.

2.  Fossil and archaeological evidence indicates that selection for running probably occurred between two and three million years ago in the face of substantial climate change in Africa. By the time of *Homo erectus*, hominins were not only carnivores but also were effective long distance runners.

3.  Because bipedal hominins, our ancestors, were intrinsically slow, selection for running favored endurance over speed to enable persistence hunting. This form of hunting takes advantage of the human ability to keep cool through sweating while simultaneously running in hot temperatures at speeds that would make animals who cool by panting overheat. Over long distances and through a combination of running and walking as well as chasing and tracking, persistence hunters drive their prey into a state of heat exhaustion. Persistence hunting, which is still practiced, albeit rarely, must have been a major method of hunting before the invention of lethal projective weapons, which was less than 500,000 years ago.

4.  An evolutionary perspective suggests that although many people think distance running is unusual, it is actually abnormal to not run on a regular basis. However, the way in which people run today is unusual compared to the way our ancestors ran, potentially leading to several kinds of mismatches. In particular, many runners today typically run at faster speeds and for longer distances; they run on flat, hard surfaces; they wear cushioned shoes with elevated heels; and many people do not run in social contexts.

# Introduction

Most present-day humans spend an inordinate amount of time sitting, and mostly locomote (move around) by walking. Running is employed almost exclusively for sport or exercise, which is hardly surprising given its greater metabolic cost and higher likelihood of injury. According to some estimates, as many as 70 percent of distance runners get injured in a given year (1), and there are numerous accounts of endurance runners who destroy their joints, succumb to stress fractures, and incur other serious medical conditions. Further, despite overwhelming evidence that regular endurance physical activity is vital for promoting overall well-being, there are widespread concerns that excess running can be unhealthy (2). Anyone who has run a marathon has probably been reminded (incorrectly) that Pheidippides died after his legendary run from Marathon to Athens. Altogether, it is hardly surprising that many people today, including runners, question the notion that humans were born to run long distances.

Until recently, scientists have been equally skeptical that humans evolved to run long distances. Compared to other mammals, humans are slow, awkward runners and early studies of the human running economy incorrectly claimed that it, when adjusted for body size, was as inefficient as penguin locomotion (3). Prior to 2004, only two scientific papers had been published on the evolution of human running (4, 5), both of which highlighted how human runners, who cool by sweating, can drive prey animals, who cool by panting, into a state of heat exhaustion—a strategy known as persistence hunting. Two decades later, Bramble and Lieberman (6) integrated fossil, archaeological, ethnographic, physiological, and anatomical evidence to make the case that the ability to run long distances evolved in the genus *Homo* around two million years ago. Since then, numerous papers have been published to explore the hypothesis that natural selection favored adaptations for long distance running in the human genus. While a majority of these papers have supported the endurance running hypothesis, the role of running in human evolution still raises questions and engenders disagreement amongst scientists. To what extent was persistence hunting employed? How much are derived features that improve human running performance actual adaptations or simply by-products of adaptations that evolved for walking? If humans evolved to run, why do we get injured so much? And, most importantly, how can an evolutionary approach to running help prevent injury and improve performance?

In this chapter, I review what scientists do and don't know about the evolution of human running and consider the relevance of an evolutionary perspective on endurance running to contemporary human running. I first review the evidence that the evolution of walking was an important, contingent event that made possible later selection for endurance running. I then consider evidence for endurance running in the genus *Homo*, and how endurance running evolved through natural selection for hunting and scavenging. I conclude by considering how an evolutionary perspective on running in our ancient past is useful for thinking about running today, including the problem of injury prevention.

## How Walking Set the Stage for Running

Although running and walking are biomechanically very different, any discussion of the evolution of running needs to begin with the question of selection for bipedal walking. This is due to the fact that evolution is a contingent process in which natural selection acts on variations present in a population that resulted from previous evolutionary events. Therefore, it is not surprising that the unusual long distance running abilities of humans would never have evolved if hominins had not previously evolved to be slow, unsteady but efficient bipedal walkers.

To appreciate this argument, consider first that humans and chimpanzees are sister species, more closely related to each other than to gorillas (Figure 1-1). This is significant for reconstructing hominin locomotor evolution because chimpanzees and gorillas are remarkably similar to each other, and numerous studies demonstrate that their differences are primarily attributable to size—female and male chimpanzees average 30 and 50 kg, respectively, while female and male gorillas average 70 and 200 kg, respectively (7). That means that unless the two species' similarities evolved independently, which is improbable to the point of being impossible, then the Last Common Ancestor of gorillas, chimpanzees, and humans (LCAgch), as well as the LCA of chimpanzees and humans (LCAch), must have been very much like a chimpanzee or a gorilla (which amounts to nearly the same thing). One implication of this logic is that in terms of locomotion the LCAch was most likely a knuckle-walker. This peculiar form of locomotion, in which forelimb weight is borne by the middle phalanges of the hands that are flexed below the palms, facilitates quadrupedal locomotion in chimpanzees and gorillas, whose forelimbs are much longer than their hindlimbs (8). The disadvantage of knuckle-walking, however, is reduced energetic efficiency. The cost of transport (the energy spent moving a unit of body mass a given distance) in knuckle-walking chimpanzees (and presumably also gorillas) is approximately four times higher than in most other mammals, including humans (9, 10). Chimpanzees and gorillas, however, live in very resource-dense environments and walk little: gorillas travel less than 1 km/day, and chimpanzees travel 2–3 km/day (11, 12). It is therefore likely that the high metabolic cost of knuckle-walking

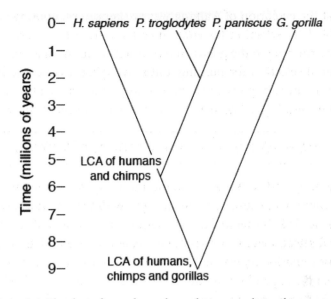

**Figure 1-1** The above figure shows the evolutionary relationships between humans and the African great apes. Although gorillas and chimpanzees are generally similar, with most of their differences the result of size, humans and chimpanzees are sister species (most closely related to each other). Consequently, the last common ancestor of chimpanzees and humans was probably chimpanzee-like and thus a knuckle-walker unless the many similarities between gorillas and chimpanzees evolved independently.

in these apes is outweighed by the benefits of having long arms and fingers that facilitate tree climbing.

Although species in the chimpanzee and gorilla lineages, including the LCAgch and the LCAch, were probably knuckle-walkers, climate change at the time the human and chimpanzee lineages split likely altered the cost-to-benefit ratio of knuckle-walking in the first hominins. Abundant evidence indicates that the world's climate at this time was cooling rapidly, causing rain forests in Africa to shrink and fractionate (13). Under such conditions, any apes, including the LCAch, living at the margins of the forest zone would almost certainly have needed to travel further on a daily basis in order to forage for sufficient fruit and other resources. In these more open environments, the high cost of transport of knuckle-walking would have become an increasing disadvantage, and would have favored selection for alternative, less costly forms of locomotion. In the case of hominins, that form of locomotion was evidently bipedalism, as documented by a range of anatomical features in all four of the oldest hominin fossil species so far known (Figure 1-2): *Sahelanthropus tchadensis* (ca. 6–7.2 Ma [million years ago]), *Orrorin tugenensis* (6 Ma), *Ardipithecus kadabba* (5.8–4.3 Ma), and

*Ardipithecus ramidus* (4.4 Ma). Although these species certainly did not walk like modern humans, they would have been able to save considerable energy during locomotion if they were able to walk with less flexed hips and knees than bipedal apes (14). Bipedalism may also have been a benefit for upright foraging on branches or the ground (15, 16). Either way, if the LCAch had not been a costly knuckle-walker, then bipedalism might never have evolved.

Although bipedalism must have been adaptive for the first hominins, habitually upright posture and locomotion does incur substantial costs that set the stage for the evolution of running. Most importantly, bipeds can produce power with only two legs rather than four, and thus the earliest hominins must have been about half as fast as their quadrupedal ancestors. In addition, running on two legs is intrinsically less stable than on four, seriously limiting agility during maneuvers such as rapid changes of direction and speed. Early hominins probably thus lost many of the high speed athletic capabilities that enable male chimpanzees to

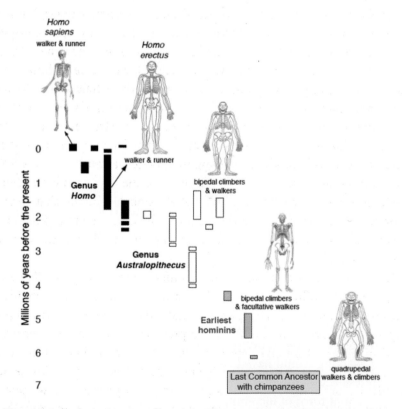

**Figure 1-2** Evolutionary tree of hominins showing major locomotor categories of the last common ancestor of humans and chimpanzees, the earliest hominins (genera *Sahelanthropus*, *Ardipithecus*, and *Orrorin*), the genus *Australopithecus*, and the genus *Homo*.

hunt colobus monkeys, and it is reasonable to hypothesize that their slow sprinting speeds made them more susceptible to predation. Regardless, early bipedal hominins survived in Africa and eventually gave rise to a radiation of a diverse group of species known as the australopiths (see Figure 1-2). These hominins, which were found in both East and South Africa and lasted from a little over four million years ago until about 1.2 million years ago, apparently experienced further selection to be effective bipedal walkers, probably enabling them to walk long distances to obtain underground storage organs such as tubers and roots (8, 17). Although australopith fossils have many adaptations for efficient striding gaits, many of the features they retained for arboreal locomotion such as long pedal phalanges and relatively short lower extremities would have compromised their ability to run (6, 18, 19).

## Origins of the Genus *Homo*

As noted above, natural selection is often driven by climate change, but is always contingent on prior events and the heritable variation present in a population. Just as selection for bipedalism in the earliest hominins was driven by climate change and was contingent on previous selection for knuckle-walking, selection for endurance running in the genus *Homo* appears to have been driven by yet more climate change and was contingent on the prior evolution of upright bipedalism.

Although many details about climate change in Africa and elsewhere over the last few million years are the subject of much ongoing research, it is clear that long-term trends of global cooling accelerated approximately 2.8 million years ago initiating the Ice Age, also referred to as the Pleistocene. Further, many independent lines of evidence indicate that Pleistocene climate change in Africa involved substantial aridification (increasingly dry), causing marginal rain forest habitats to become woodland and many former woodland areas to become open grassland habitats (20).

It is not surprising that these habitat shifts at the start of the Pleistocene in Africa apparently influenced the evolution of hominins, who probably struggled to survive in increasingly open, arid habitats. As patches of fruit and other high-quality plant resources that are the preferred foods of apes became more widely dispersed and smaller, selection most likely favored hominins who were better able to find and chew alternative resources. Two different kinds of selection evidently occurred at this time. One led to a group of new species, the robust australopiths (sometimes grouped in the genus *Paranthropus*), which became hyper-adapted to chewing tough, highly fibrous foods thanks to massive teeth and faces able to generate and withstand high chewing forces (21).

The other line of selection led to the genus *Homo*, a group of species selected to exploit higher quality foods, including meat. Although the origins of *Homo* are murky, the oldest fossils attributed to the human genus are currently dated to 2.8 Ma (22). By 1.9 Ma there were three species of early *Homo*: *H. habilis*, *H. rudolfensis*, and *H. erectus* (23) (see Figure 1-2). Since *H. habilis* and *H. rudolfensis* retain many australopith-like features such as relatively short lower extremities and larger teeth (17), it is probable that *H. erectus*, which is more derived, evolved from *H. habilis* or some as yet unknown earlier species. Regardless of exactly when, where, and from whom *H. erectus* evolved, this species exhibits a combination of distinct, novel features. Despite much variation, *H. erectus* differs from more primitive hominins, especially the australopiths, in having relatively longer lower limbs, bigger brains, smaller teeth, a vertical face without a snout, and more.

The genus *Homo* was not only anatomically different from earlier hominins, but also behaviorally different as evident from the archaeological record. A few stone tools have been proposed to be as old as 3.3 Ma (24), but butchery sites with flaked stone tools do not start to appear until 2.6 Ma, about the same time as the oldest fossils attributed to the genus *Homo* (25). Whether the butchered animals in these sites were hunted or scavenged is debated, but starting about 2 Ma these sites intensify in number and size with clear evidence for hunting of large, prime-aged animals (26). By 1.7 Ma, new kinds of more sophisticated tools such as hand axes appear (27). Although one cannot rule out the australopiths as stone tool–makers, there is little question that the genus *Homo* was highly dependent on stone tools, especially for processing meat, which is otherwise difficult to chew with human or ape-like teeth (28). Even more importantly, by the time of *H. erectus*, the genus *Homo* was engaging in full-blown hunting and gathering, which involves not only hunting but also extractive foraging, recurrent tool-use, and intense cooperation such as food-sharing (17).

## Did Early *Homo* Run to Scavenge and Hunt?

Evidence for scavenging and hunting in *Homo* raises the question of how early *Homo* was able to enter the carnivore guild. Being a carnivore requires the strength, speed, power, and fighting ability necessary not only to kill prey but also to compete with other carnivores who fight aggressively for access to any carcass (29). As noted above, human bipeds are intrinsically unsteady and slow, and even the fastest humans today are unable to sprint much faster than ten meters per second for less than a minute, about half the speed that antelopes and other African mammals can sustain such speeds for as long as four minutes

(30). Bipedal hominins also lack natural weapons such as fangs, claws, and paws. While it is commonly assumed that early hunting was made possible by stone tool technology, the archaeological record indicates that early *Homo* lacked the technology to make sophisticated weapons that would have been effective for hunting or competing with other carnivores. The only weapons available to early *Homo* were untipped wooden spears, clubs, and rocks. Stone points for spear tips were not invented until five hundred thousand years ago, and more lethal technologies such as the spear-thrower and the bow and arrow were invented less than one hundred thousand years ago (31, 32). Early *Homo* would thus have been unable to overpower any prey, and probably had to rely on untipped wooden spears, which are used safely only from a distance. Hunters today using metal-tipped spears still keep a distance of more than seven meters from their prey, too far for untipped spears to be thrown accurately and with lethal force (33).

The contingent nature of evolution appears to have made possible selection for an unusual solution to the problem of how early hominins could have become carnivores. As noted above, because hominins are bipeds, they are necessarily slow and relatively awkward runners. However, as proposed by Carrier (5), as well as Bramble and Lieberman (6), selection for carnivory appears to have favored endurance running in order to enable persistence hunting. This method of hunting involves a combination of long distance running and tracking. The fundamental principle of these hunts is that hunters, usually in a group, pursue on foot an animal in hot weather until that animal collapses from hyperthermia. In general, hunters typically initiate hunts at the hottest time of the day and they usually pick the largest animal they can because larger animals overheat faster than smaller animals (34). Pursuit is accomplished through a combination of chasing and tracking, with chasing done at a moderate running pace (about ten minutes per mile) and tracking is typically done while walking. According to Liebenberg (34), who collected GPS data on ten persistence hunts by the Bushmen in the Kalahari, the average total distance was 27.8 km, and they ran only relatively slowly for about half the time, resulting in a total average speed of 6.2 km/hr (a fast walking speed below the walk/run transition speed). Persistence hunting is obviously now rare, and probably became less common after the invention of the bow and arrow, the domestication of hunting dogs, and other relatively recent technologies. Even so, persistence hunting has been extensively documented in the ethnographic record of hunter-gatherers in Africa, North America, South America, Australia, and even in Siberia (35).

Persistence hunting takes advantage of several unique human capabilities, of which one of the most important is thermoregulation. Whereas most animals cool by panting, during which evaporation of saliva on the tongue and upper trachea cools the blood supply to these tissues, humans primarily cool by sweating in which evaporation of sweat on the body's surface cools subcutaneous blood. Human sweating is partly made possible by an elaboration of eccrine glands that are present at much lower densities in monkeys and apes (36). Effective human sweating, which requires convection of hot air near the skin surface, is also facilitated by the loss of fur over most of the body because human hair follicles produce mostly very fine vellus hair rather than long, coarse terminal hair (38). Together these derived features lead to two thermoregulatory advantages compared to panting (39). First, human sweating occurs over a vastly larger surface area than just the tongue and oral cavity, and thus can cool much more blood. Second, unlike panting, human sweating is decoupled from respiration during locomotion. Although walking and trotting animals can pant, quadrupeds cannot pant while galloping because the mechanics of this gait cause back

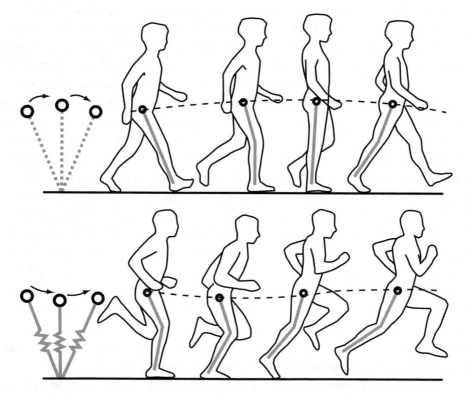

**Figure 1-3** Comparison of mechanics of walking (top) versus running (bottom). In walking the leg functions like an upside-down pendulum, raising the center of mass (circle) during the first half of stance before it falls in the second half. In running, the legs function like springs, storing up elastic energy during the first half of stance as the center of mass falls and then recoiling during the second half of stance helping to push the body up and into an aerial phase.

and forth oscillations of the viscera that interfere with the diaphragm's ability to inspire air (40). Galloping animals thus overheat more rapidly than trotting animals, especially in hot conditions, designating trotting as an endurance gait (41). Unfortunately, it is not yet known when hominins lost their fur and increased the number of eccrine glands, but developmental studies are beginning to provide clues that may lead to the identification, and subsequent dating, of the genes involved in these transformations (39, 42).

Another key set of adaptations that make persistence hunting possible are the anatomical features that enable humans to run long distances efficiently at relatively high speeds. These adaptations are too numerous to describe here in detail, but fall into three general categories. The first are features that improve economy such as relatively long legs (43), and almost a dozen tendons and other spring-like structures in the lower extremity, including the foot, which store up elastic energy (potential mechanical energy) during the first half of stance (weight-bearing) as the body's center of mass falls, and then recoil during the second half of stance helping initiate the aerial phase (non-weight-bearing) of the stride (see Figure 1-3). These structures are so effective that elite human endurance runners with legs of approximately a meter can match the stride lengths of full-sized horses (6). Importantly, these elastic structures benefit running rather than walking, a process that does not use mass-spring mechanics. Since running is an inherently less stable gait than walking, a second set of important adaptations maintain stability. These adaptations include short toes (18), an expanded cranial portion of the gluteus maximus (44), a tall waist with the ability to rotate the torso counter-phase to the pelvis (45), decoupling of the head and neck with a nuchal ligament (a tendon-like structure from the head to the back of the neck) that helps keep head stable (46), and expanded semicircular canals (tubes in the inner ear) with improved sensitivity for perceiving rapid head pitching accelerations (47). Third, since running engenders much higher and more rapid forces than walking, another set of important adaptations for running include increased joint surface areas relative to body mass in the lower extremity and lower spine (48). Larger joint surface areas are important because they minimize stresses acting on cartilage by spreading forces over larger areas. Importantly, although some of these adaptations are evident in *H. habilis*, they are all evident by the time of *H. erectus* suggesting that this species had excellent endurance running capabilities (6).

A final set of adaptations for persistence hunting are cognitive. Hunters must be alert to a wide range of sensory stimuli, and they must be superb naturalists and trackers, able to interpret a wide range of cues, especially footprints, to have an accurate mental map of their environment, and to have a theory of mind about the prey. As detailed by Liebenberg (49), tracking requires a hunter to use the hypothetico-deductive method to make and then test a series of hypotheses. How long ago were tracks formed? How fast was the animal going? What was its gait? Where is it likely to be headed? Is it wounded?

It is thus perhaps not coincidental that moderate to vigorous physical activity, such as running, upregulates Brain Derived Neurotrophic Growth Factors (BDNFs) that improve memory and other cognitive functions, especially in parts of the brain involved in mental mapping (50). Humans appear to have independently evolved the ability to upregulate endocannabinoids (psychoactive compounds similar in structure and function to those in cannabis) and their receptors during long distance running, which heighten sensory awareness and provide a sense of euphoria (the "runner's high"), possibly an adaptation for persistence hunting (51).

It is worth noting that almost all increases in brain size in human evolution follow the origin of hunting and gathering, which, as noted above, includes not only carnivory but also a reliance on tools and intense cooperation. Endocranial volumes (ECV) of fossil hominin crania attributed to the genus *Australopithecus* from the period between 3.3–2.5 Ma average approximately 450 cm$^3$, but then more than double to approximately 1020 cm$^3$ by 1 Ma (46). To be sure, multiple factors underlie this metabolically costly increase, but among them must have been the ability to hunt, presumably through persistence hunting which was made possible in part by long distance running. Although the extra energy made possible by hunting may have released a constraint on selection for bigger brains (17), it is also possible that selection on endurance increased upregulation of BDNFs and other growth factors that affect not only brain growth, but also metabolic regulation during exercise, which in turn led to increased overall brain growth and development (50).

Despite the many lines of evidence that support the endurance running hypothesis, it is (like all evolutionary hypotheses) challenging to test. Are there other explanations for the evolution of endurance running? The most commonly raised alternative possibility is that human endurance running capabilities are a by-product of selection for sprinting. This hypothesis can be rejected. Although hominins certainly must have needed to sprint on occasion when fighting or being chased by predators, human sprinting capabilities give little credence to the hypothesis that sprinting performance was under strong selection. The fastest human sprinters can attain speeds of 10.4 m/s for 100 m and 8.5 m/s for 400 m, less than half the speed of most medium-sized hoofed animals and carnivores, which can run approximately 20 m/s for at least four minutes (30). Another critique is that early butchery sites such as FLK-Zinj (a famous site in the Olduvai Gorge of Tanzania dated to 1.8 Ma) are dominated by prime-aged adult males rather than old and young prey (52). However, larger animals overheat faster than smaller ones, making them the preferred prey for persistence hunters (34, 35). Finally, if the persistence hunting hypothesis is incorrect, then scientists must produce other explanations for why humans are so superb at endurance running, and how early *Homo* was able to hunt prior to the invention of sophisticated projectile weapons.

## Contemporary Implications of Humans' Evolution as Runners

What is the relevance of humans' evolutionary legacy as endurance runners? How is an evolutionary perspective on human running useful for contemporary runners and would-be runners to help them run better and avoid injury?

The most obvious implication of the evidence that humans evolved to be endurance runners is to put long distance running into its proper context as a normal, fundamental, and natural human behavior. Although people tend to consider themselves and the world around them to be ordinary and normal, rapid cultural transformations over the last few thousand years (a blink of the eye in evolutionary time) since the invention of agriculture and industrialization have altered human environments so profoundly that many aspects of our lives today are, in fact, peculiar from an evolutionary perspective. Among other shifts, it is only during the last few hundred generations that people stopped hunting and gathering, and no longer needed to run regularly as adults. Even as recently as the nineteenth century, Native American peoples throughout North America regularly engaged in long distance running for hunting, to send messages, and for social and ritual purposes (53, 54).

Humans' legacy as runners thus suggests that is just as abnormal from an evolutionary perspective to not run on a regular basis as it is to fly in airplanes, drink soda, and sit in chairs all day. To be sure, many innovations, such as sanitation and antibiotics, have yielded substantial health benefits, but some of these environmental shifts also have negative consequences for health that cause mismatch conditions: diseases that are more prevalent or severe because our bodies are imperfectly or inadequately adapted to novel environments (17). In the same way that inadequate nutrition causes disease, inadequate levels of moderate to vigorous exercise adversely affect almost every system of the body. Low levels of such exercise—of which running is the most basic form—have especially negative consequences for the musculoskeletal, cardiovascular, digestive, immune, and nervous systems, contributing to diseases such as osteoporosis, congestive heart failure, coronary heart disease, many forms of cancer, type 2 diabetes, depression, anxiety, and more (55). Physical inactivity is a major risk factor for these diseases as the body's systems develop in response to stresses generated by running and other kinds of moderate to vigorous activity, thus matching capacity to demand (56). Since no one until recently was physically inactive there never was selection to cope with the absence of these phenotypically plastic responses. As a result, people who don't run (or engage in some modern equivalent of running) develop disease-prone phenotypes such as weak bones, hypertension, atherosclerosis, high levels of inflammation, insulin resistance, and low levels of dopamine and serotonin.

Put differently, today people mostly run for fun or fitness, and despite the success of the recent running boom in popularizing jogging, marathons, and other running events, running is widely considered an optional, even odd behavior. In reality, running and other equivalent forms of moderate to vigorous exercise slow the rate of aging and reduce the risk of countless causes of morbidity and mortality. As any runner knows, running long distances can also be an immensely satisfying and rewarding experience. Sadly, not enough people experience these pleasures that were made possible by our evolutionary history.

Another important lesson to learn from our evolutionary history of running is that the ways in which we run today are often unusual, and may contribute to mismatches. Five kinds of running mismatches merit discussion: speed, distance, surface, shoes, and running form.

**Speed and distance**. Everything is subject to trade-offs and running is no exception, especially in regards to speed and distance. As runners increase speed and distance, they increase their likelihood of injury, especially if their bodies are poorly adapted to such stresses (1, 57). High-intensity running may also stimulate cardiac remodeling that potentially leads to pathology (58). In this regard, it is illuminating to consider that many running habits today may be evolutionarily abnormal. Paleolithic runners almost certainly never trained by running fifty to one hundred miles a week, and they never stood on a painted line and then ran as fast as possible without stopping for 26.2 miles. Instead ethnographic evidence indicates that hunter-gatherers rarely ran fast, and they didn't typically run long distances without resting. Persistence hunts in the Kalahari, for example, involve a mixture of walking and slow running, rarely exceeding a half marathon in terms of running distance (34). Even Tarahumara Native Americans (farmers, not hunter-gatherers) who run long races known as *rarajipari* (for men) and *ari-wete* (for women) do so only a few times a year, and always at moderate speeds of about ten-minute-mile pace or less. Contrary to claims made in the popular book *Born to Run* (59), Tarahumara adults run long distances infrequently (60).

In short, although humans evolved to run, an evolutionary perspective indicates that we did not evolve to run long distances at fast speeds on a regular basis. As a result, it is unlikely there was selection for the human body to cope with some of the extreme demands runners place on their bodies.

**Surfaces**. Until recently, all running was done on trails and other natural aboveground surfaces that are typically more uneven, compliant, and otherwise variable than the asphalt and concrete surfaces on which many people run today. Hard, flat running surfaces were almost unknown prior to the nineteenth century, and became commonplace in the developed world only in the twentieth century. Treadmills were not available to consumers until the 1960s. These novel surfaces have likely affected running in several ways relevant to injury.

One such difference is between kinematic and kinetic variation. It is unquestionable that trail running involves considerably more substrate variation than treadmill or pavement running in which every step is essentially the same. Trail runners must constantly adjust for variations in the hardness and orientation of the ground, and they frequently have to turn, climb, descend, and cope with obstacles such as rocks, puddles, and roots. Although controlled studies (comparison study of groups) of the effects of these sources of variation have yet to be undertaken, a recent study found that runners adopted much greater kinematic variation including foot strike type when they ran on soft versus hard surfaces independent of speed, footwear, age, sex, and other factors (61). These and other sources of variation probably affect the likelihood of repetitive stress injuries that are caused by repeated stresses of sufficient magnitude, orientation, and type that cause microdamage to tissues (62). More research is needed to test if these variations affect injury rates as claimed anecdotally.

A second possible benefit of running on trails and other natural aboveground surfaces is that they are typically less stiff than asphalt and pavement. The extent to which differences in substrate stiffness affect injury is poorly established, however, because runners typically adjust lower extremity stiffness to substrate stiffness and thus run with less compliant legs on softer surfaces, both when measured in terms of overall leg stiff during stance (63) as well as during just the period of impact (64). Studies disagree whether stiffer lower extremities correlate with higher (65) or lower (66) injury rates.

A final issue is the likelihood of tripping or other perturbations that can lead to traumatic injuries such as ankle sprains. Unfortunately, there is no research on this issue and one can only hypothesize that trail running has both costs and benefits for avoiding injurious perturbations. On the one hand, trails are less predictable and have more obstacles; on the other hand, runners may be more alert on trails and thus less likely to fall when they encounter expected obstacles such as rocks and roots as opposed to unexpected obstacles such as uneven pavements.

**Shoes and Running Form.** Few topics have generated more controversy in athletics than whether or not modern running shoes contribute to the epidemic of injuries currently experienced by runners today. The debate is too large and complex to summarize here, but a few points deserve brief mention.

First, the debate over shoes has largely been framed in terms of the null hypothesis that running in modern shoes is better than running barefoot or in minimal shoes. In other words, the burden of proof for researchers has been to show that barefoot running is advantageous compared to shod running rather than vice versa. From an evolutionary perspective, this is a questionable null hypothesis (68). Just as humans have evolved to breastfeed and eat a diet high in fiber, humans also have evolved to run barefoot or in minimal shoes. The modern running shoe with cushioned and elevated heels, arch supports, toe springs, motion control, and other sophisticated features was invented only in the 1970s. That said, the argument that running barefoot is more "natural" than running in shoes doesn't mean that the former is necessarily healthier. An evolutionary perspective therefore suggests that researchers should consider different types of footwear, including the absence of footwear, in terms of competing costs and benefits.

Viewed in terms of trade-offs, the obvious benefits of shoes are to protect the sole of the foot, and provide cushioning between the foot and the ground thus slowing the rate of loading as well as damping forces (69). In addition, shoes may decrease work by the foot muscles (70, 71, 72). However, these benefits may also come with four costs that require further study:

First, and most obviously, shoes limit sensory information from the glabrous surface (bottom) of the foot, the only part of the body that regularly comes into direct contact with the ground. One well-studied consequence of reduced sensory feedback is that shod runners are more likely to collide with the ground on their heels, causing an impact peak with a high rate and magnitude of loading (force) (64). Even individuals in minimal shoes are more likely to rearfoot strike (land heel-first) than those who are barefoot (73). Currently, there is a vigorous debate about the effect of impact peaks on injury among shod individuals (67, 74, 75), but no one can rearfoot strike consistently on hard surfaces without eliciting considerable pain. Although habitually barefoot runners sometimes land on their heels on soft surfaces (61), it stretches credulity to imagine that humans evolved to run long distances on hard surfaces on their heels while barefoot.

Second, heel counters (inserts) move the initial center of pressure of the heel relative to the ankle, thus increasing the forces that together cause the foot to pronate (69). Shoes also increase forces around the knee (76). Cushioned shoes thus decrease stability and may sometimes increase potentially injurious forces in the ankle and knee.

Third, habitual use of shoes appears to cause feet to become weaker (60, 77, 78). It is a reasonable, but untested, hypothesis whether a weaker foot is more prone to injury.

Finally, several studies have shown that barefoot individuals tend to run differently than shod individuals, especially those who are untrained. In addition to landing more often on their forefoot, barefoot runners tend to have a higher cadence with relatively shorter strides at a given speed (61, 70, 79, 80)—kinematic patterns that have been argued to reduce injury rates (74, 75, 81).

Unfortunately, reliable evidence to test the effect of many of these trade-offs on injury rates is lacking. High quality, prospective, physician-diagnosed injury studies of long-term habitually barefoot individuals have not been undertaken. Instead, most comparisons of barefoot and shod running have used habitually shod people that were asked to run barefoot and thus cannot account for lack of training or adaptation. It probably takes months if not years for people to adapt their anatomy and kinematics to barefoot running.

**Social context of running**. A final mismatch to consider is the social context of running. Many people report that they do not run as much as they like because they cannot overcome their disinclination (82). This aversion is normal. Although humans evolved to run long distances, almost all endurance running was either in the context of play as children or of necessity as adults. When surplus food is scarce—as it often must have been prior to the invention of farming—spending extra energy on needless exercise such as running is not only challenging but also a selective disadvantage because it diverts energy from reproduction, on which natural selection operates. In other words, no adults in the Stone Age ran long distances just for fun or because it was prescribed for their health, but instead ran because it helped them to survive. People also ran in social contexts. Persistence hunters typically ran in groups, and it is likely that Paleolithic hunters were no exception. An evolutionary perspective thus suggests that to help more people run, we should not expect education or prescriptions alone to be effective. Instead, people are more likely to run when it is fun and social, and they are either incentivized, nudged, or obliged.

## CHAPTER 2

# Injury and Illness Rates

## BY BRIAN J. KRABAK AND EREK LATZKA

## Key Points

1. Ultramarathon runners are healthier overall than the general population. They have lower rates of many of the deadliest diseases in the general population, including cancer, heart disease, and diabetes.
2. Compared to the general population, runners miss less time from work and school and they require less overall outpatient medical visits per year.
3. Despite the high incidence rates of injury, most runners experience minor injuries or illnesses that often resolve soon after completion of a race.
4. Many of the most serious medical illnesses—exercise-associated collapse, heart attack, heat stroke, and exercise-associated hyponatremia—have non-specific presentations and need to be addressed quickly when they do occur.

## Introduction

Running—it's more than just a sport, a hobby, or a way to lose weight—it's a part of who human beings are; a unique species that evolved not only to sprint, but to run great distances for survival (1, 2) (Figure 2-1). Over the past half-century, more men and more women are running for longer distances for more years than ever before. Between 1976 and 2014, the number of Americans who participated in marathons increased from 25,000 to 550,600 (3). Shortly thereafter, half marathons in the United States grew in popularity from 303,000 participants in 1990 to over two million

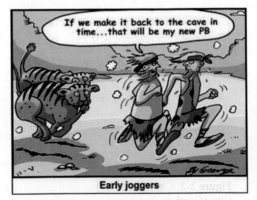

**Figure 2-1** From Out There By George. Reprinted with permission.

from 2014 (3). More recently, as runners continue to push the limits of the human body, ultramarathon (defined as any race with distance greater than 26.2 miles or 42 km) participation has rapidly increased with over seventy thousand runners per year worldwide (4, 5).

As more people participate in long distance running, there is a greater opportunity to understand the risks of running related injuries or illnesses and opportunities for prevention. But first one must understand the factors that impact the running athlete. This chapter will focus on our current understanding of rates of injury or illness and risk factors for musculoskeletal injury and medical illnesses for runners during training and races of various lengths. The chapter will provide the foundation for subsequent chapters throughout the book.

## Gender

As running has grown in popularity, there has been a shift in the number of female and male race participants. In the 1980s, women comprised only 5 to 12 percent of marathon runners in the United States (6, 7). By 2015, the number of female runners had steadily increased to comprise 44 percent of marathon runners (8). In the New York City Marathon, female participation is even higher, with a female-to-male ratio of 1:1 in 2007, up from 1:6 in 1983 (Figure 2-2) (9). Even more women run half marathons, and they made up 61 percent of participants in 2015 (3). Despite these changes in gender demographics, the majority of ultramarathon runners remain men with the disparity in direct correlation to

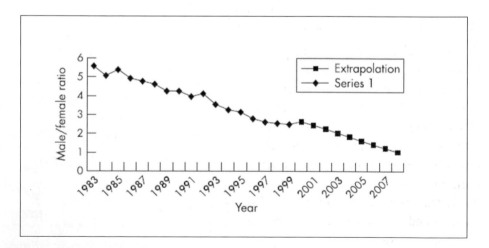

**Figure 2-2** Comparison of the number of male and female runners over time in the New York City Marathon. Reprinted from Peter Jokl Citation: Jokl P, Sethi PM, Cooper AJ. Br J Sports Med. 2004;38(4):408–412 with permission.

the distance of the race. Women represent 21 to 32 percent of single-stage ultra-marathon runners (10, 11), and 12 to 30 percent of multi-stage ultramarathons (12, 13).

## Age

There has been an increase in the average age of male and female runners across all race distances. The proportion of marathon runners in the Masters division (age less than forty years) increased from 26 percent to 49 percent between 1980 and 2015; during that same time, the mean age of male runners increased from thirty-four to forty years and female runners from thirty-one to thirty-six years (3). This trend is even more pronounced in ultramarathons, where Masters runners are the majority (14), with a mean age of forty to fifty-three years (15, 16).

## Performance

Regardless of the demographics, some factors have been shown to influence performance across all types of races. First, finishing rates of races are inversely related with both total distance and temperature. When controlling for variables—such as temperature, elevation gain, and running surface—by looking at events with both half and marathons, 88 to 91 percent of runners finished a half marathon and 78 to 84 percent finished a marathon (17). Finishing rates for ultramarathons are even lower, but tend to be less predictable due to the more extreme race environment impacted by terrain (e.g. mountains, deserts, tundra), surface (e.g., dirt, grass, sand, track, pavement), temperature, distance, and nutritional demands (e.g., self-supported or provided at interval aid stations). In the longest ultramarathons, only 38 percent of participants finished a 153-mile (246 km) single stage race and 44 percent of participants finished a 994-mile (1,600 km) multi-stage event (16, 18). Optimal performance has been shown to occur during temperatures of 40 to 59 degrees Fahrenheit (19), average humidity of 52 percent (17), and under 100 percent sky-cover (20). Other factors including older age, belonging to the female sex, and decreased caloric intake on race day are associated with higher dropout rates and slower finishing times (11, 21, 22).

## Injury and Illness

With changing runners' demographics and multiple variables at play in any endurance race, it is important to recognize the most common injuries and illnesses that affect this population. To understand these comparisons, one does not need to be a statistics major, but should be familiar with the difference between prevalence and incidence rates. Prevalence rates represent the proportion of a population with a disease or injury, typically at a specific point in time or cumulatively over one year. Incidence rates represent the number of new cases of a disease of injury over a given time period, typically ranging from a single event to one year. Or more simply, prevalence describes how common an injury is, while incidence describes risk of it occurring. These definitions will be utilized throughout the rest of this chapter.

The first step to understanding injury and illness rates in runners is to understand the overall risks and risk factors involved. As shown in Table 2-1 and Table 2-2, there is an increase in the number of race participants that require medical care with the increased distance of a race. Research suggests that on average 1 percent of all half marathon participants undergo a medical encounter during the event compared to 8 percent of marathon runners and 66 percent of ultramarathon runners (23). The direct relationship of increased injury rates and distance is also true during training. Studies suggest a one-year prevalence of injury among runners increases steadily from 32 percent, to 52 percent, to 65 percent for half, full, and ultramarathons, respectively (23). Removing distance as a variable, the risk of injury or illness in marathons significantly increased with later start times (17), higher temperatures (19), first-time participation, concurrent participation in other sports, and recent injury (24). Similarly, in ultramarathons, the risk of injury and illness increased with less experience and younger age (11, 15). Despite the reported higher rates of injury and illness in ultramarathon runners, they appear to be a relatively healthy group. Compared to the general population, these athletes have lower rates of comorbidities including cancer, heart disease

**Table 2-1** Comparisons of the Overall Rates of Injury and Illness in Distance Running Events.

| Overall Injury Rates | Half Marathon (16–21 km) | Full Marathon (42 km) | Single-Stage Ultramarathon (56–165 km) | Multi-Stage Ultramarathon (165–1600 km) |
|---|---|---|---|---|
| **Incidence** *Impacting Performance or Requiring Medical Encounter* | 0–4% | 1–18% | 40% | 57–85% |
| **Incidence** *Self-Reported After Event* | 40% | 65% | Unknown | 72–90% |
| **Incidence** *Pooled per Systematic Review* | 1% (N=97,490) | 8% (N=82,776) | Unknown | 66% (N=539) |
| **Prevalence** *One Year per Systematic Review* | 32% (N=6,206) | 52% (N=1,650) | 65% (N=1,212) | Unknown |

**Table 2-2** Proportion of Total Injuries by Type for Various Distance Running Events.

| Type of Injury or Illness | Half Marathon 16–21 km | Full Marathon 42 km | Multi-Stage Ultramarathon 219 km | Multi-Stage Ultramarathon 250 km |
|---|---|---|---|---|
| Musculoskeletal | 46% | 17% | 22% | 19% |
| Medical | 27% | 63% | 27% | 10% |
| Dermatologic | 27% | 21% | 45% | 71% |

(coronary artery disease or CAD), diabetes DM, and HIV; not to mention less outpatient medical visits and fewer missed days of work or school per year (11).

## Musculoskeletal Injuries

Musculoskeletal (MSK) injuries in the distance runner are often an overuse injury affecting the muscles, bones, connective tissues, and joints (11, 25). MSK injuries typically involve the lower extremities with reported incidence rates between 19 to 79 percent (26). When comparing different race lengths, there are patterns between MSK injury rates and race distance. There is an inverse relationship between race distance and overall MSK injury rates as a proportion of total injuries. Half marathon injuries are 44 to 46 percent MSK (6, 27), compared to 19 to 22 percent in ultramarathons (13, 15) (Table 2-2). The location of MSK injuries reverses with increased distance, with a ratio of knee-to-ankle injuries of 2:1 in half and full marathons (7, 23, 27), but 1:2 in single-stage and multi-stage ultramarathons (11, 13, 28). In multi-stage ultramarathons, MSK injury rates peak on days 3 and 4 of the race (13, 15).

Research has attempted to identify risk factors for MSK injury in the long distance runner. Prior injury within twelve months, quadriceps angle greater than twenty degrees, running seven days per week, and less experience in years running all increase the odds of MSK injury (11, 29, 30). On the other hand, neither BMI, warm-up time, stretching, running surface, terrain, shoe age, nor pace have been found to impact the overall MSK injury rate in any of these races (26). Although for some variables, the data isn't quite clear. As an example, studies have shown that both training more—greater than 64 km per week (29)—as well as training fewer miles and hours per week have been found to be significant risk factors for injury (6, 31). One study showed female gender significantly increasing the odds of encountering a lower extremity injury by 4.7 (32), while others do not support this conclusion (26, 29). Similarly, the relationship between age and MSK injury is unclear, as both younger and older age have each been found to increase risk of injury (33, 34).

# Knee Injuries

The knee is the most commonly injured joint in the general running population (26, 35). Studies suggest significant risk factors for knee injury include older age, female sex, quadriceps angle greater than 20 degrees, and inexperience (26). Increased training per week appears to lower the risk of knee injury but increases the risk of hamstring and quadriceps injuries (24, 26).

The most common knee injury is Patellofemoral Pain Syndrome (PFPS), or "runners' knee" (25, 35). The one-year prevalence of PFPS in half-marathon runners is 6 percent (36), and 10 percent in marathon runners (6, 31). Race-day incidence rates of PFPS appear to be similar across all distances (Table 2-3), occurring in 13 percent of half-marathons (27), 0.2 percent to 26 percent of marathon runners (24, 38), and 7 to 20 percent of single and multi-stage ultramarathon runners (28, 39, 40).

The second most common cause of knee pain in runners is Iliotibial Band Friction Syndrome (ITBFS) (35). It involves pain at the outside (lateral) knee, due to friction of the iliotibial band (ITB) where it runs over the lateral prominence of the upper leg bone (femoral condyle) especially at thirty degrees of flexion, running up or downhill, changing speeds, and increasing mileage (14, 41). ITBFS is particularly common in longer distances and extreme terrains, with an annual incidence in ultramarathon runners of 16 percent (11), compared to 14 percent in marathon runners (41), 11 percent of half-marathon runners (36), and 2 to 11 percent of recreational runners (35, 42). Race day incidence rates in both single-stage and multi-stage ultramarathons range from 7 to 9 percent (10, 39). ITBFS is more common in women, with a lifetime prevalence of 7 to 10 percent (35), compared to 5 to 7 percent in men (43). The most significant risk factor is hip abductor weakness (14), which in a prospective study of marathon runners was found to be present in 100 percent of those who developed ITBFS (41).

Table 2-3 Knee Injuries: Patellofemoral Pain Syndrome and Iliotibial Band Fraction Syndrome in Distance Running Events.

| Knee Injury | Half Marathon | Full Marathon | Single-Stage Ultramarathon | Multi-Stage Ultramarathon |
|---|---|---|---|---|
| Patellofemoral Pain Syndrome | 6–13% | 0–26% | 20% | 7–16% |
| Iliotibial Band Friction Syndrome | 11% | 14% | 7–16% | 9% |

Another common knee injury in runners is patellar tendinopathy. Patellar tendonitis has a general running population prevalence of 5 to 23 percent (35, 42), and in half-marathon runners 13 percent (36). The race-day incidence in multi-stage ultramarathon runners is similar, at 7 percent to 19 percent (16, 28).

## Ankle Injuries

Ankle injuries are more common in longer distance races such as single-stage and multi-stage ultramarathons. They can involve a variety of diagnoses but are typically due to overuse injuries involving the tendons or acute trauma leading to ligament sprains. Achilles tendon injuries occur in 6 to 10 percent of all runners (42), 10 percent of half-marathon runners (36), and 11 to 24 percent of marathon and ultramarathon runners (6, 11, 16). Of note, Achilles tendinitis has been noted to be the most common ankle diagnosis within multi-stage ultramarathons (28, 39).

The term "ultramarathoner's ankle" was coined by Bishop in 1999 due to the high rates of this injury in ultramarathons and extremely low rates within the general running population as well as half and full marathons (40, 44). It is a catchall diagnosis for injury to the tendons on the top, or front, of the ankle. A study of single-stage ultramarathon runners noted a one-year prevalence of 15 percent (10), and race day incidence in multi-stage ultramarathons of 14 percent to 30 percent (28, 39). One theory for the increased frequency in ultramarathon races is an altered gait pattern, which has been described as a "propulsive shuffle," with increased movement at the ankles and decreased movement at the knees and hips (39).

The ankle sprain is a common injury not just in runners, but in all athletes. It is often secondary to trauma from an awkward landing, and leading to injury of the ligaments around the ankle joint. The rates in the general running population are 10 to 11 percent (42), and similar to 10 percent half-marathon runners (36), 12 percent of marathon runners (37), and 9 to 11 percent of single-stage-ultramarathon runners (10, 11) (Table 2-4).

**Table 2-4** Ankle Injuries: Sprains, Achilles Tendinopathy, and "Ultramarathoner's Ankle" in Distance Running Events.

| Ankle Injury | Half Marathon | Full Marathon | Single-Stage Ultramarathon | Multi-Stage Ultramarathon |
|---|---|---|---|---|
| Sprain | 6–10% | 12% | 9–11% | |
| Achilles Tendinopathy | 1–10% | 24% | 11–12% | 8–19% |
| "Ultramarathoner's Ankle" | | | 9–15% | 14–30% |

## Foot Injuries

Similar to ankle injuries, foot injuries are often due to overuse injuries involving the soft tissue (i.e., plantar fasciitis) or bones (i.e., metatarsal stress fractures). Plantar fasciitis is one of the most common soft tissue injuries in the lower extremity (14). The overall risk appears to be higher in runners with flat feet (pes planus) or high arches (pes cavus). The one-year prevalence for plantar fasciitis is 5 to 8 percent in the general running population (35, 42), but increasing in distance runners to rates of 18 percent in half marathoners (36), and 10 percent in single-stage ultramarathon runners (10).

## Back and Hip Injuries

Low-back pain (LBP) and hip pain are common chronic problems in men and women, but most studies agree that it occurs less in distance runners than the general population. The annual incidence of LBP is reported as 6 percent in recreational runners (42), 3 percent in marathon runners (37), and 12 percent in single-stage ultramarathon runners (11). Hip injuries are mostly diagnosed as greater trochanteric pain, which occurs in 4 percent of the general running population (42) and 3 percent of multi-stage ultramarathon runners (13, 16). Other hip injuries have comparable rates, with hip flexor strain incidence of 1 to 4 percent in single and multi-stage ultramarathon runners (10, 13).

## Bone Injuries

Bone injuries in long distance runners involve a variety of disorders ranging from edema (swelling) to broken bones (fractures). Medial Tibial Stress Syndrome (MTSS) (aka "shin splints"), presents as a dull aching pain at the posterior-medial (behind and inside) border of the shin bone. MTSS has an incidence of 14 to 15 percent in the general running population (42). The one-year prevalence of 10 percent in half-marathon runners (36), and 8 to 11 percent in ultramarathon runners are comparable to the general population (16, 28), while one-year incidence within marathon runners is 20 percent (37).

Stress fractures are less common, and as a proportion of all recorded injuries and illnesses make up less than 1 percent of encounters in half and full marathons (27, 38). The one-year prevalence of stress fracture is 5 percent in half-marathon runners (36), but increases to 8 percent in single-stage ultramarathon runners (10). They are more likely to occur in the tibia in the general running population, as opposed to the hip or foot (42). However, the typical location changes in ultra-marathon runners, where 45 to 48 percent of stress fractures occur in the foot and a lifetime prevalence rate is 12 percent (11). Within ultramarathons, risk factors for stress fractures include younger age, female sex, less experience, increased running intensity, and less resistance training (11).

## Muscle Injuries

Of all MSK injuries in long distance runners, the most common is a muscle strain, which represents a stretch or tear of the muscle fibers (38). The most susceptible muscle in runners appears to be the quadriceps, which has been reported as the most common site for muscle pain in both single-stage and multi-stage runners (10, 13). Its risk is in direct proportion to days of training per week (24). Hamstring injury rates are steady among all runners, even comparing half-marathon and ultramarathon runners (11, 36). Risk factors for hamstring pain in marathon runners include male sex, first time participation, and aerobic cross-training (24). Risks for calf pain include male sex and younger age (24).

Another common type of muscle injury is Exercise Associated Muscle Cramping (EAMC). The etiology of EAMC has for years been thought to be due to sodium deficiency and dehydration, but more recently studies have shown that cramps are likely due to neuromuscular excitability and abnormal reflex activity in fatigued or damaged muscles (22, 45, 46). EAMC makes up a high proportion of race-day medical encounters, occurring in 21 to 26 percent of runners in half marathons, and 32 to 46 percent in marathons (17), but only 3 percent in multi-stage ultramarathons (13, 21). Though not entirely clear, the lower rates in longer distances may be related to a slower pace during the ultramarathon races (45).

## Illnesses

A variety of medical injuries can affect distance runners. Some are life-threatening, such as heart attacks or heat stroke; others like heartburn and nausea may seem relatively trivial, but still have major impacts on performance. The overall incidence of injury and illness in runners is directly related to distance (Table 2-1), but as a proportion of total injury and illness, medical diagnoses make up a smaller piece of the pie at distances longer than a marathon: they comprise up to 63 percent of all marathon encounters (38), but only 10 to 27 percent of all multi-stage ultramarathon encounters (13, 15) (Table 2-2). Medical encounters for illness are most likely to occur during the first stage of a multi-stage event, highlighting the importance of heat and altitude acclimatization (15). Other risks for increased medical illness in distance runners include higher humidity (27), and ambient temperature over 60 degrees F (16 degrees C) (19). See Chapter 21 for more details.

## Exercise-Associated Collapse (EAC)

EAC is a term for any illness that causes a runner to collapse during or after a race. The causes of EAC vary from benign and self-limiting to life-threatening. The rates of EAC per 1000 runners are 1.06 in half marathons, 11.25 in marathons, 2.8 to 7.2 in single stage ultramarathons (21, 47), and 43 to 196 in multi-stage ultramarathons (13, 15). EAC prior to the finish line is most concerning as it more likely secondary to cardiac arrest, heat stroke, severe exercise-associated hyponatremia, or low blood sugar (47, 48). EAC after the finish line is typically benign and is often due to transient low blood pressure caused by pooling blood in the lower extremities and the engorged muscles stop pumping blood back up to the heart (14). EAC is more likely to occur at certain times, including 3.5 hours after starting the marathon when most runners are finishing (38), and near race closure or stage cutoffs (47), possibly due to changing levels of exertion.

## Heart Attack and Sudden Death

The first recorded sudden death in a distance runner was that of Athenian soldier Pheidippides in 490 BC after he ran approximately 25 miles (40 km) from the battlefield at Marathon to Athens to announce their victory over the Spartans. Although Pheidippides's death came after running the distance that has become known as a marathon, he was actually more of an ultramarathon runner, as earlier that same week he had run 300 miles round-trip from Athens to Sparta, requesting their allegiance in the war.

The largest study of heart attacks (cardiac arrest) was examined in 6.9 million half-marathon runners and 3.9 million marathon runners over ten years (8). The authors reported half-marathon incidence of 0.27 per 100,000 runners, and marathon incidence of 1 per 100,000 (for a combined incidence of 1 cardiac arrest per 184,000 runners). Male runners were at a significant risk for a cardiac event, which was more likely to occur during the latter miles of a marathon or half-marathon. Of the cardiac arrests reported in this study, 63 percent were fatal (1 death per 259,000 runners), and of those who died 65 percent had an enlarged heart compared to 17 percent with ischemic heart disease (poor blood flow to the heart). Thus, survivors of running heart attacks tended to have characteristics associated with ischemic heart disease, meaning they were older, with known coronary artery disease (CAD) risk factors (e.g., high blood pressure, diabetes, family history). The rates for single-stage and multi-stage ultramarathons are unknown.

## Heat and Cold Illness

Heat illness is a spectrum of disease, increasing in severity from heat exhaustion to exertional heat stroke (EHS). In general, risks include increased temperature, humidity, and sunshine (or a lack of shade, water, or rest), ages greater than fifteen and less than sixty-five, and a lack of acclimatization (40). Heat acclimatization is particularly important, as the cardiovascular system accommodates for increased temperature by expanding plasma volume and increasing cooling via sweating (40). Controlling for terrain and temperature, one study of half and marathon runners reported heat illness rates of 0–0.5 per 1000 runners and 0–1.4 per 1000 runners (17). Comparing ultramarathons, 7 percent of single-stage dropouts reported inadequate heat acclimatization as their reason for dropping out (10), and 3 percent of runners required medical attention in a multi-stage race (13). See Chapter 12 for more details.

Alternatively, runners can suffer injuries due to cold temperature, including frostbite and hypothermia. Despite risk factors like altitude, wet clothing, and wind, which are more common in ultramarathons, there is scant evidence describing cold injuries in the literature. Controlling for terrain and temperature, one study reports increased risk in the marathon versus the half, with 0 to 8 percent of marathon runners versus 0 to 1 percent of half marathon runners presenting to finish line tents with hypothermia (17). See Chapter 13 for more details.

## Exercise-Associated Hyponatremia (EAH) and Encephalopathy (EAHE)

EAH is a relatively recently described illness in the running world. It is a low salt (sodium) level in the blood, defined as less than 135 mmol/L (normal is around 140 mmol/L), which can present as a range of symptoms from nausea, vomiting, and dizziness to altered mental status, seizures, and even death. Its origins may relate to a 1969 study that presumed race-day weight loss to be a risk factor for heat stroke, and recommended "the ideal regimen of water drinking is to take about 300 ml every 20 minutes or so" (49). The incidence of hyponatremia varies per race, but is as high as 4 percent in half marathons (50), 0 to 22 percent in marathons (51, 52, 53), 0 to 51 percent in single-stage ultramarathons (54, 55), and

8 to 11 percent in multistage ultramarathons (16, 52). Fortunately, only 0.23 per one thousand half-marathon runners, 0.23 per one thousand single-stage ultra-marathon runners (21), and 0.85 per one thousand multi-stage ultramarathon runners (15) actually require medical attention for symptomatic hyponatremia. See Chapter 11 for more details.

## Hypoglycemia

Hypoglycemia (low blood sugar) is another illness that is considered life threatening if not diagnosed and treated quickly, especially in diabetic runners. Fortunately, its incidence is extremely rare, with only one case in 91,750 half-marathon runners (27), 1 case per 81,277 marathon runners (38), and three cases in 6,344 single stage ultramarathon runners (47). Of note, all three ultra-runners with hypoglycemia presented as EAC prior to the finish line, making up 38 percent of the pre-finish line EAC runners (47).

## Acute Kidney Injury (AKI)

AKI is a medical illness caused by decreased blood flow (perfusion) to the kidneys, as the body prioritizes perfusion of the lower extremity musculature and attempts to cool through blood shunted to the extremities and skin of the body. Incidence of AKI has also been found to be directly related to worsening dehydration (56, 57). Incidence rates of AKI generally increase with race distance, with 24 percent of half marathon runners (50), 40 percent of marathon runners (58), 34 percent of single-stage ultramarathon runners (59), and 55 to 80 percent of multi-stage ultramarathon runners (56). Fortunately, these injuries usually resolve shortly after these races, usually within twenty-four hours of finishing. That being said, there have been multiple cases of runner's AKI progressing to renal failure resulting in prolonged hospitalization. Within multi-stage ultramarathons, runners appear to recover between stages (Figure 2-3) (56). Aside from race distance, risk factors for AKI include belonging to the male sex (50), older age (59), and NSAID use (57).

## Exertional Rhabdomyolysis

Rhabdomyolysis is the breakdown of muscle fibers into proteins that then enter the circulation, and at high concentration can cause kidney damage. The diagnosis is usually based on a laboratory value of muscle enzyme creatinine kinase (CK) at five to ten times the upper limit of normal. Marathon runners have an

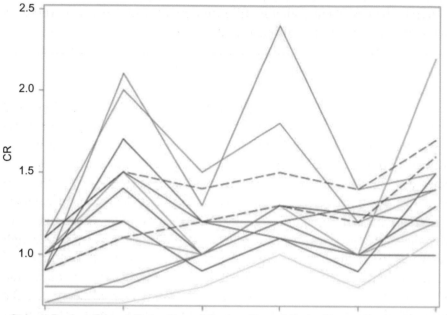

**Figure 2-3** Changes in Serum Creatinine (Kidney Function) during an Ultramarathon. Reprinted from Lipman GS, Krabak BJ, Waite BL, Logan SB, Menon A, Chan GK. A prospective cohort study of acute kidney injury in multi-stage ultramarathon runners: the Biochemistry in Endurance Runner Study (BIERS). Res Sports Med. 2014;22(2):185–192.

average rise in CK of 540 percent (48), and single-stage ultramarathon runners have an average rise of up to 2,450 percent, with start to finish values increasing from 178 to 43,763 units/liter (18).

## Respiratory Illness

Respiratory illnesses in distance runners include allergies, asthma, exercise-induced bronchospasm (EIB), and fluid in the lungs (pulmonary edema). Overall, distance runners have higher rates of these illnesses than the general population. Allergies, or hay fever, have been found to be four times more prevalent in single-stage ultramarathon runners than the general population (11). EIB, which is the constriction of airways five to fifteen minutes after exercise onset caused by hyperventilation's cooling and drying effects (60), has been found to be two to five times more prevalent in marathon runners than the general population (48, 61), and may be even more common in the ultramarathon runner (62). Pulmonary edema on the other hand is very rare, with no events recorded in half marathon runners, and 0.08 events per 1000 single-stage ultramarathon runners (21). Despite the low likelihood, it is still recommended that any new wheezing be evaluated, especially if it occurs at altitude.

## Altitude Sickness

Altitude sickness occurs at elevations greater than 2,500 meters (8,250 feet), and is more likely to occur during a marathon or ultramarathon in an extreme location. Although incidence rates are rarely reported in the literature, the potential for altitude sickness should be respected given its potentially fatal consequence. The spectrum of altitude sickness starts with acute mountain sickness that can range from uncomfortable to debilitating with headache, anorexia, nausea/vomiting, dizziness, fatigue, and insomnia, which onset typically within twelve to twenty-four hours after ascent. Altitude sickness can progress in severity to high altitude cerebral edema (HACE) with an altered mental state, altered gait, and can culminate with coma and death. There is also the potential for fluid in the lungs (high altitude pulmonary edema, HACE), which often presented on the second or third day after ascent (40). Risk factors include rapid ascent, living at low altitude, younger age, and a history of altitude sickness (40). See Chapter 14 for more details.

## Gastrointestinal (GI) Symptoms

GI symptoms are common in long distance running, but incidence rates vary widely with rates of 3 to 87 percent (13, 63, 64), depending on study methodology. Up to 69 percent of runners will experience exercise-related transient abdominal pain (ETAP), colloquially referred to as cramps or "side stitches" that typically improves with conditioning (65, 66). Nausea and vomiting has been reported as the most common cause of dropping out of elite single-stage ultramarathons (10). Other causes of GI pain may relate to the upper GI tract (e.g., reflux, heartburn, belching, bloating, nausea, vomiting) or lower (flatulence, side-stitch, urge to defecate, diarrhea, intestinal bleeding). In general, lower GI tract symptoms are more common among half-marathon and marathon runners (67, 68, 69), while upper tract symptoms, especially nausea, are more common in ultramarathon runners (10, 70, 71). Significant risk factors include a history of symptoms (72), being of the female sex (67), younger age, recent illness (24), race-day weight loss (73), and increased carbohydrate intake (72). The relationship between NSAID use and GI symptoms is unclear, as studies have provided conflicting results (70, 74). Finally, GI bleeds are surprisingly commonplace, with 16 percent of marathon runners reporting bloody diarrhea after race (48), and positive stool blood testing in 87 percent of ultramarathon runners (64). The etiology of these bleeds is theorized to be repetitive gut trauma in the setting of decreased blood flow to bowel from reduced perfusion, as some studies report reductions in perfusion of up to 80 percent when running (48). See Chapter 16 for more details.

## Dermatologic Injury

Dermatologic injury incidence rates vary widely based on the distance of a running race. As shown in Table 2-2, dermatologic injuries make up 45 to 71 percent of all diagnoses in ultramarathons (13, 15), compared to only 21 to 27 percent in half and full marathons (27, 38). Blisters (Figure 2-4) are the most common dermatologic injury with incidence rates of 4 to 9.4 per 1000 runners in the half marathons (17), 3.8 to 17 per 1000 runners in the full marathons (17, 38), and 1.6 per runner in a multi-stage ultramarathon (15). Unique to multi-stage ultramarathons, the risk of dermatologic injury increases during stages 3 and 4 of a race, highlighting the cumulative trauma that occurs from running long distances over consecutive days (15). Chafing or painful dermatitis due to repetitive friction affect 2 to 16 percent of marathon runners (75) and make up 9 percent of all medical encounters during a race (13). Subungual hematomas have been reported in 3 percent of marathon runners, and 3 to 10 percent of ultramarathon runners (13, 75). See Chapter 8 for more details.

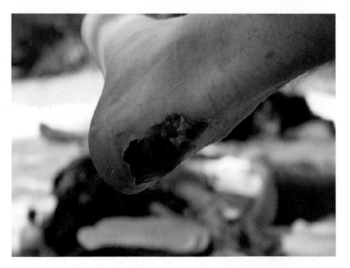

**Figure 2-4** Posterior heel blister during a multi-stage ultramarathon.

CHAPTER **3**

# Footwear Matters: Interplay of Footwear, Mechanics, Injury, and Performance

## BY IRENE S. DAVIS AND WEIJIE FU

## Key Points

1. Running shoes have gone through significant changes over the past fifty years, beginning with very minimal shoes and evolving into highly supportive and cushioned shoes, back to very minimal, and then on again to highly cushioned.
2. Despite the technological advancements that have been made in running shoes, the incidence of injury in runners remains high.
3. Our most natural running state is barefoot, which promotes a different foot strike pattern than when running in conventional shoes.
4. Shoes with cushioning promote a rearfoot strike pattern. Minimal shoes, which lack cushioning, promote a forefoot strike pattern and the closest running pattern to barefoot running.
5. Transitioning to minimal footwear takes time and patience. The calf and foot muscles should be strengthened and mileage should be progressed gradually.
6. Starting children in minimal footwear may allow a more natural development of their arch and will eliminate the issues related to transitioning.

## Introduction

Shoes are the only piece of equipment that a runner needs for his or her sport. The recent and varied footwear trends have spanned from no cushioning to highly-cushioned shoes, and from no control to highly controlled shoes. This has left many runners wondering just which running shoes are best for them. Therefore, the purpose of this chapter will be to help clarify the different classifications of footwear and to review the evidence regarding the effect of each of these types of shoes on mechanics. We will begin with a brief review of the history of running shoes. We will then discuss the development of motion control and cushioning shoes, with a focus on differences between them. This will be followed by a review of barefoot running, as this is considered our most natural running state. As barefoot running was the motivation for the re-emergence of the minimal shoe, it will be the topic that is next discussed. The various types of minimal shoes will be then described along with the mechanics associated with this type of footwear. As minimal footwear places significantly different loads on the foot and lower leg, safe transition programs will be reviewed. Additionally, an important interaction of foot strike and footwear will be discussed. In the end, we will make suggestions to assist runners in choosing the optimal footwear for them.

## A Brief History of Running Shoes

Anthropological evidence suggests that humans began running approximately two million years ago (1). According to this evidence, the modern human form reflects adaptations that have facilitated bipedal running. Some of these adaptations occurred in the foot and ankle. These features include a longitudinal medial arch and long Achilles tendon, both of which were not present in our pre-running ancestors. Along with these features, the human foot has twenty-six bones with thirty-three articulations. Each of these joints has six degrees of freedom of movement to allow the foot to move in many ways, allowing it to function in a variety of ways such as serving as a rigid lever, a mobile adapter, and having spring-like characteristics. Thus, the human foot appears to be well adapted for both walking and running gait without any footwear at all.

The first recorded shoes appear to have had the prime function of protecting the plantar surface of the foot. These shoes were found in the caves of Fort Rock, Oregon and have been dated back 10,000 years. They were constructed of sagebrush bark and were comprised of a flat surface to cover the sole of the foot with straps to hold it onto the foot (Figure 3-1). The prime purpose of this shoe was to protect the sole of the foot from injury.

Leather athletic shoes appeared in the early 1800s (2). Rubber soles were added to them around 1832 to enhance their durability and were called plimsoll shoes. In 1895, J. W. Foster & Sons (later to become Reebok) added spikes under the forefoot of the athletic shoe and developed the first running shoes. In 1926, Adolf Dassler introduced the first customized running shoe. This shoe had customized spikes depending upon whether it was to be used as a sprinting or distance running shoe. Runners such as Jesse Owens wore Dassler's shoes in 1936, and his shoes' success later led to the formation of Adidas.

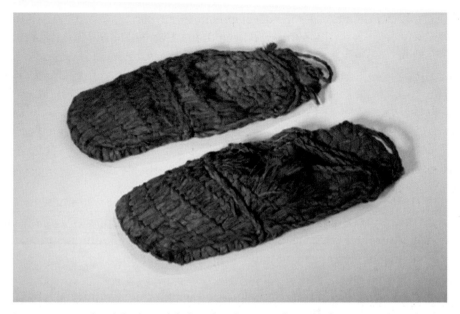

**Figure 3-1** Sagebrush bark sandals found in the caves of Fort Rock, Oregon, dating back 10,000 years. Copyright University of Oregon Museum of Natural and Cultural History, photograph by Jack Liu.

In 1961, the New Balance Company, originally an orthopedic shoe company in Boston, using input from runners such as Johnny Kelly, developed a new type of running shoe called the Trackster. It had an elevated heel wedge, a wide toe box, and a rippled sole. Simultaneously, the Onitsuka Company of Japan (later to become Asics) produced another shoe with a cushioned heel called the Onitsuka Tiger (Figure 3-2a). The Onitsuka Tiger was marketed in the United States by Bill Bowerman, a University of Oregon track coach, and Phil Knight, one of his disciples. However, Bowerman and Knight soon decided to form their own company, called Blue Ribbon Sport, which eventually became Nike. In 1972, they developed their own version of the Tiger that they named the Nike Cortez (Figure 3-2b). It was an instant success.

## Motion Control, Neutral Stability, and Cushioning Shoes

Over the next few years, numerous athletic footwear companies emerged and a variety of running shoes began to appear on the market. Along with standard cushion-heeled shoe, two new classifications of conventional running shoes appeared. These were the motion control and the cushioned shoe. This development began with Nike in response to a rise in running injuries noted in the early

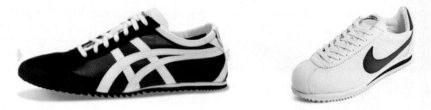

**Figure 3-2** Introduction of the cushioned heel into running shoes. A. Onitsu Tiger. B. Nike Cortez.

1970s (2). The founders of the company consulted with some well-known sports podiatrists who believed excessive pronation and excessive impacts were the culprits. Based on their feedback, Nike developed shoes with additional pronation control as well as shoes with additional shock attenuation. Additionally, a third category evolved into a neutral stability shoe.

Most conventional shoes are constructed with a midsole thickness of 22 to 24 mm and a heel-to-toe drop (difference between height of the heel and ball of the foot) of 10 to 12 mm. However, motion control and cushioning shoes have different structural characteristics than the neutral stability shoe. The motion control shoe is designed specifically to support and control the foot, and was aimed at individuals with flexible flat feet that excessively pronate. Therefore, it is generally constructed with stiff, reinforced heel counters, significant arch supports, and a higher density of the medial midsole compared to the lateral midsole. They tend to be stiffer and heavier than either a neutral or a cushioned shoe. The cushioned shoe, on the other hand, is designed specifically to assist with shock attenuation, particularly for individuals with high-arched, rigid feet that excessively supinate. They are constructed with an overall lower-density midsole, and are lighter and more flexible. The neutral stability shoe falls in between the motion control and cushioning shoe with some characteristics of each, but to a lesser degree. With time, the motion control and cushioned shoes have become increasingly supportive and increasingly cushioned with the extremes being shoes such as the Brooks Beast and the Hoka One One (Figure 3-3).

Biomechanical studies of these shoe types have been conducted to determine whether they function as they are designed. Recently, Lilley et al. (3) reported significant reduction in peak rearfoot eversion (back of foot turning out) in a motion control shoe compared to a neutral shoe. This finding has been supported by others in the past (4, 5, 6). Additionally, while eversion increases under fatigued conditions in a neutral stability shoe, it is reduced when using a motion control shoe (7). The downside to increasing motion control is that impacts (forces) tend to increase, as measured by tibial shock, as foot pronation is limited (8).

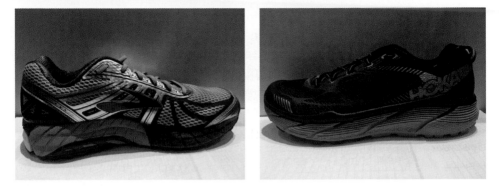

**Figure 3-3** Extreme Footwear. A. Brooks Beast control shoe. B. Hoka One One cushioned shoe.

As these shoes were designed for different foot structures and function, Butler et al. (9, 10) examined the interaction of foot type and shoe type on impact loading and foot pronation. No interactions were noted for most of the variables tested, indicating that matching arch type to shoe type has no effect. But a main effect of footwear was noted, whereby the motion control shoe reduced variables associated with foot pronation to a greater degree than the cushioned shoe. Additionally, the cushioned shoe reduced variables associated with cushioning to a greater degree than the motion control shoe.

## Conventional Shoes and Injury

The purpose of prescribing footwear based on foot type and mechanics is to reduce injuries. However, support for this type of running shoe prescription is limited. Knapik et al. (11) recently reported on meta-analysis (analysis of multiple studies) of three large studies that included over 7,000 military recruits. Participants were randomly placed into either a control or an experimental group. The experimental group had their footwear prescribed based on foot type. Those with flat, pronated feet were given a motion control shoe, those with high-arched, supinated feet were given a cushioning shoe, and those with normal arches were given a neutral stability shoe. Participants in the control group were all given a neutral stability shoe regardless of foot type. Injuries were monitored over the course of basic training. The authors concluded that prescribing footwear based on foot type had no influence on injuries. Ryan et al. (12) also studied the effect of matching footwear to foot type based upon the foot posture index. Participants were classified as having neutral, moderately pronated, and highly pronated feet. Motion control, neutral, and cushioned shoes were randomly assigned to these runners. Overall, they found greater missed days due to injury in the motion control shoe with the least days missed in the neutral shoe. The authors conclude that providing motion control shoes to runners with neutral or pronated feet may increase the risk for running-related pain. This finding was supported by a systematic review that concluded that the prescription of motion control shoes for runners was not evidence-based. However, in contrast, a study by Malisoux et al. (13) reported that runners with pronated feet would benefit the most from motion control shoes. Regarding cushioning shoes, Theisen et al. (14) concluded that midsole density has no influence on running injury risk. Based upon these studies, it is understandable why the consumer remains confused about how to buy their shoes. However, the propensity of literature suggests a neutral stability may be best choice of these categories.

## Barefoot Running: Our Most Natural Form

As we evolved to run barefoot, we discovered that it is our most natural state and one that has been used as a model for the development of minimal shoes. While there has been a group of underground runners who have shed their shoes since the 1960s, it was Christopher McDougall's *Born to Run* that reignited the barefoot movement when published in 2009. Advocates of barefoot running suggest that running without shoes provides important sensory input and allows the foot to function as it is adapted to function. Opponents believe that the foot needs additional cushioning and support to sustain the repetitive loads of running. Interestingly, both groups believe their approach will lead to the fewest injuries.

One of the clearest differences between barefoot and conventionally shod running is the way the foot strikes the ground. Approximately 90 percent of runners habituated to conventional cushioned running shoes land on their heels (15) and are classified as rearfoot strikers (RFS). These runners typically display a very distinct impact transient in their vertical ground reaction force (Figure 3-4) that is associated with their heel contact.

The higher rate of loading associated with this impact transient, measured as the slope of this first rise to peak, has been associated with many common running-related injuries (16). One percent of conventionally shod runners land on the ball of their foot and classified as forefoot strikers (FFS). This pattern is not associated with an impact transient, therefore having vertical rates of loading that are significantly less than RFS (17). The remaining 10 percent land with a flat foot and are classified as midfoot strikers (MFS). These runners exhibit vertical force patterns that are between a RFS and a FFS runner. The impact peak is typically reduced from a RFS pattern, and can be missing as in a FFS pattern. Most habituated barefoot runners do not land on their heels (18, 19) as it would cause

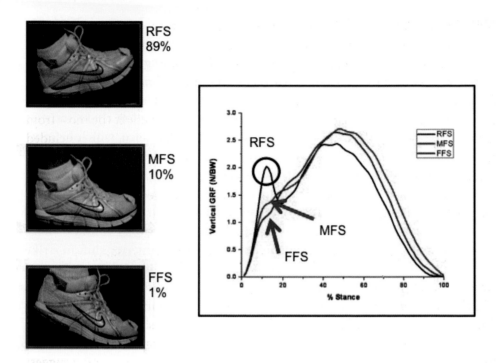

**Figure 3-4** Effect of footstrike pattern on the vertical ground reaction force. A RFS pattern results in a distinct impact peak (black circle), a FFS typically eliminates the impact peak (blue arrow), and a MFS typically falls between a RFS and a FFS pattern.

pain. The human heel pad is adapted to attenuate the loads of walking, but not running (20). Therefore, barefoot runners land predominantly with a FFS pattern. This results in reducing or eliminating vertical impacts resulting in vertical rates of loading that are half that of a RFS (21). Additionally, there is a reduction or elimination of the lateral ground reaction force peak that also occurs early in stance (Figure 3-5a).

The reduction of the vertical and lateral ground reaction force peaks in early stance during barefoot running and reduces the external pronatory force on the foot. Additionally, the lever arms to the vertical and lateral forces are reduced when the elevated heel and lateral flare of a shoe are removed. This can clearly be seen in Figure 3-5b. With reductions in both the vertical and lateral forces, as well as their lever arms, the resultant pronatory torque on the foot is reduced in the barefoot condition. In fact, Bonacci et al. (22) reported that rearfoot pronation was significantly reduced during barefoot running compared with running in traditional shoe.

The FFS landing typically associated with BF running increases the load on the Achilles tendon (23). Greater load, combined with high stretch velocity

(24), induces greater stiffness within the muscle-tendon unit. Greater tendon stiffness is associated with greater energy storage and overall tendon health. This is supported by reports that the Achilles tendons of the jump leg in athletes exhibited greater mechanical (stiffness) and material (Young's modulus) properties (25). In contrast, a study of runners with varying foot strike patterns (12 FFS, 12 MFS, 17 RFS) found no difference in Achilles tendon characteristics (26). However, these runners were tested at an 18 km/hr pace, which by most standards would be considered sprinting. As strike pattern shifts anteriorly with speed, the MFS and FFS patterns of some runners in this study may not be their usual ones at distance running speeds. In a related study, it was reported that runners who were habituated to minimal footwear exhibited stronger, stiffer Achilles tendons than those habituated to conventional running shoes (27). The authors suggested that this might be due to an anterior shift in strike pattern resulting in greater loading of the calf and Achilles. While strike pattern was not monitored in this investigation, other studies have shown that running in minimal shoes does facilitate a more anterior strike pattern (28). The cross-sectional nature of this study limited the authors' ability to determine that strike pattern caused the changes in the Achilles tendon. Therefore, they

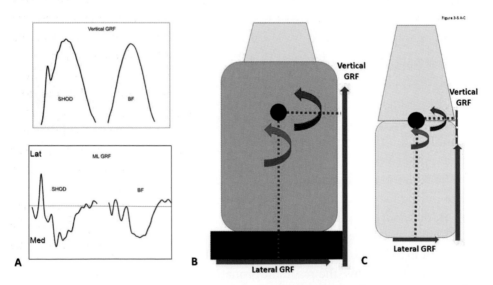

**Figure 3-5** A. Reduction in vertical (top panel) and lateral (bottom panel) impact transients of the ground reaction force during running with shoes (shod) and barefoot (BF). B. Shod running: The contribution of these early vertical and lateral impact force transients (straight arrows) and their lever arms (dotted lines) on the pronation torque (curved arrows) about the subtalar joint axis of the foot. C. Barefoot running: Note the reduction of the vertical and lateral forces and their lever arms when shoes are removed (or footwear is minimal).

conducted a prospective study where runners transitioned from a conventional shoe to a minimal shoe with instructions on using a FFS pattern (29). Their findings were consistent with their cross-sectional study, with Achilles tendons becoming significantly stronger and stiffer following the six-month transition. There is a 52 percent lifetime incidence of Achilles tendinopathy in runners (30) and approximately 90 percent of runners today are RFS in conventional shoes (15). Therefore, it is plausible that the incidence of Achilles tendinitis might be significantly reduced in runners adopting a more barefoot style of running which would increase tendon stiffness and strength. Another benefit of barefoot FFS running is that it leads to significant reductions in patellofemoral contact stresses (31). This is due to the combination of lower vertical force and higher contact area (due to greater knee flexion). High contact stresses are one of the proposed causes of patellofemoral pain, one of the most common injuries runners sustain. If we assume being barefoot is our natural state, then forefoot striking may be a fundamental component of our normal running mechanics that we have lost with the advent of cushioned shoes.

There are numerous other benefits to running in our most natural state. There is important sensory input that helps to control our posture. Simply wearing a thin pair of socks has been shown to cause a statistically significant decrement in our static postural stability (32). Additionally, sensation from the foot provides important information to modulate the stiffness of the leg spring that is dependent upon the surface the foot is encountering. For example, single leg landings in bare feet result in less stiff, more compliant landings than in cushioned shoes (33). More compliant landings result in lower impact loads to the musculoskeletal system. Another benefit of being barefoot is that it promotes strength of the arch musculature (34). Chronic support of any muscle will lead to muscle weakening. In the foot, this can lead to a compromised arch structure. In support of this, a study of 2,300 Indian children between four to thirteen years (35) found that flatfoot was most common in those who wore closed toed shoes. It was less common in those who wore sandals and least common in the unshod. The authors concluded that shoe wearing in early childhood might be detrimental to the development of the longitudinal arch of the foot. More studies are needed to truly understand the impact of shoes on this age group.

## Minimal Shoes

While the benefits of being unshod are many, current societal norms require individuals to be shod for most of their daily activities. Additionally, there are

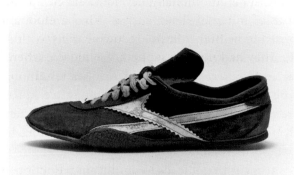

**Figure 3-6** Shoes of Ron Hill who won the Boston Marathon in 1970. These shoes are more minimal than the minimal shoes of today. Courtesy of Amby Burfoot.

times when the foot needs to be protected from environmental hazards such as sharp objects and extreme heat or cold. Therefore, the ideal shoe might be one that provides these protections while allowing the foot to function as close to barefoot as possible. However, this brings us full circle to where shoes began as simple flat surfaces to protect the sole with a means of holding them onto the foot. For most of our running history, shoes have been quite minimal, such as those worn by Ron Hill when he won the Boston Marathon in 1970 (Figure 3-6).

Over the next forty years, shoes became more supportive and cushioned. However, with the barefoot running explosion in 2009, the minimal shoe re-emerged. The first minimal shoe on the market was the Vibram FiveFingers shoe that was originally developed for boating (Figure 3-7a). The barefoot community

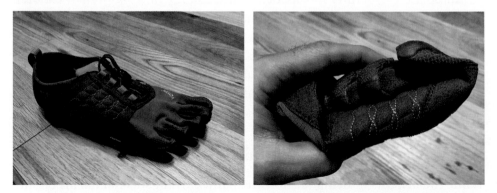

**Figure 3-7** Full minimal shoes. A. Vibram FiveFingers Shoes. B. SoftStar Minimal Shoes.

quickly adopted this shoe. Additionally, new footwear companies appeared with their own versions of minimal shoes, such as Vivobarefoot and inov-8. These shoes were designed to be highly flexible allowing the shoe to be rolled up in a ball (Figure 3-7). They had no arch support, no midsole (therefore no heel-to-toe drop), and a flexible heel counter. Therefore, they were neither supportive nor cushioned. Because there is no midsole, these minimal shoes do not need to be replaced until the outer sole wears out, which may be in thousands of miles. For example, the Xero shoe company guarantees their minimal shoes for 5,000 miles.

The goal of a minimal shoe is to mimic barefoot running mechanics (Figure 3-8). Warne and colleagues (36) conducted a six-week transition program to minimal footwear that included strengthening as well as gait training for adopting a FFS pattern. Loading rates were significantly higher in the minimal shoe compared to the conventional shoe condition at baseline. This provides caution regarding early use of minimal footwear. However, loading rates were significantly reduced in the minimal shoe condition following training suggesting that a gait adaptation had occurred. A study by Squadrone and Gallozzi (28) compared running mechanics in the Vibram FiveFingers shoes to that of barefoot running and running in conventional shoes (Nike Air Pegasus). All participants were experienced barefoot/minimal footwear runners. They assessed variables of stride length, cadence, and ankle angle at footstrike, and

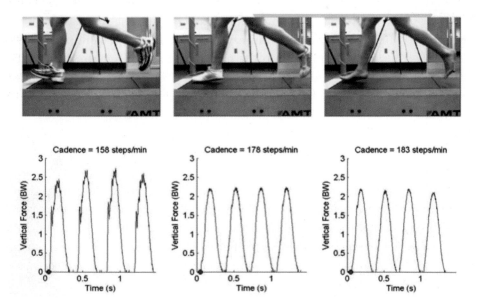

**Figure 3-8** Ground reaction forces of a runner with a RFS pattern in conventional shoes, a FFS pattern with minimal shoes, and a FFS pattern in bare feet.

knee and ankle moments. They found that the mechanics of minimal shoes were similar to those while running barefoot, but different from the conventional shoe.

## Partial Minimal Shoes

As time progressed, some of the established running shoe companies entered the minimal shoe market. However, these shoes were not quite as minimal as the original ones. They were designed with less cushioning (typically 11 to 22 mm), less arch support, and less heel-to-toe drop (typically 4 to 8 mm) than a conventional shoe, but more than a full minimal shoe. A shoe classification scheme has been suggested that ranks shoes from minimal to maximal on a scale of 0 (total maximal) to 100 (total minimal). The ranking is based on a variety of shoe characteristics (37), with these new partial minimal shoes falling somewhere between 50 to 100 percent index. Partial minimal shoes were designed to be a compromise between a full minimal shoe and a conventional shoe. However, an important question is whether running in either type of shoes mimicked barefoot running. Bonacci and colleagues (22) compared two partial minimal shoes (Nike Free, Nike Lunar Racer) to a conventional shoe (Nike Air Pegasus). Using similar variables to Squadrone and Gallozzi, these authors concluded that running in the partial minimal shoe replicates running in the conventional shoe, and is significantly different from running barefoot. This is likely due to the midsole cushioning in the partial minimal shoes that promotes a heelstrike running pattern. Full minimal shoes, lacking any cushioning, make it much less comfortable to land on the heel, thus promoting a more anterior strike pattern. Recently, Squadrone and colleagues (38) went a step further and compared barefoot and conventional shoe mechanics to those across a variety of running shoes, from minimal to partial minimal. All participants were experienced minimal footwear runners. Their results suggested that the two full minimal shoes were most like the barefoot condition, and most different from the conventional shoe. As shoes became more cushioned, mechanics became more like those associated with the conventional shoe. Taken together, these two studies suggest that cushioning significantly influences mechanics, and that full minimal shoes are the best for adopting a barefoot running style. This is supported by a recent study by Rice et al. (17) that reported that load rates, in all components of ground reaction forces, are reduced to the greatest degree when running with a FFS pattern in full minimal shoes. Therefore, footwear really matters.

## Minimal Shoes and Injury

The changes in mechanics associated with running in a full minimal shoe alter the loading to the lower leg. Landing with a FFS increases the demands placed upon the calf and Achilles, as well as the medial and plantar foot musculature. Muscles are critical to the strain profile of the bones they support. Muscular fatigue has been shown to be associated with increased bone strain (39). Consequently, weakness of the foot musculature places the metatarsals at increased risk for injury. Therefore, transitioning should be progressed slowly to allow the musculoskeletal system adequate time to properly adapt. The studies reporting on minimal footwear injuries have all incorporated overly aggressive transitions (40, 41). For example, one study reported on a series of ten cases of foot injuries associated with minimal footwear, where the average transition to full running mileage was three weeks (41). However, studies have shown that transitioning to minimal footwear that involves a slow progression can be done safely without injury (42) twenty-four hours apart, in both CRS and MFW (pre-test). A slow transition to minimal footwear has also been shown to result in significant hypertrophy of both the intrinsic and extrinsic muscles of the foot as measured with MRI (43).

It is often assumed that a partial minimal shoe will be associated with a lower injury risk than a full minimal shoe. However, a study by Ryan et al. (44) seems to counter this assumption. These authors randomized ninety-nine conventionally shod runners who were training for a 10K race into one of three footwear groups: full minimal (Vibram FiveFingers), partial minimal (Nike Free), and neutral (Nike Air Pegasus). Running progressed gradually and injuries were monitored over the twelve-week training period. These authors noted that there were twice as many injuries in the partial minimal versus the full minimal shoes. Based on previous studies (22), runners in the partial minimal shoes are more likely to continue to land on their heels. But partial minimal shoes have reduced cushioning under the heel, thereby reducing the ability to dampen the impacts of heelstriking and increasing the risk of injury. Runners in the full minimal shoes did have a greater incidence of calf and Achilles pain. This suggests that they may have transitioned to a more anterior strike pattern. It also suggests that the transitioning program may have benefited with the addition of a strengthening program to better prepare the calf and Achilles.

## Transitioning to Minimal Footwear

With a very slow progression, one may be able to transition to a FFS pattern in minimal shoes without injury. Unfortunately, we currently don't know exactly how slow that progression needs to be for individual runners, and most runners don't have patience for slow progressions. Implementing a strengthening program that helps to fortify the key areas undergoing additional load helps to augment the transition process. These areas include the muscles of the posterior lower leg as well as the medial and plantar foot muscles. Exercises should address both the intrinsic and extrinsic foot muscles. They should begin with static exercises and progress to more dynamic ones. Foot doming (Figure 3-9a), or the short foot exercise, is one of the fundamental exercises that provides stabilization of the foot core (45). The runner is instructed to stiffen their toes and press them towards the ground without flexing them. Then they are asked to draw the ball of their foot back towards the heel, shortening their foot while squeezing their arch. This exercise can be progressed to doming and hopping in place, first on two feet, then one foot (Figure 3-9b), and then from foot to foot. It can then be progressed to doming and hopping off a four-inch step with two feet, then one foot, maintaining the dome during the landing. Other foot exercises such as toe abduction (spreading) and adduction (squeezing) (Figure 3-9c, Figure 3-9d) and towel curls should be added. Double heel raises can be progressed to single heel raises (Figure 3-9e, Figure 3-9f). One-minute bouts of jump roping can also be added to include a power and endurance component to the training. Exercises are progressed in terms of both repetitions and difficulty over an eight-week period (Figure 3-10).

Stretch feet before and after each session. Sitting with one leg crossed over the other, point your foot and stretch your toes into flexion. Hold for 5 seconds and repeat 5 times. Then pull your ankle back and your toes back stretching your arch. Hold for 5 seconds and repeat 5 times. Move each of your five long foot bones with respect to each other.

## *Minimal Footwear and Performance*

The overall benefits of minimal shoes have been to promote a barefoot style running that is associated with softer landings, reduced joint torques, and patellar contact stresses and stronger feet. All of these should factors should help to reduce injury risk. But runners are also often interested in how this change in running will influence their performance. There have been a number of studies comparing the economy of barefoot running with other shoe conditions (46, 47, 48). A systematic review of these studies has concluded that running economy is improved

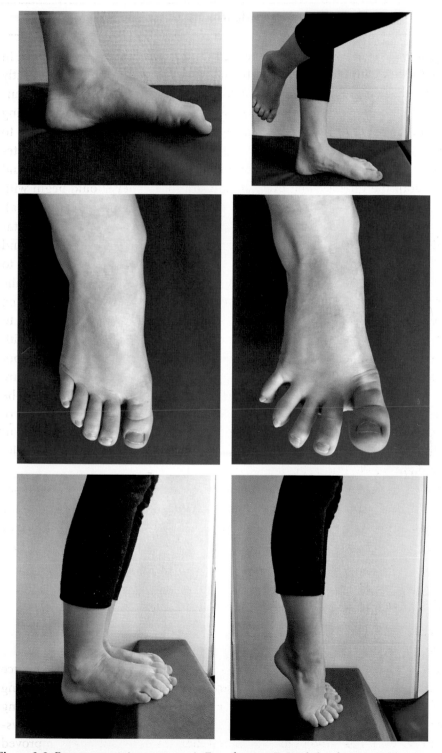

**Figure 3-9** Foot core exercise program. A. Foot doming. B. Single leg doming and hopping. C. Resting. D Toe spreads. E. Toe spreads (left) and squeezes (right). F. Calf raises.

**Figure 3-10**  Spaulding National Running Center: Daily Foot/Ankle Exercises

Stretch feet before and after each session. Sitting with one leg crossed over the other, point your foot and stretch your toes into flexion. Hold for 5 seconds and repeat 5 times. Then pull your ankle back and your toes back stretching your arch. Hold for 5 seconds and repeat 5 times. Move each of your 5 long foot bones with respect to each other.

| | Week 1 | Week 2 | Week 3 | Week 4 | Week 5 | Week 6 | Week 7 | Week 8 |
|---|---|---|---|---|---|---|---|---|
| Double leg heel raises on flat surface | 3 sets of 10 to 3 sets of 20 | 3 sets of 20 to 3 sets of 30 | | | | | | |
| Double leg heel raises off edge of step | | | 3 sets of 10 to 3 sets of 20 | 3 sets of 20 to 3 sets of 30 | | | | |
| Single leg heel raises on flat surface | | | | | 3 sets of 10 to 3 sets of 20 | 3 sets of 20 to 3 sets of 30 | | |
| Single leg heel raises off edge of step | | | | | | | 3 sets of 10 to 3 sets of 20 | 3 sets of 20 to 3 sets of 30 |
| Towel curls | 3 sets of 10 to 3 sets of 20 | 3 sets of 20 | 3 sets of 20 to 3 sets of 30 | 3 sets of 30 | 3 sets of 30 | 3 sets of 30 | 3 sets of 30 | 3 sets of 30 |
| Toe Spread | 3 sets of 10 to 3 sets of 20 | 3 sets of 20 | 3 sets of 20 to 3 sets of 30 | 3 sets of 30 | 3 sets of 30 | 3 sets of 30 | 3 sets of 30 | 3 sets of 30 |
| Toe Squeeze | 3 sets of 10 to 3 sets of 20 | 3 sets of 20 | 3 sets of 20 to 3 sets of 30 | 3 sets of 30 | 3 sets of 30 | 3 sets of 30 | 3 sets of 30 | 3 sets of 30 |
| Doming | 3 sets of 10 to 3 sets of 20 | 3 sets of 20 | 3 sets of 20 to 3 sets of 30 | 3 sets of 30 | 3 sets of 30 | 3 sets of 30 | 3 sets of 30 | 3 sets of 30 |
| Doming Hopping in place | | 3 sets of 30 | 3 sets of 30 | | | | | |
| Doming Hopping Square | | | 3 sets of 10 forward and back | 3 sets of 20 forward and back | 3 sets of 10 side to side | 3 sets of 20 side to side | 3 sets of 10 diagonal and back | 3 sets of 20 diagonal an back |

when running either barefoot or in minimal shoes compared with conventional shoes (49). Economy was similar between barefoot and minimal footwear conditions. The improvement in economy with minimal shoes was also shown to also result in improved speed as measured over a 5K run (50). Therefore, it does appear that minimal footwear may also help to improve performance over conventional running shoes.

## Maximal Shoes

Maximally cushioned shoes are the newest shoe type on the market today. These shoes have soft durometer, (hardness) thick soles, typically between 30 to 40 mm in height (Figure 3-3). They are designed to provide maximal cushioning and are the antithesis of the minimal shoe. These shoes have become extremely popular as they are purported to soften landings. However, there is only one published study comparing the mechanics of these shoes to conventional running shoes (51). These authors found that vertical load rates and tibial shock were higher, but not significantly different between the maximally cushioned shoes (Hoka One One) compared with a conventional shoe (Nike Air Pegasus). While this counters the shoe claims of providing cushioned landings, it is not surprising in light of previous research, which suggests that humans stiffen their leg when landing on soft surfaces (33, 50). Therefore, runners adapt to the additional cushioning of these shoes by landing harder, with a net result of no overall change. However, it should be noted that runners in this study were not habituated to this footwear. Additional studies are needed to determine if mechanics change once runners have become adapted to the footwear.

# Summary: How to Choose the Right Shoe

Running shoes have gone through a wide range of changes throughout the past five decades. They began as minimal and then progressed into shoes that became increasingly more supportive and cushioned. Runners have been conditioned to believe that this additional cushioning and support was needed to run safely. However, despite the technological advances in footwear, up to 79 percent of runners still get injured in any given year. Large scale studies have suggested that injuries are not reduced when supportive or cushioned shoes are prescribed based upon foot type. Minimal shoes re-emerged with the barefoot explosion of 2009. Runners quickly gravitated towards these shoes to adopt a barefoot style of running. However, they did not realize that they were not just running in a different pair of shoes; they were running with different mechanics that takes time to adjust to. Without proper adaptation, many experienced calf and foot injuries, and the market responded by producing partial minimal shoes. However, evidence suggests that runners maintain a RFS pattern in partial minimal shoes, and may be at greater risk for injury due to the reduced cushioning.

So how does one best choose their running shoe? Minimal footwear has been associated with many benefits including softer landings, reduced joint torques, reduced patellar contact stresses, greater sensory input, stronger foot and arch muscles, and stronger Achilles tendons. However, transitioning too quickly without allowing the foot and lower leg to adapt can cause injury.

Therefore, the following recommendations are made based upon the available current evidence.

1.  If you are happy with your footstrike pattern and footwear, and are not experiencing running-related injuries, there is no reason to change anything.
2.  If you are a rearfoot striker, are not experiencing injuries and do not want to transition to different running mechanics, then choose a neutral stability running shoe. Look for shoes that have an outsole that is not significantly wider than the upper portion of the shoe. Outsole flaring can result in increased torques to the foot and lower extremity. Neutral stability shoes will have adequate heel cushioning to accommodate the impacts of rearfoot striking. However, it is important to replace these shoes every 300 to 500 miles of wear as the midsole begins to lose its ability to dampen the impacts over time. This is when runners can begin to experience injuries, which can often be remedied with new shoes. Proceed cautiously if choosing a partial minimal shoe. Research suggests that running mechanics will not change, but support and cushioning will be reduced. This may increase your risk for injury.
3.  If you have been experiencing injuries, and/or want the benefits of full minimal footwear, be prepared to take time with it. This transition takes many months for a runner to return to their typical running mileage. Fortifying the structures of the lower leg and foot with a strengthening program will help augment this transition. Progress running slowly. One way to accomplish this is to use a walk-run program where you begin with thirty minutes of walking briskly in the minimal shoes and then gradually replace the walking with running. Once running thirty minutes continuously, increase your time by 10 percent per week. Let pain be a guide in your progression.
4.  Allow your children to spend time barefoot and consider choosing minimal footwear for them. Starting your children with a minimal approach will help to strengthen feet and lower legs and will eliminate the issue with transitioning altogether!

## CHAPTER 4

# Training for Long Distance Running

## BY JONATHAN DUGAS

## Key Points

1. The physical stresses of long distance running greatly increase the risk of injury or acute illness.
2. Understanding and managing the stresses you place on your body is crucial to remaining healthy and able to train.
3. OTS is rare, but athletes stricken with OTS require many months of rest of greatly reduced training loads before they can return to pre-OTS training levels.
4. High-intensity training improves running economy, which can enhance running performance across all distances.

## Introduction

In running, "success" can mean many things. For most, it can be remaining injury-free, achieving performance goals, or just being able to continually enjoy the sport throughout the lifespan. No matter how you choose to define success, however, the journey involves doing the "right" training that triggers specific physiological changes in your body that will help you run faster and longer.

The common enemy of runners everywhere is injury. When stricken down by a running injury, we can't complete the requisite training that will produce the physiological adaptations that make success possible. So at the outset of a running career, all runners face a dilemma: How do I train to achieve success? How do I maximize my training time so that I can push myself as hard as I can, to produce the largest adaptations, but without going over the edge and getting injured? This is a topic of central importance for every distance runner. We won't explore every single approach here, but instead the aim of this chapter is to help you understand the principles at play, and more importantly, how to apply them to your running so you can be successful—no matter how you define it.

## Principles of Training

Although a young profession, exercise physiology has made great advances in unlocking the mechanisms that lead to improved exercise performance. As such, a technical lexicon surrounds these topics, and it is helpful to work with these terms outlined in Table 4-1.

**Table 4-1**

| | |
|---|---|
| Frequency | The number of training sessions, normally in a week |
| Duration | The length in distance or time of each training session |
| Volume | The product of frequency and duration |
| Intensity | The relative physiological difficulty of exercise, measured as a fraction of $VO_2$ max, maximal heart rate, or peak running speed |
| Training load | The product of volume and intensity, and an indicator of stress placed on the runner |
| Law of Specificity | A training principle stating that physiological adaptations are specific to the training activity |
| Overload | Increasing training load over a period of time |
| Overreaching | A state of very heavy training load associated with a temporary performance decrement |
| Recovery | A period of reduced or lowered training load that permits the body to repair, regenerate, and produce beneficial adaptations |
| Overtraining syndrome | A special condition in which hormonal and physiological responses to training are disrupted, producing an inability to train and perform without symptoms |

Quantifying Training Stress (Load)
(Frequency x Duration) x Intensity = Training Load

"We can't manage what we don't measure." This quote is most often attributed to management expert Peter Drucker. It is not clear who actually uttered these words, but the point is clear: if we want to manage our training and increase our odds for success, we need to quantify the stress our running is inflicting on us. This means we must apply a systematic and scientific approach to our training.

As you are well aware, running is hard. It places significant stress on your body depending on how far or how hard you run. But because it is the stress that helps us get better, it is helpful to describe it in a standard way. In much the same way that we can quantify the physical stress exerted on a piece of steel, we can also quantify the training stress we exert on our bodies when we run. This is called the training load, and is described as a simple product of two variables:

Volume x Intensity = Training Load

Since training load is a product, increasing either volume or intensity results in an increase in load, and that means only one thing: more stress on your body. Therefore our aim is to be conscious of the training load we are placing on systems, being careful not to place so much on them that they "break," which in our world of distance running can be an injury or illness, but always means time off from training so we can recover.

## Overload, Specificity, and the Legend of Milo

We have long known that adaptations and changes occur with training, however the field of Exercise Physiology is a young one, and our understanding of the exact mechanisms behind the physiological adaptations came about only in the latter half of the twentieth century. An oft cited example of how the body adapts, and one used in most exercise physiology courses, is the legend of Milo of Croton, an ancient Greek wrestler in the sixth century BC. Part of his legend states that Milo carried a four-year-old bull on his shoulders (prior to slaughtering and eating it!), which is an impressive feat of strength by any standard. He is said to have achieved this by lifting a newborn calf above his head as a young boy, and repeating this task each day—until eventually he was able to lift the grown bull. We will never know if Milo really did lift a four-year-old bull above his head, but we can most certainly use what we know about the physiological adaptations to training to explain how it could have happened.

Milo's legend is a simple but accurate example of two key training principles: overload and specificity. Overload is just what it sounds like: adding more load (or stress) than what is presently applied. Specificity is also what it sounds like, and is most often referred to in training as the Law of Specificity. It means that the physiological adaptations are specific to the training stress applied. In Milo's story, the reason he could lift the four-year old bull is that he lifted said bull every day until it was grown, thus applying specificity to his training by lifting a bull. He also applied the principle of overload by lifting the ever growing bull. Each day as the bull grew only slightly bigger, he lifted it, thus adding some weight (but not too much, and more on that later) to the mass he was lifting.

As runners trying to improve, we overload our systems by increasing the training load, and that can be accomplished by modulating the volume, intensity, or both. Doing this sets off a series of physiological mechanisms that ultimately improve our performance.

## General Adaptation Syndrome

The foundation of what we know about physiological adaptations to exercise training is from the work of Dr. Hans Selye, an endocrinologist who studied the physiological response to "stress" in the early and middle twentieth century. Selye studied an organism's physiological responses to noxious agents. In a defining experiment, he injected the tissue of different organs into mice and observed that, no matter what he injected, the physiological response was the same. That might seem self-evident today, but Selye hypothesized that the different injections would cause different responses. Observing that the response was independent of the type of injection, he concluded that it was non-specific in nature, meaning that no matter what the stimulus, the body responded in the same manner. He is also credited with introducing the biological connotation of stress, which until that time was applied almost exclusively in a physical sense of "stress and strain" on an object or person.

But in the context of exercise training, Selye is best known for introducing the general adaptation syndrome, or GAS (Figure 4-1). Selye developed this model to describe not only how we respond to stressors, but also that we can adapt to those stressors, and even reach a state of exhaustion if the stressors are chronic in nature. Early exercise physiologists who had studied Selye's work applied his GAS model to explain how exercise training causes adaptations.

In Selye's model, a stressor disturbs homeostasis. This causes an "alarm phase," which represents the mobilization of non-specific hormonal and other

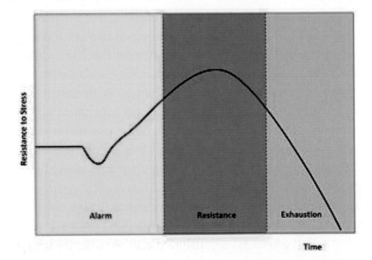

**Figure 4-1** Example of general adaptation syndrome in context of stress.

physiological responses to cope with the stressor. The mounting of these physiological processes helps us maintain homeostasis. However if the stressor is of sufficient frequency and duration—for example, running four to six times each week—we will begin to adapt to it so that what was initially a shock to our system becomes a more normal situation, resulting in a lesser physiological response to maintain homeostasis. It is during this "resistance phase" that the effect of the physiological responses is adaptations that enhance our ability to cope with the stressor. Should the stressor continue at too high a frequency or duration, however, "exhaustion" arrives, which for Selye meant the inability to continue to cope with the stress, and not a literal state of physical exhaustion.

## Modern Application of the GAS

In Selye's paradigm, stress was a good thing. Stress represented a state in which the body was coping with an external stimulus, and even producing adaptations to better cope with that stress in the future. If we drop Selye's GAS model into a distance running context, it looks like this:

In application, we want to perturb our physiological systems by overload. Ideally we are very specific in the way we do this, for example we increase our distance gradually, which will improve our endurance, or we start a period of speed work (high-intensity training), which will help us run faster. If the frequency of this training is appropriate, we enter Selye's resistance phase, and sooner or later become overreached, at which point we reduce the training load and recover, thus permitting our body to produce the adaptations that improve our performance.

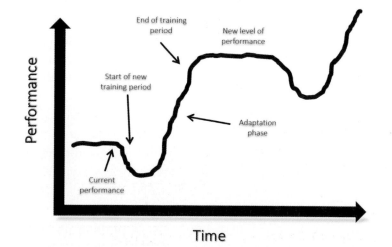

**Figure 4-2** Selye's general Adaption Syndrome in a training context.

# Running Economy

The ability to be economical in our movement has been a key to the evolution of humans over the millennia. On the African savannah, when humans existed as hunter-gatherers, conserving energy in an environment of scarce resources was a determinant of survival. Our ancestors faced a significant challenge as they sought to move from a current location to a distant place, where there might be more water or more food. But traveling by foot costs energy, which was often scarce. Hence, we evolved to be extremely good walkers, using relatively little energy to travel at walking speeds across flat land, and also relatively good runners when compared to other four-legged mammals.

As a species, humans are not quite as good as runners as we are walkers, and running costs us around 10 percent more energy per unit of distance we cover. Regardless, the principles are the same: economy of movement determines success, for our ancient ancestors but also for the modern runner, because given a finite ability to go between Point A and B, the runner who can cover that distance using as little fuel as possible will have greater odds at success. Therefore when we run at any given speed, we want to use as little energy as possible to maintain that speed.

# How to Improve Running Economy

In sports science, we say that the first step to becoming a world champion is to choose your parents wisely, because, while many factors predict your running economy (and performance), your genes are the most important indicator of your athletic success. Genetically inherited traits like your body mass, the distribution of that body mass, and other variables all work to determine how economical a runner you can be. But many physiological characteristics can be improved with training, and the evidence is clear that when we increase the training load in an appropriate and specific manner, one of the outcomes is improved running economy.

When exposed to slow long distance running, we produce adaptations that are specific to that activity. These are mostly cardiovascular in nature and are listed in Figure 4-3. In real life what we see is that at a given running speed, our effort level is lower, and that is because we are using less oxygen to do the same amount of work. It's easier for us. So how do we get there?

Technically we refer to this as sub-maximal training, since it occurs at intensities that are below your $VO_2$ max, heart rate, or running speed. In more colloquial terms this is known as "base training." Novice runners will benefit most

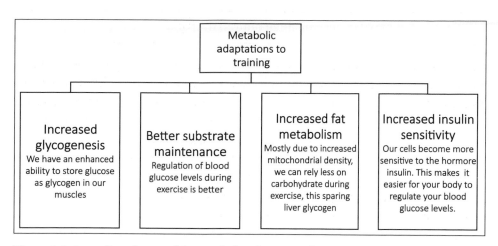

**Figure 4-3** An outline of some of the metabolic adaptations that occur with endurance training.

by engaging in this type of training, but experienced and already well-trained runners have little to gain by engaging in it. The exception is that if your goal is to perform over longer distances, then you must apply the law of specificity to your training and complete some running at slower speeds (over longer distances) so that you adapt to being on your feet for many hours.

The common trap many runners fall into is the "more is more" paradigm, where very high-mileage weeks are seen as the ultimate training stimulus. In many ways it's easy to clock high-mileage weeks, especially for the experienced runner, yet doing so not only represents relatively low-quality training, but can also lead to an unmanageable increase in training load if the distance increases too quickly, or if the volume and intensity are not modulated in an appropriate manner to create the right progression. Even if manageable, however, longer distances are associated with more muscle damage, and that can either prevent a planned increase in training load due to more recovery time, or even result in injury.

The law of specificity states that the adaptations humans produce (and that ultimately improve performance) are specific to the training. Therefore, if your aim is to run faster, then doing more miles at a sub-maximal pace violates this principle of training. Instead the most effective way to improve your distance running performance is by engaging in high-intensity interval training (HIIT).

## High-Intensity Interval Training

While slow long distance running is always completed at sub-maximal intensities, HIIT can be performed at higher than maximal (supra-maximal); maximal

(100 percent of max); or sub-maximal but relatively high intensities (greater than 90 percent VO$_2$ max). The adaptations produced from this type of training are more specific to our desired outcome—running faster! Consequently, these adaptations tend to be more neuromuscular in nature, as opposed to the cardiovascular adaptations that result from long slow distance running, although further metabolic adaptations can occur with HIIT.

Experienced runners will know HIIT as speed work or interval training, both of which are accurate terms to describe the nature of the activity. What runners might not be familiar with are the well-understood principles behind HIIT and how to apply them best to improve performance. Because training load increases when intensity goes up, it is absolutely crucial to modulate volume so that the overall load, while increased, is not too high. In other words, you can't violate the law of specificity and train at high volumes and high intensity. That is a certain recipe for failure.

## Quality versus Quantity

Prescribing HIIT is easy, even if the actual execution is difficult. Typically, you should replace no more than 10 to 15 percent of your weekly volume with HIIT. It is better to err on the 10 percent or less side than trying to do too much. When approaching HIIT, you must decide on the focus of each training period. Performing intervals at sub-maximal running speeds in which the work to rest ratio is higher (for example 2:1), or intervals in which you are running closer to 100 percent of VO$_2$ max and the work to rest ratio is lower, for example 1:2.

A typical example of the sub-maximal intervals is the classic 400m interval workout. In one version, you complete the appropriate number of reps at a pace slightly faster than your 5K race pace and rest for 60 to 90 seconds between reps. This helps teach your neuromuscular system how to run more economically at these faster running speeds, while also building "fatigue resistance," which in turn will help maintain running speed during a race. Depending on your experience and fitness, this workout can be modified and completed at faster running speeds and adjusting the work to rest ratio by increasing the rest time between reps.

The other approach is completing workouts in which your running speed is close to—or even faster than—the speed at which you achieve VO$_2$ max. It is best to complete a maximal treadmill test to exhaustion to determine that speed, but if that is not possible then for most runners the pace at which you can complete a 1K time trial will be very close, and sufficiently intense to produce adaptations. The optimal duration of these intervals is 60 to 75 percent of your 1K time trial

**Table 4-2** An example of one week from a HIIT training period. To ensure you make adaptations, you must apply the principle of overload by completing the intervals at a speed faster than which you can currently run for a given distance. Exactly how much faster is tolerable will depend on the athlete, but 5 percent faster than current 5K race pace is provided here as a starting point.

| Monday | Tuesday | Wednesday | Thursday | Friday | Saturday | Sunday |
|---|---|---|---|---|---|---|
| Easy to moderate | HIIT | Easy to moderate | HIIT | Easy to moderate | Long run or rest | Long run or rest |
| 30–60 min at 50–60% VO$_2$ max | 8 x 400 m, at ~5% faster than your 5km race pace, resting 60 s between reps | 30–60 min at 50-60% VO$_2$ max | 8 x 400 m, at ~5% faster than your 5K race pace, resting 60 s between reps | 30–60 min at 50–60% VO$_2$ max | 30–60 min at 50–60% VO$_2$ max | 30–60 min at 50–60% VO$_2$ max |

time, but regardless, two to three minutes should be sufficiently hard to cause meaningful adaptations to occur.

Because the nature of these workouts is maximal, it is impossible to overestimate the importance of an extended rest period. For these training sessions, the work to rest ratio must be structured so that the recovery period is twice the duration of the reps. Therefore, if the interval duration is two minutes, the rest period following each interval must be four minutes. In addition, it is worth repeating the importance of controlling your weekly volume during a very hard training period such as this. Running at such high intensities places undue amounts of stress on your body, because in addition to the high intensity, the type of exercise is a novel activity that your body needs to learn how to cope with.

## Overtraining Syndrome (OTS)

**Runner A:** "How'd the race go on the weekend? Did you get your PR you have been training so hard for?"

**Runner B:** "I thought I was very well prepared, but on the day I just didn't have the form, I must have been overtrained."

Distance running can sometimes create a confluence of variables that lead to overtraining syndrome. It is extremely important to clarify the technical definition of overtraining syndrome, because many runners, as in the example above, often use it incorrectly. What the runner above described is fatigue, or more specifically overreaching, which is an accumulation of fatigue resulting from too

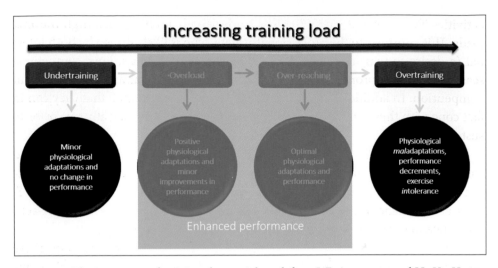

**Figure 4-4** The continuum of training phases. Adapted from L.E. Armstrong and J.L. VanHeest, 2002, "The unknown mechanism of the overtraining syndrome," *Sports Medicine* 32(1): 185-209.

much training relative to too little recovery, but that can be resolved in a matter of days by implementing appropriate recovery. Overreaching certainly creates a performance decrement, as will overtraining syndrome—although they are entirely different mechanisms.

In their position statement on OTS, the European College of Sports Science describes OTS as "an accumulation of training and/or nontraining stress resulting in long-term decrement in performance capacity with or without related physiological and psychological signs and symptoms of maladaptation in which restoration of performance capacity may take several weeks or months."

OTS is relatively rare, although in elite athlete populations the prevalence (the proportion of athletes who have OTS) is thought to be higher compared to recreational populations. But because OTS cannot be reproduced in the lab, it remains understudied. However, there is agreement among experts that OTS is related to a state in which the athlete can no longer cope with even daily training stress, and that it is likely caused by too heavy a training load (which can be heightened by competing too often) with inadequate recovery. It most often involves psychological as well as physical symptoms.

Although a real condition, the risk of OTS in nearly all recreational athletes remains low if only for the fact that an athlete is more likely to sustain an injury prior to arriving at an official diagnosis of OTS. Because the training loads required to produce OTS are so high, and must be sustained, most competitive, recreational runners will avoid OTS simply by being required to engage in daily activities like work and family life that inadvertently prohibit such high training loads. This contrasts to the professional athlete, who is likely driven by both internal (a desire to win) and external factors (contract renewals, long competitive seasons, etc.) that promote extremely high training loads, amplified by frequent competition. In addition, these athletes are so effectively trained that they can in fact cope with these high training loads longer than recreational athletes prior to sustaining injury.

Preventing OTS is crucial, because recovery from it can take months, and sometimes athletes never return to their past performances after being overtrained. And although most of us are highly unlikely ever to get close to OTS, there are tools and techniques that can help identify when an athlete is approaching a state of extreme overreaching and might be on a path to OTS.

Since recovery can be long, avoiding OTS altogether is crucial, and there are some tools available that help athletes and coaches. Psychological symptoms often precede and worsen as OTS develops, and mood state questionnaires like the Profile of Mood States (POMS) can be used to track an athlete over time. Originally developed in 1971, the POMS questionnaire consists of a list of sixty-five items such as "Lively," "Angry," and "Fatigued." The individual is instructed to read each item and choose how they have been feeling in the past week about that particular item by choosing from several options: Not at all, A little, Moderately, Quite a bit, or Extremely. Also, although less studied but still sensitive to life stresses, the Daily Analysis of Life Demands in Athletes (DALDA) questionnaire can be used to understand when both training and life stresses might be approaching unsustainable levels. Sample DALDA questions are in Table 4-3.

There are also physiological tests that have been shown to detect overreached states, and can therefore guide an athlete and coach on when it is appropriate decrease the training load. The Heartrate Interval Monitoring System (HIMS) is a short running test that uses heart rate, specifically the heart rate recovery, to detect changes in training status (Figure 4-5). It is practically feasible for both runners and team sports since it requires only a 20m shuttle run and takes

Table 4-3 Sample DALDA questions.

| Topic | Description | Response |
|-------|-------------|----------|
| Muscle Pains | Do you have sore joints and/or pains in your muscles? | The individual chooses to response with: A: Worse than normal B: Normal C: Better than normal |
| Weight | How is your weight? | |
| Enough sleep | Are you getting enough sleep? | |

only thirteen minutes to complete. It was designed to be used by team sports prior to a practice session, and as such works effectively as a warm up, too. The test itself requires participants to run for two minutes at four different running speeds; the recovery heart rate between stages and at the end of the test is the primary outcome measure. Coaches can also teach athletes how to complete this test on their own, and simply review heart-rate monitor files over time to track training status.

It should be noted, however, that none of these tools have been proven to prevent OTS, but rather have been developed to detect spikes in training stress that indicate overreaching and thus warrant a reduction in training load. Because of the limitations to studying overtraining, we do not yet have a proven tool to detect exactly when it will occur, and thus the "art" aspect of coaching pairs well with the "science" aspect as coaches and athletes use these tools and training principles to cautiously walk the path hard training while avoiding failure—be it injury, illness, or OTS.

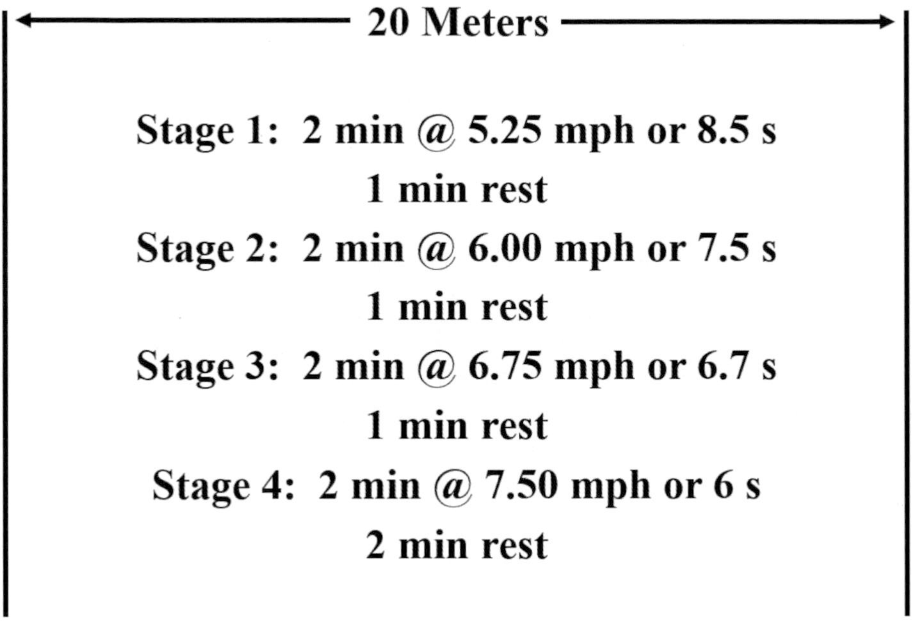

---

**◄────── 20 Meters ──────►**

**Stage 1:  2 min @ 5.25 mph or 8.5 s**

**1 min rest**

**Stage 2:  2 min @ 6.00 mph or 7.5 s**

**1 min rest**

**Stage 3:  2 min @ 6.75 mph or 6.7 s**

**1 min rest**

**Stage 4:  2 min @ 7.50 mph or 6 s**

**2 min rest**

---

**Figure 4-5** The Heart Rate Interval Monitoring System (HIMS) protocol, from Lamberts et al., *J Strength and Conditioning*, 2004. After measuring out a 20 meter shuttle run, the runner completes each shuttle at the given speed, or in the number of seconds in the diagram. Between intervals, the runner stands quietly to capture heart-rate recovery (HRR). Deviations in HRR can then be used to help detect overreaching or increased training stress, and help an athlete and coach understand when to consider modifying a training program.

# Summary

Training for distance running is about connecting multiple training periods in the absence of injury. Applying the basic training principles outlined in this chapter can help you avoid injury, primarily by taking a systematic and objective approach to your training techniques. Although real, OTS is a rare injury, and most runners remain at low-risk for OTS even when completing peak training periods. As a recreational runner, your time is much better spent carefully mapping out an annual plan that balances hard training periods with competition, and always listening to your body so that you can remain injury and illness free.

## CHAPTER 5

# Hydration Recommendations for Training and Competing

## BY ERIC K. O'NEAL AND TAMARA HEW-BUTLER

## Key Points

1. Hydration needs are dynamic and highly specific to each individual and running scenario.
2. Drinking according to the dictates of thirst while running is sufficient for most cases and protects against the perils of both dehydration and overhydration because the body regulates blood sodium concentration and circulating plasma volume through stimulation and inhibition of thirst and anti-diuretic hormone.
3. A scheduled drinking plan versus drinking to thirst is likely only necessary when sweat losses of approximately 4+ percent of body mass are expected and starts with a rough estimation of fluid needs based on predicted sweat losses and then guided by thirst, stomach fullness, and palatability.
4. Normal thirst stimulus will result in euhydration for runs separated by twenty-four hours or longer. However, under training scenarios with shorter bouts between recovery periods, particularly in the heat, a goal of replacing 115 to 120 percent of sweat losses incurred will help runners to ensure the next bout is initiated in an euhydrated state. Urine specific gravity can be a helpful in identifying runners that regularly fail to rehydrate adequately between runs.

## Introduction

The act of running generates heat from repetitive muscular contractions, which enable us to move forward (metabolic heat production). If cooling mechanisms are not activated, in response to metabolic heat production from working muscles, then our body temperature can rise to dangerously high levels and cause heatstroke. In humans, sweat production promotes heat loss through a process called "evaporative cooling." Because sweat water is continually lost to the environment during running, runners need to replace lost fluids during and following exercise. Thus, hydration guidance is of critical importance to long distance runners.

The purpose of this chapter will be to: 1) examine the basic physiology of fluid balance; 2) provide a brief review of the two most prominent viewpoints on hydration strategies in the scientific community and examine recent research related specifically to hydration and running; 3) offer a simple, self-diagnostic test to determine if you need to develop a hydration strategy based on your running scenario; and 4) cover the steps you should take if you plan on implementing your own formal hydration strategy. While understanding the physiology of hydration is likely a little overwhelming for the average runner, developing a sound hydration strategy (or choosing not to develop a hydration strategy, see below) does not have to be overly complex.

## Overview of the Physiology of Fluid Balance

The body is designed to protect both plasma osmolality (the amount of solute particles in a liter of water) and plasma volume (the amount of blood flowing within the circulation or vascular space). Although the body senses and defends plasma osmolality, for practical purposes, we will use plasma osmolality and plasma sodium concentration [Na+] interchangeably because sodium is the main solute particle which contributes to plasma osmolality (Plasma osmolality = 2 x plasma [Na+][mmol/L] + glucose [mmol/L] + blood urea nitrogen [BUN in mmol/L]) (1). As such, the physiological significance of abnormally low or high blood sodium concentration relates to "tonicity" balance which is an important regulator of cell (and tissue) size.

Here is how "tonicity" balance works: sodium ions are primarily located in the fluid that is found outside of the cells (called the extracellular fluid, or ECF fluid, space). Potassium (K+) ions are mostly found within the fluid that is located inside of the cells (called the intracellular fluid, or ICF, space). Neither sodium nor potassium ions can passively cross the cell membrane. However, both ions can equally attract water molecules, which causes water to move back and forth across the cell membrane to equilibrate the ratio between water and ions (both inside and outside the cells). This (passive) water movement across the cell membrane—to equilibrate water and ionic balance both inside and outside of cells—is called osmosis. Therefore, due to this osmotic process, hyponatremia (low blood sodium) will cause body water to flow into the cells while hypernatremia (high blood sodium) will cause body water to flow out of the cells. The medical significance of either a high (hyper) or low (hypo) blood sodium concentration (natremia) relates to either cellular and tissue shrinkage (hypernatremia) or cellular and tissue swelling (hyponatremia). Therefore, normal blood sodium concentrations (normonatremia; 135–145 mmol/L) produce a liquid and ionic environment that cells and tissues are of a perfect size and can function optimally. This is the main reason why the body strives to protect normal blood sodium concentrations at all times: to maintain optimal cell size.

Blood sodium concentration is continuously monitored within the brain via osmosensors that are located within highly vascularized brain structures called circumventricular organs (CVO) (2, 3). The CVOs are both sensory and secretory and lack a blood brain barrier; thereby permitting the central nervous system to communicate directly with tonicity changes within circulating blood (2, 3). When blood sodium concentrations are too high, these CVOs respond by stimulating the secretion of anti-diuretic hormone (ADH) from the posterior pituitary gland into the circulation. The body's main anti-diuretic hormone, more formally referred to as arginine vasopressin (AVP), prevents urinary water loss by facilitating water absorption at the kidney, thereby promoting fluid retention. If blood sodium concentrations continue to rise despite water retention via AVP (anti-diuretic hormone) stimulation, then the sensation of thirst is activated. Thirst stimulation motivates fluid intake that is physiologically designed to promptly deliver water back into the body, when needed. Thus, the combination of water retention and fluid intake effectively serves to dilute elevated blood sodium concentrations back into the normal range. Conversely, if blood sodium concentrations become too low, both AVP and thirst are suppressed (not stimulated). So, if the body does not need water (and it is diluting the sodium), then the extra water promptly exits the body as urine. This urinary-free water excretion, coupled with the absence of fluid intake, will essentially concentrate blood sodium levels back up into the normal physiological range by pouring off extra fluid.

The regulation of water within the circulation (plasma volume) is largely driven by the amount of sodium circulating within the blood vessels. Under-replaced sodium can decrease the amount of circulating water, forcing tissues to work without an adequate blood supply to deliver nutrients and eliminate wastes (under-perfusion), while also causing low blood pressure (cardiovascular instability). Decreases in plasma volume are detected by specialized volume/pressure receptors that are called baroreceptors, which are located within the carotid bodies of the aortic arch. Stimulation of these baroreceptors, from an 8 to 10 percent drop in blood pressure or plasma volume (4), will stimulate sodium to be retained in the body. Sodium retention occurs mostly in the kidneys (i.e., salt is retained by the kidney rather than excreted in the urine) by activating the hormonal system known as the renin-angiotensin-aldosterone system, or RAAS, for short. The RAAS system facilitates reabsorption of sodium at the kidney (i.e., not excreted in urine) and increases the palatability for sodium-rich foods (4, 5). Sodium conservation and subsequent ingestion of salt alone or in combination serves to increase circulating plasma volume back to baseline levels over time (nineteen to twenty-four hours) (6, 7) while maintaining plasma tonicity through integrated coordination with the osmoregulatory system (6).

## Optimal Hydration Advice? Depends on Who You Ask . . .

A dichotomy of opinions has emerged within the scientific community in regard to hydration and endurance exercise performance/safety. The origin of this split began when the highly regarded American College of Sports Medicine (ACSM) organization published a position stand that included the statement, "During exercise, athletes should start drinking early and at regular intervals in an attempt to consume fluids at a rate sufficient to replace all the water lost through sweating (i.e., body weight loss)" (8). The premise of this statement is clearly at odds with real world application, as the most successful endurance athletes often lose the most weight in endurance competitions (9, 10, 11). A concerted effort from scientists opposed the promotion of this assertion when runners began to drink too much fluid (12). However, the perils of dehydration have remained prominent in textbooks (13) and continue to persist within the running community (14).

An excellent window into the origins of both arguments (dehydration versus over-hydration) has been debated elsewhere (15). As such, the ACSM has amended their original position stand by proposing a goal of fluid ingestion that does not exceed sweat losses but limits loss in body weight to less than 2 percent (16). This position has been repeatedly verified in laboratory settings when a 2 percent decrease in body weight (usually by heat exposure or severe restriction of fluid) from baseline before exercise has been repeatedly shown to impair performance, heat dissipation, and cardiovascular function, especially in hot and humid environments (17). While the exercise science laboratory allows for very tight controls in regard to conditions between performance trials (internal validity), these studies often fail to represent real world race conditions (ecological validity). The artificially controlled environments incorporated are often much more severe in regard to the majority of race environments, particularly in comparison to marathon distance events which are predominantly scheduled in cooler months. Another debated aspect concerning studies that support the less than 2 percent loss in body mass strategy is the frequent incorporation of time to exhaustion performance tests that require participants to cycle or run at a single intensity and end when the intensity cannot be maintained versus time trials (10). Two recent studies (described in Table 5-1) both failed to show that intentionally drinking to maintain less than 2 percent body mass loss is advantageous to drinking to thirst alone (often referred to as ad libitum) during runs in high thermal stress conditions.

While these two approaches (drink to limit body mass loss to less than 2 percent or drink to thirst) continue to be debated, the authors of this chapter promote a position that leans more heavily toward the latter with a few extra considerations. Drinking to reduce body mass loss to less than 2 percent is too conservative to be promoted, as the top marathon runners in the world are predicted to lose 6 to 11 percent of their body mass during competition while drinking for less than sixty seconds over the entire race distance (18). Observations of the hydration practices of some of the world's most elite runners in Kenya also suggest that very little, if any, fluid intake takes place during training and that ad libitum fluid intake between training bouts is all that is needed to promote day-to-day euhydration (19). However, comparing the habits of the world's elite athletes to the average runner may not be highly transferable. Elite athletes are less affected by extreme environments and likely can overcome greater fluid deficits than the average runner, without compromising performance. Likewise, conclusions observing behavior of the Kenyan running cohort are drawn from group means, not individual data. The variance reported with these means suggests very different hydration habits exist between runners in the study cited. Drinking to thirst provides the proper stimulus for the majority of running situations, but there are individuals and certain race or training scenarios where incorporating a formal hydration strategy may potentially improve performance (see next section).

## Do You Need a Hydration Plan?

Running creates unique obstacles in regard to fluid intake during exercise. Swimmers can place a water bottle next to the pool while swimming laps, and cyclists can carry multiple water bottles on their bikes. Carrying any substantial volume of fluid for runners, typically means wearing a belt full of water bottles or a backpack with a bladder system. Neither of these options is desirable for runners seeking to maximize running economy and can present a new set of problems in regards to chafing. During long runs on hot days, access to chilled

> **Box 5-1** Determining sweat loss volume for fluid prescription
>
> Directions
>
> 1. Before you run, weigh yourself on a digital scale in the nude. Make sure your scale is accurate and reliable (always measure more than once). Weigh yourself using the metric mode (1 liter of water = 1 kg of mass; converting using pounds and ounces is not as easy). This makes prescription fairly easy as most water bottles are demarcated by 0.1 liters. Typical race aid station cups are a little under 0.25 liters when filled to the top for a visual reference.
> 2. Choose a time of day where environmental conditions will come closest to matching conditions you expect to experience during competition. Run for 1 hour at the pace you expect to maintain during your event.
> 3. After drying off post-run, weigh yourself again in the nude.
>
> Tips for the most accurate assessment
>
> - We recommend not drinking or using the restroom during this process for simplification. However, if you choose to do so, you need to add the volume of fluid you ingested after initial weigh-in to your difference in body mass from pre- to post-run. Voids must be subtracted from difference in body mass or an overestimation of sweat losses will occur.
> - Pace and environmental conditions can drastically alter your sweat losses. It is not necessary to conduct these steps for every run, but assessing sweat losses once or twice a month and keeping a log that includes pace, weather conditions, and duration can really help you establish a good conception of what your sweat losses will look like across a variety of conditions.
> - Weigh in and out in the nude. Sports bras and running shorts and shirts can retain up to a liter of water when fully saturated resulting in considerable underestimation of actual sweat losses.
> - We highly recommend using the 1 hour time frame so you can easily extrapolate the total sweat loss you expect to experience in your event.
>
> How to use this information
>
> - *How much should I drink during my run example*: You lost 1.25 liters of sweat during a 1 hour run matching your expected race day environment/pace for a marathon. Your expected marathon finishing time is 4 hours resulting in an estimated 5 liters of total sweat loss. If you weigh 60 kg and your target weight loss is 4% of body mass your goal would be to finish with approximately 2.4 kg (or 2.4 liters) of sweat losses that will not be replenished). Your goal is to replace 2.6 liters of your 5.0 total liters of sweat loss. This number can be divided into your finishing time (i.e. 4 hours) to determine your hourly fluid intake (0.65 liters/hour).
> - *How much should I drink between heavy training bouts during hot weather example:* You just completed a 75 minute morning run that resulted in a 2.1 kg of body mass change (or ~2.1 liters of sweat loss). Before your run at 4:00 this afternoon your goal should be to replace ~120% of your sweat losses with beverage fluid intake if you are going to also be eating between your training bouts. Simply multiple your sweat losses (2.1 liters) by 1.2 (i.e. 120%). The result would be 2.52 liters. To optimize fluid retention, spread your fluid intake out over the day. This will reduce urinary losses. All beverages count as fluid intake, not just water! Milk in your cereal, soup, and fruits and vegetables all provide additional fluid intake. Unless directed by your doctor, don't avoid salty foods when training heavily in hot weather as sodium is a key to fluid retention.

water quickly disappears, decreasing beverage palatability. Runners can drink from paper cups passed out by aid station workers to keep from carrying fluids during races. However, some skill is required to ingest a significant volume of fluid when drinking from a paper cup while running at faster paces without slowing down. Fortunately (despite popular opinion), significant fluid ingestion is only needed or beneficial in very few running scenarios (see Figure 5-2). Most runners who begin races that result in significant sweat losses likely optimize running performance, and can minimize time and effort spent drinking by losing 3 to 4 percent of body mass. However, runs that produce sweat losses within the

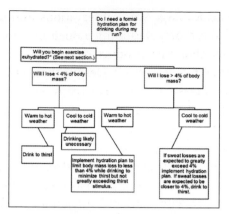

**Figure 5-2** Hydration strategy implementation decision tree.

3 to 4 percent range also result in the grayest area in regard to whether or not a hydration schedule/plan is needed. Regardless, and this cannot be emphasized enough, runners should always lose and never gain weight during a run. On runs in which sweat losses are expected to greatly exceed 4 percent body mass (see Box 5-1), a hydration plan allows for optimal fluid loss while also insuring overdrinking does not occur.

You will notice that the first subheading in Figure 5-2 addresses pre-run hydration status as the initial consideration on deciding to a schedule during your run. If you have ever competed in a large distance running event, you may have painfully learned that the most difficult task during the day is often not the race to the finish but the race to get into an outdoor, portable bathroom facility before the starting gun is fired. Many runners have developed an exaggerated fear of dehydration, resulting in impaired performance or health risks and have likely consumed fluids well beyond thirst before the race. Combine this factor with previous day tapering (no sweat losses) and sodium-rich, thirst inducing pre-event meals and you will encounter the most hyperhydrated groups of individuals on the planet converging on a relatively small area. As you can see in Box 5-1, most investigations that conclude "modest" dehydration impairs performance require participants to begin runs in very hot environments preceded by a significant state of dehydration from pre-performance tasks sweat losses followed by severe fluid restriction, a much different scenario than is experienced on race day. An explanation detailing how to estimate your race day sweat losses is available in Box 5-1, but it is suffice to state that on cool to cold race days, fluid intake is unlikely necessary in race distances of half marathon distance or shorter for most runners.

Obviously longer, competitive runs in the heat warrant more consideration for implementing planned hydration strategies. An excellent field study by Lee et al. in 2010 (20) provides large-scale observations examining directly measured fluid intake and thermoregulation of trained but non-elite male runners competing in a half-marathon race conducted under high humidity (81 percent) and warm temperatures (26.4 degrees C). Despite these environmental stressors, average ad libitum fluid ingestion was only slightly greater than 400 mL during the race (less than 20 percent of the 2.6 ± 0.6 liters sweat losses incurred) resulting in body mass loss easily exceeding greater than 2 percent body weight. More importantly, this modest fluid ingestion resulted in core temperatures exceeding 40 degrees C (marker often associated with heat stroke) for ten of the twenty-five runners assessed. All runners were asymptomatic of heat illness and these results have been further supported with similar investigations conducted in even hotter environments accompanied by no symptoms of heat illness (21). Fluid consumption during much longer races (longer than 100 km) also support that most runners will exceed 2 percent loss in body mass from sweating and again that greater loss in body mass is correlated with faster finishing times and no greater risk of heat-related injury (11).

Contrast the race day scenario above with runners engaged in a heavy summer training period that includes multiple training sessions in a single day, evening runs, and training bouts the subsequent morning. Attention to hydration demands are likely given less consideration in these situations. This is despite the fact that the importance of proper hydration for optimizing training performance is likely more crucial than in the day leading up to the fall and winter races for which the runners are preparing. The results of the second two studies described in Table 5-1 highlight the importance of (i.e., recovery) fluid intake between training bouts. Few scientific observations of ad libitum fluid intake between training bouts for runners have been conducted. A recent investigation (22) found three of thirteen runners completing a one-hour run in a warm environment (26 degrees C) failed to replace even 90 percent of their sweat losses (approximately two liters) with ad libitum fluid consumption in twelve hours following an afternoon run even when dinner and breakfast were consumed (Figure 5-3). More interestingly, the same runners showed nearly identical trends of low recovery fluid replacement percentage in comparison to fellow runners when the running bout was replicated by intensity and duration but in a cool (18 degrees C) environment that induced less sweat losses. This is the only quantitative evidence we are aware of that supports the existence of a hydration behavior pattern that we have frequently observed anecdotally (i.e., a minority of the running population likely self-selects a less than optimal level of fluid intake between training bouts to elicit the best training bout quality, but those who do are habitual offenders). Again, it should be emphasized that normal thirst stimulus (see the other

**Table 5-1** Review of recent studies examining role of hydration on running performance, thermoregulation, and heart rate.

| Reference | Participants and Protocol | Results |
|---|---|---|
| (Dion et al. 2013)[38] | Male runners (n = 10) completed a treadmill half marathon in hot (30 °C; 42% humidity) while drinking ad libitum (3.1 ± 0.6% loss in body mass) or drinking on a schedule to keep body mass loss less than 2% (1.3 ± 0.7% loss in body mass). | Final rectal temperature was 0.3 °C higher and mean heart rate was elevated by 4 beats/min while drinking to thirst. Finishing time (89.8 ± 7.7 min) was not different from drinking to schedule (89.6 ± 7.7 min). |
| (Lopez et al. 2016)[40] | Male (n = 8) and female (n = 5) runners completed 5 laps on a 4-km single track trail in hot weather (WBGT = 28.3 ± 1.9 °C) while drinking ad libitum (2.6 ± 0.5% loss in body mass) or on a schedule to keep body mass losses under 2% (1.3 ± 0.5% loss in body mass). | No differences were found in final core temperature and minimal differences in heart rate. Finishing time did not differ for ad libitum intake (104.2 ± 9.2 min) versus drinking to a schedule (104.6 ± 10.6 min). |
| (Casa et al. 2010)[39] | Male (n = 9) and female (n = 8) runners completed 3 laps on a 4-km single track trail in the heat (WBGT 26.5 °C) while beginning in either a euhydrated or dehydrated state. Runners completed around an hour of exercise in the heat the day before time trials to induce dehydration. During the euhydrated trials runners drank liberally while beverage consumption was restricted for the 22 hour period before the time trials in the dehydrated treatment. Runners were only allowed to drink while running during the euhydrated trial. | Core temperature was not statistically different at the end of the first or second loop, but was higher by 0.3 °C at the end of the third loop when runners started time trials dehydrated and were not allowed to drink. Heart rate did not differ at the end of any loops. However, pace was improved for all 3 laps individual and overall time (euhydrated = 53.2 ± 6.1 min; dehydrated = 55.7 ± 7.5 min) was improved when runners began euhydrated and were allowed to drink while running. |
| (Davis et al. 2014)[25] | Male (n = 11) and female (n = 2) runners completed morning 10-km time trials on a challenging outdoor running course in the heat (WBGT ~23 °C) after replacing either 75 or 150% of their sweat losses from a run the previous evening in the heat (WBGT ~27 °C) that resulted in ~3% loss in body mass. | Heart rate and final core temperature did not differ between fluid replacement treatments. However, running performance was increased with 150% recovery fluid replacement (45.9 ± 6.0 min) versus 75% recovery fluid replacement (47.3 ± 6.6 min). |

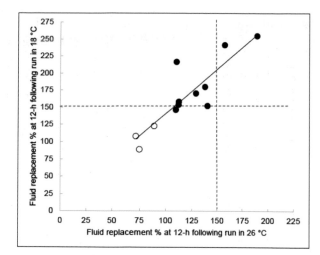

**Figure 5-3** Scatterplot for fluid replacement volume by percentage of sweat loss at twelve hours (intraclass correlation = 0.89; p < 0.001). Each marker represents an individual runner. Markers with no fill represent the three participants described in discussion. Dashed lines represent 150 percent fluid replacement as suggested by ACSM guidelines. (Reproduced with permission from authors.)

participants' fluid replacement patterns in Figure 5-3) is likely all that is needed for the majority of runners to adequately rehydrate, but recognizing (see section below on USG) these chronic hypohydraters is where the focus of individuals giving hydration advice should be concentrated. The explanation for the differences rehydration efforts by outliers on both ends of the spectrum is not well understood and likely multifaceted (e.g., differences level of concern for dehydration, food, and beverage selection), and may even have a genetic component that has yet to be strongly elucidated (23, 24).

The impetus for the latter study was earlier findings that replacement of 75 percent of sweat losses of runners beginning a seventy-five minute evening run in a euhydrated state resulted in a decrease of performance of 3 percent in a 10K time trial the following morning compared to 150 percent replacement of sweat losses with beverage fluid intake over the same time period (25). Session rate of perceived exertion was also rated higher despite the slower finishing times with 75 percent fluid replacement. It must be noted, however, that decreased performance was not accompanied by change in final core temperature or an increase in heart rate (i.e., no health or safety risks were incurred). Runners simply chose to decrease their pace to offset potential cardiovascular drift (increase in heart rate that occurs with significant loss in body water) or thermal strain.

Similar to the responses displayed in Figure 5-3, a small portion of runners reported that replacement of only 75 percent of their sweat losses was not that different from the volume of fluid they would normally expect to consume.

On the other hand, most participants reported 150 percent replacement during a twelve-hour time frame as greatly exceeding what they considered would be their normal fluid intake volume under the same training scenario. The authors concluded that while 150 percent replacement provided improved performance compared to modest recovery fluid under replacement, a target somewhere in the middle ground (115 to 120 percent replacement) is likely optimal as total fluid retention between the two fluid intake volumes differed minimally after urinary voids were accounted for.

In summary, when serious training bouts separated by less than twelve hours are taking place in warm environments, meals should be consumed regularly and a concerted effort should be made to ensure that a level of beverage fluid intake greater than or equal to 115 percent but not greatly exceeding 150 percent of sweat losses (accomplished by simply drinking ad libitum for most runners) is achieved to promote pre-run euhydration, optimizing training quality and minimize risk of EAH.

## Determination of Hydration Status

Beginning exercise in a fully hydrated state is crucial in minimizing the need to ingest fluid while running and optimizing performance. As described earlier, plasma osmolality/sodium concentration is the regulated variable that is monitored by the brain (osmoreceptors) and fiercely protected by the body's redundant physiological mechanisms (AVP secretion and thirst stimulation). Plasma osmolality is considered the "gold standard" biomarker for representing fluid balance within the body (1, 3, 26, 27). The normal range for plasma osmolality is 282–298 mOsmol/kgH2O (28) while the normal range for sodium concentration is 135–145 mmol/L (12). While useful in the laboratory, it is difficult to imagine a scenario in which plasma osmolality could actually be incorporated by the recreationally competitive runner. Unless you have the capability to draw your own blood, centrifuge it to separate red blood cells from plasma, and then use an osmometer to determine osmolality level of the separated plasma, this measurement is of little practical value.

There are many surrogate measures of hydration status of various levels of validity that are quick, cheap, and easy to perform. However, we recommend the following two considerations for runners. The first is to use change in body mass to determine sweat losses. While not 100 percent accurate (29) the difference in weight after simply weighing yourself in the nude before and after a run will get you within 90 percent or more accuracy of the volume of sweat you have lost under most conditions. In a survey of close to 300 half- and full-marathon runners (30), less than 3 percent reported using this method when assessing hydration status. It is impossible to accurately prescribe fluid intake during or between runs as outlined above if a ballpark estimate of sweat loss cannot be determined. We like to use the analogy that developing a drinking schedule without understanding your sweat loss volume is akin to trying to determine when you need to get gas while driving around in a car with a broken gas gauge. Fortunately most drivers would not routinely run out of gas after a little experience driving under such conditions. However, there would undoubtedly be a small percentage of drivers who were too cautious and pumped gas way more often than needed (i.e., runners at risk for hyponatremia) and drivers who occasionally ran out of gas (i.e., runners experiencing significant enough dehydration that performance may be hindered). A recognition of actual sweat losses can help runners determine fluid needs to prevent excessive dehydration, but more importantly can prevent extreme hyperhydration and hyponatremia during exercise.

Multiple investigations have repeatedly found recreationally competitive runners have no idea of how much sweat loss they incur on a typical run and almost always underestimate actual sweat losses, likely due to the immense volume of sweat that is never seen due to evaporation (body's primary mechanism to cool itself). First noted by Passe et al. in 2007 (31), runners completing a ten-mile run on a track with ample opportunities to drink were able to estimate their fluid intake with precision, but underestimated their sweat losses by over 40 percent. Perplexingly, the authors devoted most of their attention to the fact that the

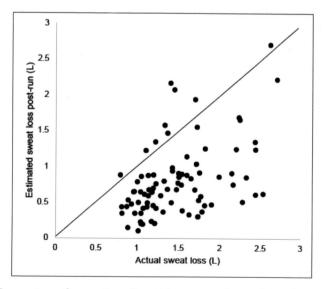

**Figure 5-4** Comparison of perception of sweat loss to actual sweat loss volume in male and female runners. Each marker represents an individual. All runs lasted sixty minutes and were conducted under a variety of environmental conditions.

runners only replaced around 30 percent of their sweat losses. When compared to incorrectly estimated sweat losses, the runners were not actually that far off from fully replacing what they perceived (again incorrectly) to be their sweat loss volume. Figure 5-4 displays the combined data from multiple studies (22, 32, 33) conducted in our laboratory in which we have asked runners of both genders to estimate their sweat losses after runs of sixty minutes in varying environments. The first item of note in the figure is how much sweat loss variability (range from ~0.75 to almost 3 L per hour) exists between runners, highlighting the vast differences in hydration needs during and between running bouts. The second trend to note is that while in general, heavier sweaters estimated greater sweat losses, almost all runners underestimated their sweat losses (markers below the 45-degree angle line) with many underestimating by a wide margin (some by as much as two liters in a single hour!). Box 5-1 details steps on how to accurately determine your sweat loss volume and common mistakes that we have seen runners make when attempting to use this method.

Understanding your true sweat loss volume can answer almost any hydration strategy related question. However, for runners that do not want to constantly calculate sweat losses and measure fluid intake, we recommend using a refractometer to occasionally spot check yourself before runs. Refractometers are fairly inexpensive (around 30 dollars), easy to use, and provide an objective assessment tool. Urine specific gravity (USG), the density of urine relative to distilled water, is assessed by establishing the magnitude of refraction of light passing through a drop of urine placed on the refractometer. While some have debated the validity of USG (34), and it is by no means a perfect assessment measure, we have found it to be a useful tool when determining if low fluid intake has taken place between runs separated by approximately twelve hours (e.g., evening run followed by run the next morning or twice-per-day training). Figure 5-5 displays the individual responses of morning USG from the study by Davis and colleagues (25) described in Table 5-1. When a mixed variety of beverages and two meals were served with 75 versus 150 percent of sweat loss replacement from an evening run, morning USG was increased with low fluid replacement for every runner with an average difference of twelve units. A USG of less than or equal to 1.020 is often cited as a marker of euhydration, but may be a little bit of a conservative criterion for runners training in the heat. Shift from "normal" USG should also be considered if your log reveals you regularly exhibit lower USG (e.g., less than 1.010). Urine color is also a popular assessment technique (35) but the difficulties in duplicating accurate assessment of urine color between researchers is well-documented (36). Again, it is important to stress that neither of these techniques (USG of urine color) are as accurate, reliable, or useful as using measured sweat losses,

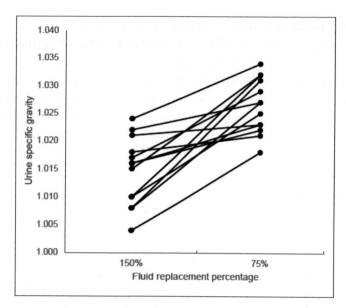

**Figure 5-5** Comparisons of urine specific gravity (USG) at twelve hours after replacement of 75 versus 150 percent of sweat losses incurred during a seventy-five-minute evening run in the heat. Sport beverages, juice, and water were consumed during recovery and a standardized dinner and light breakfast were served.

fluid intake, and urine output in establishing hydration status/fluid intake needs, but they might be useful as secondary measures of establishing if your normal thirst stimulus does not promote optimal fluid consumption between training bouts. Above all, physiology strives to protect plasma osmolality and volume; thus all excreted and secreted fluids represent the body's response to the preservation of osmotic balance and circulating blood volume and not always an accurate real-time measure of total body hydration status.

## Conclusions

Because water is essential to life, evolutionary pressures to maintain circulating water and preserve osmolality are encoded within the DNA of all vertebrates (and some invertebrate) species (37). The amount of water that each individual needs at any given time, in any situation, to protect plasma volume and osmolality is centrally dictated in real-time by linear alterations in the physiological sensation of thirst (3, 28). The more water that the body needs, the thirstier animals become (and vice versa) (28). The dire consequences associated with both underdrinking and overdrinking have been sensationalized and are rare. However, misguided drinking (not in response to thirst) can have fatal consequences if unexpected variables exceed maximum compensatory capabilities associated with habitual tendencies (often from well-intentioned advice). Therefore, under the vast major-ity of running scenarios hydration advice should be simple: drink to thirst. Any overshoot or under-replacement of fluid will be continuously corrected by redun-dant physiological systems. In situations where this may not be the case (e.g., ultramarathons in the heat) or if you simply are unsure about your hydration needs, a proper understanding of your sweat losses can help you to be confident that you are not making a significant error in either direction.

## CHAPTER 6

# Performance Nutrition

## BY LESLIE BONCI

## Key Points

1. Optimizing sports nutrition practices can maximize performance, recovery, and health.
2. Food rules: elimination, extreme eating, and timing mistakes can impact short- and long-term performance goals.
3. Fuel substrates need to be customized with regards to quantity, quality, form, and timing.
4. Recommendations for fluid must consider resting needs, activity, sweat loss, and sodium loss.
5. Screening for Relative Energy Deficit in Sports is essential to safeguard health and optimize performance.

## Introduction

Distance running is a compilation of training consistency, perseverance, and dedication. Fueling for distance requires strategic planning for consistency, quantity, and quality of ingested foods and fluids to optimize training performance, recovery, and events. In a 2005 study, 90 percent of ultra-endurance runners felt that nutrition impacted performance (1). Endurance exercise puts physiological stress on the body resulting in a constant state of preparation for the next training session/race or reparation from the previous workout/event. Being proactive and anticipatory with regard to food and fluid timing, selection, and amount can optimize performance and minimize the risk of injury, digestive distress, and delayed recovery post-runs. Most importantly, nutrition strategies need to be customized and practiced in training to fine tune.

Many runners are more mindful of their pace than their plate. Unintended consequences of improper fueling, elimination without justification, or overconsumption affect not only performance, but also health. Athletes without lactose intolerance who eliminate dairy may find it more difficult to meet protein and calcium needs. Athletes who eliminate gluten without justification may consume inadequate amounts of protein, whole grains, fiber, vitamins, and minerals.

It is a health-care practitioner's responsibility to help athletes safeguard health and optimize performance. The Internet is rife with sports nutrition recommendations and runners may be influenced by other runners, coaches, or trainers, none of whom are experts in sports nutrition. Evidence-based sports nutrition recommendations rather than sensationalism should be the rule, not the exception.

# Basic Nutrition Facts for Endurance Runners

## How Does Endurance Sport Impact Nutritional Status?

In general, the longer one is physically active, the greater the energy demands and the need for additional calories above those required for resting energy expenditure. In addition, exercising at temperature or altitude extremes can also increase energy and fluid requirements. For many athletes, the physical gut jostling associated with running presents a set of unique challenges in finding on the run nutrition that is both tolerable and palatable. As distance increases, intake does not always keep pace with the additional miles, or conversely, during tapers, there is no justification in consuming more calories than what is needed. Constant modification, evaluation, and contemplation are required by both health-care practitioners and the athlete to achieve a plan that can be realistically implemented.

## What Are Some Common Sports Nutrition Mistakes?

Many runners follow self-imposed food rules. This may include the list of foods that have caused GI distress during training or races, or food consumed during a particularly bad race outcome, where the food becomes the scapegoat and is then relegated to the never-to-consume-again pile. In addition, there are athletes that choose to eat green, or clean, or lean, not realizing that what they give up may be the foods that optimize performance. It is important to get an overall assessment of nutrition and hydration status, best done by a sports dietitian to get a better picture of the athlete's food beliefs, anxieties, and concerns so appropriate recommendations can be made.

---

### Elimination without Justification

---

Food fads are trendy, sexy, and quite appealing, and when a successful distance runner proclaims that gluten free, Paleo, or non-GMO is the secret to success it is hard not to be enthralled. However, the downside is that those foods and nutrients eliminated may not be adequately replaced, resulting in a deficit which can negatively impact strength, speed, stamina, and recovery. Certainly runners with foods allergies, food intolerances, and food sensitivities should be cautious about what they choose to eat, but if a food is taken away from the plate, there needs to be a comparable replacement.

In attempt to eat healthfully, some runners are extremely rigid with their food choices, opting to minimize fat intake, trying to avoid all sugars, consuming only organic, and keeping processed foods to a minimum. Avoidant behavior can result inadequate calorie consumption, which may contribute to impaired performance and increased risk of injury.

## Too Little Fuel or Excessive Consumption Pre-, During, or Post-Training or Races

GI distress is a deal breaker for most runners, resulting in sometimes being overly cautious with food and fluid intake around the time of exercise in the hope of preventing digestive discomfort. Inadequate fueling may negatively impact performance and may also result in muscle protein breakdown during a run. Conversely, overconsumption can cause GI distress and is also an excess calorie load for the body, which could result in unwanted weight gain. Runners need to personalize and customize food choices, form, and volume to find what works well.

## Inadequate Recovery

The only way to become a great runner is to put in the miles. This may be one daily training run, two-a-days, interval training, hill training, and resistance training sessions. Inadequate fueling and hydration post-exercise delays muscle glycogen and protein resynthesis, and may negatively impact the immune system and central nervous system functioning. That being said, there is absolutely no need to consume copious amounts of calories post-training runs and many runners find they don't have a large appetite after a hard workout. Post-training fueling can be a small amount of food and/or fluid, not a meal. For more information on recovery nutrition, see Chapter 22.

## Reliance on Engineered versus Real Food

Those who spend several hours a day training, in addition to work and/or school, find themselves with minimal time or desire to cook. Although shakes and bars may be of use, reliance on them solely can leave a runner fiber deficient and phytonutrient insufficient. In addition, these items can be quite costly. Runners appreciate suggestions for easy and inexpensive food alternatives.

| Instead of | Choose |
|---|---|
| Gels | Honey sticks |
| Sports drinks | Diluted juice with added salt |
| Electrolyte packets, pills | Sea salt |
| Chomps | Dried fruit |
| RTD protein shakes | Smoothie made with Greek yogurt, frozen fruit, milk |
| Protein bars | Peanut butter, oats, honey, whey protein isolate rolled into balls |

## Gut Issues

Gastrointestinal issues can be some of the most pervasive and persistent problems for many distance runners. What works in practice does not always work in an event due to nerves or underfueling during training runs. Blood flow to the abdominal organs, including the intestines, is reduced 30 to 40 percent during exercise at 70 percent $VO_2$ max (2). The impact of this on carbohydrate absorption is inconclusive, but what is known is that dehydration ensues, gastric emptying slows, and then the runner is much more vulnerable to the thermic impact of running.

Although there is no need to eliminate foods unless one has a food allergy or intolerance, there are certain foods that are more likely to cause GI distress during training runs and races:

- Sugar alcohols in sugar-free gums, mints, and some low-carb foods
- Carbonated beverages
- Fried foods
- Concentrated sources of carbohydrates such as gels/blocks taken without adequate fluid
- Excessive amounts of fruit
- High fiber foods before training runs/races
- Caffeine

## It's All About Timing

While it is critically important for runners to meet hydration, macro, and micro-nutrients needs, optimal timing of ingestion has a huge impact on performance. One recommendation is to "book end" training sessions with food and fluid (i.e., before and after training), and scheduling this as part of workout time. For example, if a runner is training from 5 to 7 p.m., then ideally the pre-run fueling and hydration starts at 4 p.m., and post-run recovery eating starts as soon as possible after the run. This helps runners to prioritize both their fueling and training to optimize performance and health. Volume does not have to be enormous for either pre- or post-runs, more an appetizer than an entrée. A small amount of fuel is less likely to cause GI discomfort pre-run and a small amount post-run may be more appealing, especially when training has been intense and exhausting.

Runners need to schedule fueling into their day, rather than playing catch up. This helps to optimize carbohydrate availability, muscle protein synthesis, and energy levels.

## Fuel Substrates for Distance Running

The longer the run, the higher the calorie requirements. Ultra-endurance athletes may expend 6,000 to 8,000 kcal/d. Caloric intake needs to provide optimal calories for sport as well as overall body function. But, the challenge is to meet calorie goals with meaning—ingesting the right amount of macro and micronutrients at the right time and in the right form.

For distance runners the primary energy system utilized is the aerobic system, the efficiency of which is governed by ATP availability. For this to occur, energy needs must be met on a daily basis.

## How to Calculate Energy Requirements

See Table 6-1 for values of REE (resting energy expenditure) based on sex and age. These can be used to do calculations to find ideal energy requirements as follows:

(Sex/age matched REE) x (activity factor) = ideal caloric intake.

For example, a female ultra-runner aged 35, weighing 120 pounds (120 lbs/2.2 lbs per kg = 54.5 kg), running 60 miles/week, calorie needs would range from (8.7 x 54.5) + 829 = 1,303.5 kcal x 1.6–2.4 = 2,085–3,128 kcal/day. On heavier training days, calorie needs, especially carbohydrate requirements will be higher (3). Of

**Table 6-1** Using the REE (resting energy expenditure) calculations.

| Gender/Age | REE equation (BW in kg) | Activity Factor |
|---|---|---|
| Female, 10–18 | (12.2 x BW) + 749 | 1.6–2.4 |
| Females, 18–30 | (14.7 x BW) + 496 | 1.6–2.4 |
| Females, 30–60 | (8.7 x BW) + 829 | 1.6–2.4 |
| Males, 10–18 | (17.5 x BW) + 651 | 1.6–2.4 |
| Males, 18–30 | (15.3 x BW) + 679 | 1.6–2.4 |
| Males, 30–60 | (11.6 x BW) + 879 | 1.6–2.4 |

Adapted from: World Health Organization. Energy and Protein Requirements. Report of a Joint FAO/WHO/UNU expert Consultation. Technical Report Series. 724.

note, these energy requirements are for the total day. The logistics of optimally fueling during runs is challenging so effort needs to be put into total day as well as exercise specific fueling recommendations.

## Carbohydrates

### *How Can One Fuel without Feeling Overly Full?*

Carbohydrate is the primary fuel source for endurance exercise so those runners who have higher muscle glycogen availability and also consume carbohydrates during training runs and races tend to perform better (4, 5, 6, 7, 8). In addition, adequate carbohydrate enhances fat oxidation during exercise. Runners may be all too familiar with the physical fatigue associated with inadequate energy stores, but concomitant mental fatigue due to inadequate carbohydrate intake for nerve cells can be just as debilitating. However, carbohydrate recommendations must be personalized to take into account periodization of training, demands of completion, gut tolerance, and personal preference (9). Carbohydrate recommendations are about one gram of carbohydrate/minute during exercise or about six grams of carbohydrate per hour.

See Table 6-2 (10), Table 6-3 (10), and Table 6-4 for specific carbohydrate recommendations for sport.

### *Does the Type of Carbohydrate Matter?*

Studies have demonstrated that a mixed carbohydrate solution of glucose and fructose rather than glucose alone increased the rate of carbohydrate oxidation (11, 12). Increased exogenous carbohydrate oxidation can spare endogenous glycogen stores thus delaying the onset of fatigue. The advantage of a glucose /fructose combination is that high levels of glucose alone may result in digestive distress

**Table 6-2** Carbohydrate Requirement by Activity Intensity.

| Type of Activity | Situation | CHO Recommendations |
|---|---|---|
| Light | Low intensity/skill-based | 1.36–2.27 g/lb/d |
| Moderate | 1 h/d | 2.27–3.18 g/lb/d |
| High | Endurance-1–3 h/d, Moderate-high intensity | 2.7–4.54 g/lb/d |
| Very high | >4–5 h/d, Moderate-high intensity | 3.6–5.45 |

Adapted from: Burke et al, J Sports Sci 2011 29(suppl1):S17-S27

**Table 6–3** Carbohydrate Requirement by Specific Activity.

| Type of Activity | Situation | CHO Requirements |
|---|---|---|
| General fueling for sport | Prep for events < 90 min | 3.18–5.45 g/lb/24 h |
| CHO loading | For > 90 min of sustained, intermittent exercise | 36–48 h or 4.54–5.45 g/lb |
| Speedy refueling | < 8 h recovery between 2 –a-day training sessions | .45–.54 g/lb/h for first 4 hrs |
| Pre-event fueling | Before ex > 60 min | .45–1.8 g/lb 1–4 g pre-exercise |
| During brief exercise | < 45 min | Not needed |
| During sustained HIT | 45–75 min | Small amts (mouth rinse) |
| During endurance and stop and go sports | >1–2.5 h | 30–60 g/h |
| During ultra-endurance exercise | > 2.5–3 h | Up to 90 g/h |

Adapted from: Burke LM, Hawley JA, Wong SH, Jeudenfrup AE. Carbohydrates for training and competition. J Sports Sci. 2011; 29 Suppl 1: S17-27 (10)

**Table 6-4** Carbohydrate content in food sources.

| Food | Carbohydrate (grams) |
|---|---|
| Packet of gel | 28 |
| Raisins, 1 ounce | 22 |
| Chomps/Bloks, 4 | 33 |
| Banana, 1 medium | 30 |
| Fruit Newtons, 2 | 20 |
| Honey, 2 packets | 34 |
| Sugar cubes, 6 | 30 |
| Sports drink, 8 ounces | 14 |
| Sports bar, not low-carb, 1/2 | 24 |

without increased absorption. It is important to keep in mind that too much of any carbohydrate can result in GI distress. In addition, products with maltodextrin may result in a higher carbohydrate availability without subsequent GI distress. Occasion-specific carbohydrate can offer a two-pronged advantage: fewer GI concerns and less fatigue. The buffet approach to carbohydrate ingestion is better offered post-training runs and races where gut tolerance may be better (13).

Some coaches and athletes are intrigued by the Train LOW strategy to minimize carbohydrate to allow the body to better use fatty acids as a fuel substrate (see Chapter 22 for more information on Train LOW). Although intriguing, the unintended consequence may be impaired performance due to earlier onset fatigue (14). This does not mean runners should consume carbohydrate to excess, but under-consumption may not optimize performance. Occasional bouts of training in a carbohydrate-depleted state may stimulate performance enhancing biochemical adaptations. However, there can also be a deleterious impact on training and race day performance. The rate of perceived exertion may increase in the presence of low muscle glycogen stores. A high fat, low carbohydrate diet can negatively impact glycogenolysis and can adversely impact strength, speed, and stamina (15). For runners who choose to train low and compete high with more than one training session per day, endogenous and exogenous carbohydrate availability will be lower for the second training session, potentially impacting performance as well as immune and central nervous system functioning (14).

As more and more runners engage in carbohydrate manipulation and restriction strategies, it is important for them to be aware of the consequences of their actions. For those who train after an overnight fast, there is less available exogenous carbohydrate and potential decrease in endogenous carbohydrate availability if glycogen stores were not depleted from prior training sessions. For those who do not consume carbohydrate during training sessions that last longer than one hour and train more than once a day, carbohydrate availability for the second training session may be reduced along with decreased carbohydrate availability for immune and central nervous system functioning.

Runners who self-select a low-carbohydrate diet may notice not only reduced muscle glycogen stores impacting strength, speed, and stamina, as well as diminished immune and central nervous system functioning as noted above.

As training intensity increases, GI tolerance may decrease, rendering the body unable to tolerate fluid/foods. A carbohydrate mouth rinse may favorably impact performance as the brain perceives the presence of carbohydrate, thus delaying fatigue. Although this is an interesting concept, it is a temporary fix used primarily to allow the gut to rest. Swishing and spitting does not put fluid or fuel into the body and though this strategy may temporarily "trick" the brain into sensing that carbohydrate stores are plentiful, and delaying fatigue, prolonged exercise will require addition fluid and fuel ingestion to optimize performance. Experimentation with exogenous carbohydrate form and amount, as well as optimizing endogenous carbohydrate stores, can positively impact performance.

# Protein

Protein is not typically used as an energy source during running, but can provide up to 15 percent of the calories utilized during training runs. Runners need to consider quantity, quality, and also timing of protein intake. See Table 6-5 for protein recommendations for athletes with various goals.

Of note, it is not just important for runners to meet daily protein requirements, but distribution of protein intake is equally important. The recommendations to get at least 25 to 30 grams of protein per meal to attain 2.5 grams of leucine at each eating occasion optimizes muscle protein synthesis. As eating plans become more complicated and food choices are based not just on fuel but ethics, environmental concerns, cost, and personal preferences, meeting protein needs may sound easier than it is to achieve.

Calories in protein foods vary by fat and what may be added (i.e., fruit/sugar in yogurt). Note as well that the amount of protein in plant foods is less, requiring higher volumes to meet protein needs. For vegetarian and/or vegan athletes, it is strongly recommended they work with a registered dietitian who can help develop a meal plan to meet protein and other macronutrient needs.

See Table 6-6 (16) for animal protein sources and Table 6-7 for plant protein sources.

**Table 6-5**  Protein Recommendations by Activity.

| Type of athlete | Protein, gms/lb/BW | Daily protein needs for 150-pound athlete |
|---|---|---|
| Endurance-training > 20 hrs/week | 0.7–0.9 | 75–120 |
| Teenage athlete | 0.7–0.9 | 105–135 |
| Building mass | 0.6–0.9 | 90–135 |
| Restricting calories | 0.9–1.0 | 135–150 |
| Maximum usable amount | 0.9–1.0 | 135–150 |

Adapted from: Phillips Sm, Moore DR, Tang JE. A Critical Examination of Dietary Protein Requirements, Benefits, and Excesses in Athletes
IJSNEM 2007;17(suppl) S58-S76 (16)

**Table 6–6**  Animal Protein Sources.

| Food | Protein (gms) | Calories |
|---|---|---|
| iPhone-size serving of meat, poultry, fish | 21 | 90–210 |
| 3 oz can of tuna | 21 | 100–158 |
| 3 oz hamburger | 21 | 163–230 |
| Greek yogurt, 6–8 oz | 9–23 | 100–210 |
| Regular yogurt, 6–8 oz | 5–9 | 100–230 |
| Eggs, 3 whole or 6 whites | 21 | 210 (whole), 51 (whites) |
| Cottage cheese, ¾ cup | 21 | 135–165 |
| Cheese, 3 slices or 3 oz | 21 | 216–339 |
| Deli meat, 3 slices or 3 oz | 21 | 90–125 |
| Bacon, 7 slices | 21 | 258 |

**Table 6-7**  Plant protein sources.

| Food | Protein (gms) | Calories |
|---|---|---|
| Quinoa, 2 cups cooked | 16 | 444 |
| Whole wheat toast, 6 slices | 20 | 480 |
| Broccoli, 5 cups | 20 | 150 |
| Brown rice, 4 cups cooked | 20 | 864 |
| Black beans, 1.5 cups cooked | 20 | 340 |
| Lentils, 1.25 cups cooked | 20 | 345 |
| Tofu, 6 oz | 20 | 155 |
| Hummus, 1.25 cups | 20 | 544 |
| Edamame, 1 cup | 17 | 240 |
| Cashews, 1 cup | 21 | 785 |
| Almonds, 1/2 cup | 15 | 413 |
| Peanuts, 2/3 cup | 23 | 571 |
| Peanut butter, 5 tbsp | 20 | 470 |
| Sunflower seeds, 2/3 cup | 19 | 558 |

There have been some studies recommending the use of branched chain amino acids (BCAAs) during endurance exercise as a way of preventing central fatigue. As endurance training increases, so does the use of BCAAs (17). However, BCAAs may cause GI distress and taste terrible. As with everything else, runners are going to need to experiment with what feels comfortable in training. In addition, there are food safety concerns with protein so acceptable protein sources during exercise may include:

- Protein bars
- Protein chomps/chews

- Protein gels
- Nuts/seeds
- Nut butters
- Roasted soy nuts
- Roasted chickpeas

# Fat

Endurance training allows the body to favorably use fat as an energy substrate earlier in exercise. But it is important to note that consuming a high fat diet does not replace carbohydrates as carbohydrate availability has the bigger role to play in delaying onset of fatigue. That being said, is there any advantage to fat loading? The studies conducted to this point have not shown a benefit in performance in endurance sports (18, 19). See Table 6-8 for fat content in common foods and their caloric density.

In general, runners will require somewhere between 20 to 35 percent of daily calories from fat. From our earlier example, a 120-pound runner requiring between 2,085 to 3,128 calories/day would require somewhere between 46 to 122 grams of fat/day. So should one always strive for the lowest possible fat intake? Not necessarily. Fat is a concentrated source of calories, so for runners who are having trouble meeting energy needs, consuming a diet with more fat may provide the additional calories without leaving one feeling stuffed,

Table 6-8  Fat content in common foods.

| Food | Amount | Fat (gms) | Calories |
|---|---|---|---|
| Oil | 1 tbsp | 13.5 | 119 |
| Mayonnaise | 1 tbsp | 10 | 90 |
| Salad dressing | 2 tbsp | 8–14 | 80–140 |
| Peanut butter | 2 tbsp | 16 | 188 |
| Almond butter | 2 tbsp | 18 | 202 |
| Peanuts | 1 oz | 14 | 166 |
| Almonds | 1 oz | 14 | 164 |
| Sunflower seeds | 1 oz | 14 | 165 |
| Avocado | 1/4 ounce | 7 | 80 |
| Coconut oil | 1 tbsp | 13.6 | 117 |
| Butter | 1 pat/tsp | 4 | 36 |
| Bacon | 1 slice | 4 | 46 |

## Should Runners Be Advised to Consume Fat During Training Sessions?

Fat containing foods digest slowly, and may contribute to diarrhea or nausea during runs. Earlier studies looked at the use of medium chain triglycerides (MCTs) during exercise to provide more rapidly absorbed fatty acids to spare glycogen stores. However, MCTs can contribute distress and studies have shown that the MCTs did not spare glycogen (20).

Although both proteins and carbohydrates should be consumed in post-exercise fueling choices to expedite recovery, fat stores are not depleted during exercise and there is no need to consume fat post-exercise. That being said, fats adds flavor to food, so adding some nuts to a trail mix or spreading nut butter with honey on a bagel can be a way to add protein, calories, and taste to a post-training run.

# Fluid

Runners need to maintain optimal fluid balance to prevent sub-hydration, dehydration or over-hydration and subsequent hyponatremia. Intense exercise can blunt thirst, plus not all runners consumer enough liquid to meet baseline requirements, let alone fluid needs for running.

The Institute of Medicine's Guidelines for fluid intake are as follows:

Ninety-one ounces of liquid/day for females and 125 ounces of liquid/day for males. This can come from both foods and beverages including:

- water
- coffee
- tea
- juice
- milk
- carbonated beverages
- soups
- fruits
- vegetables

In addition to meeting baseline fluid requirements, to optimize performance, runners should develop a hydration strategy for training and races.

Sample fluid strategy:

- 2 to 3 hours before training: 16 ounces of fluid (water is fine)

- 10 to 20 minutes prior: 8 ounces of fluid
- Every 10 to 20 minutes during: 8 ounces of fluid
- Post-runs: 20 to 24 ounces of fluid for every pound lost during the run

From a gut comfort standpoint, tolerance is roughly 24 to 48 ounces of fluid/hour, so fluid intake should not be a one size fits all approach. The 2002 International Marathon Medical Directors Association guidelines recommend a fluid intake of 400 to 800 mL/h with more for faster and heavier runners, up to a maximum of 800 mL/h (21). Fluid strategies needs to be determined and practiced in training runs to gauge logistics of consumption, quantity, frequency, and selection.

# Sodium

Sodium has long been perceived to be the public health villain, with nutrition recommendations that intake not to exceed 2,300 mg/day. However, from a sports nutrition perspective, exogenous sodium intake during training and events may prevent exercise-associated hyponatremia and also exercise-associated muscle cramping. This is not to say the sodium intake should be excessive, however, in studies that have looked at exercise-associated muscle cramping, those who are prone to cramping tend to have lower serum sodium levels post-events than those who do not experience cramping (22). The risks of additional sodium ingestion during exercise may be nausea, so practicing with sodium ingestion during training sessions is advised. In addition, delivery of sodium can be through sports supplements, beverages, or salt itself rather than salt tablets which tend to increase GI distress. Recommendations for sodium during long training sessions and races may be 500 to 1,000 mg/hour (13).

Those who are salty sweaters (i.e., sweat that burns the eyes, tastes salty, and/ or leaves a gritty residue or salt stains on skin or clothes), may need to pay particular attention to sodium, and are recommended to learn how to calculate their sweat rate to prevent fluid excesses during runs.

See Table 6-9 for sodium content of common salty foods/fluids.

To prevent over-hydration and the subsequent risk of hyponatremia, it is important for runners to learn how to calculate their hourly sweat rate. A good formula to use follows:

Weight pre-run (in as little clothes as possible) – Weight post-run (in ounces [16 ounces in 1 pound]) + Number of ounces of fluid consumed during runs ÷ Number of hours of exercise = Hourly sweat rate

**Table 6-9** Sodium Content of Common Salty Foods/Fluids.

| Food/Fluid | Sodium (mg) |
|---|---|
| Club soda, 8 oz | 40 |
| Sports drink, 8 oz | 140 |
| Blue cheese, 1 oz | 400 |
| Cottage cheese, 1/2 cup | 450 |
| Parmesan, 1 oz | 528 |
| Bouillon, 1 cube | 1152 |
| Soy sauce, 1 tbsp | 1029 |
| Pickles, dill, 1 | 928 |
| Right Stuff, 1 packet | 1700 |
| Tomato juice, 8 oz | 878 |
| V8 juice, 8 oz | 887 |
| Salt, 1 tsp | 1928 |
| Pedialyte, 8 oz | 240 |
| Gatorlytes, 1 pouch | 780 |
| NUUN, 1 tablet | 360 |

Example:

A female runner weighs 135 pounds pre-run and 132 post-run, drinks 20 ounces of fluid during her run, and runs for 2 hours.

135 – 132 = 3 x 16 = 48 ounces + 20 ounces = 68 ounces ÷ 2 = 34 ounces of fluid/hour

# Micronutrients

Micronutrient requirements are taken to correct nutritional deficiencies. Iron deficiency is corrected through iron supplementation. Vitamin D deficiency is corrected with vitamin D supplementation. B vitamins in excess of need do not provide an edge. See Table 6-10 (23) for micronutrient tolerance in males and females

Note that Table 6-10 reflects Recommended Dietary Allowances but those values will be inadequate in the presence of deficiency or excess losses during exercise (i.e., sodium).

## Caffeine

Coffee house, energy drinks, caffeine pills, and caffeine-infused sports supplements are quite popular. However, is it always an ergogenic aid? Caffeine can

**Table 6-10** Micronutrient tolerance in males and females.

| Micronutrient | Males | Females | Tolerable |
|---|---|---|---|
| Vitamins | | | Upper Limit |
| Vitamin Aμg | 900 | 500 | 3,000 |
| B vitamins | | | |
| Thiamin mg | 1.1 | 1.3 | ND |
| Riboflavin mg | 1.1 | 1.3 | ND |
| Niacin mg | 14 | 16 | 35 |
| Choline mg | 425 | 550 | 3 g/d |
| Folate μg | 400 | 400 | 1,000 |
| B6 mg | 1.5 | 1.7 | 100 |
| B12 | 2.4 mcg | 2.4 mcg | ND |
| Pantothenic Acid mg | 5 | 5 | ND |
| Biotin μg | 30 | 30 | ND |
| Vitamin C mg | 75 | 90 | 2,000 |
| Vitamin D μg | 15–20 | 15–20 | 100 |
| Vitamin E mg | 15 | 15 | 1,000 |
| Vitamin K μg | 90 | 120 | ND |
| Minerals | | | |
| Boron mg | ND | ND | 20 |
| Calcium mg | 800–1,000 | 800–1,000 | 2,000–2,500 |
| Chloride g | 1.8–2.3 | 1.8–2.3 | 3.6 |
| Chromium μg | 20–25 | 30–35 | ND |
| Copper μg | 900 | 900 | 10,000 |
| Fluoride mg | 3 | 4 | 10 |
| Iodine μg | 150 | 150 | 1,100 |
| Iron mg | 8–18 | 8 | 45 |
| Magnesium mg | 320 | 420 | 350 |
| Manganese mg | 1.8 | 2.3 | 11 |
| Molybdenum μg | 45 | 45 | 2,000 |
| Phosphorus mg | 700 | 700 | 3–4 g/d |
| Potassium mg | 4,700 | 4,700 | ND |
| Selenium μg | 55 | 55 | 400 |
| Sodium mg | 1,200–1,500 | 1,200–1,500 | 2,300 |
| Zinc mg | 8 | 11 | 40 |

ND = Not determined.
Adapted from: Dietary Reference Intakes for Calcium, Phosphorous, Magnesium,
Vitamin D, and Fluoride (1997); Dietary Reference Intakes for Thiamin, Riboflavin,
Niacin, Vitamin B6, Folate, Vitamin B12, Pantothenic Acid, Biotin, and Choline (1998) (23)

reduce the onset of fatigue in endurance activity and time trial performance, but the efficacy for ultrasports is unknown. Caffeine can increase mental focus, which may be an advantage in longer duration exercise. It is important to note that caffeine can have GI side effects including nausea and diarrhea, as well as headaches, jitteriness, insomnia, elevated blood pressure, and anxiety. The suggested dosages of caffeine are 3 to 6 mg/kg BW along with carbohydrate fifteen to sixty minutes before workouts/races, followed by repeated caffeine ingestion every two to five hours may be beneficial. This does require experimentation during training not only with amount but form to determine gut tolerance and performance impact.

## Alcohol

After a hard training session or great race, a cold beer may sound incredibly appealing. However, alcohol should not be the only food/fluid choice after exercise as it can delay muscle glycogen resynthesis and healing from any exercise-associated injury. Although not a diuretic, alcohol is not a high source of carbohydrate and does not contain protein, so a better option as an accompaniment to a beer, consider pretzels and peanuts to provide the much needed carbohydrate and protein to expedite recovery. For runners who are weight focused, alcohol itself is a source of calories and can also stimulate appetite.

# Relative Energy Deficiency in Sports

Not consuming enough calories can be a problem for both male and female runners. In the short term, it can impact performance. In the long term, energy deprivation may have an impact on peak bone mass. In 2014, the International Olympic Committee developed a consensus statement on Relative Energy Deficiency in Sports (RED-S) (24). For additional information on RED-S, see Chapter 22.

Although exercise is critical to optimize health, too much activity coupled with too little fuel can cause an energy drain, where the calories consumed are less the calories expended during exercise—or energy output—amounts to the energy a person has available. So a runner who ingests 1,500 calories a day, but burns 1,500 during exercise, has no fuel leftover for basic body requirements.

## What Are the Consequences of Low Energy Availability?

In addition to immediate effects on performance—being slower, weaker, and quicker to tire—low energy availability can lead to a weakened immune system and lowered bone mineral density, which can definitely impact health. Inadequate fueling can reduce strength, endurance, speed, coordination, and concentration, while increasing one's risk for injury, illness, and stress fracture.

## What Are Some of the Signs of Chronic Energy Deficit?

It may not be obvious that the body is in a state of deprivation, and changes don't happen overnight. But with prolonged subpar intake, there can be adverse impacts on health. Here are some examples:

- Hypometabolism—reduced resting energy expenditure (fewer calories burned)
- Reduced thyroid functioning
- Bradycardia—slowed heart rate
- Hypothermia—lowered body temperature
- Hypotension—low blood pressure
- Constipation
- Decreased testosterone
- Decreased estrogen
- Decreased growth hormone production

Less is not always better when it comes to calorie intake and more is not always recommended with exercise. Being fit is a goal, being overly fatigued and underfed is not. The athlete with RED-S will benefit from consultation with a sports dietitian to develop an eating plan to optimize energy availability, health, and performance.

# Practical Issues for Runners

Once goals have been set, the issue of practicality and logistics need to be determined. During heavy training periods, runners may find that they are losing weight and don't always have a big appetite so energy output outpaces energy intake. Encouraging energy dense foods can provide the necessary calories without the volume.

## Energy Dense Foods

- Granola
- Risotto
- Cheese
- Juice
- Nuts/nut butters
- Seeds/seed butters
- Avocado
- Bagels
- Unflavored Protein isolate added to oatmeal, nut butter, soups

## Taste Fatigue

As the mileage increases and runs become longer, taste fatigue may ensue. Most products are sweet: gels, chomps, sports beans, beverages, fruit. This can become unappealing over time. Here are some suggestions to diversify the taste portfolio:

- Rice balls with soy sauce
- Candied ginger
- Taco-flavored popcorn
- Pickle slices
- Adding turmeric and ginger to a sports drink

## Food Safety Concerns

One of the challenges in endurance events is having non-perishable protein foods for the duration. Granola, cereal, sports drinks, and gels are not a worry, but what other foods are shelf stable that can be used either during or after training sessions or races? Since protein is a vital component of exercise recovery and animal protein such as yogurt, cheese, milk, eggs, may not always be practical, readily available or safe, here are some plant-based options:

- Nuts
- Roasted chickpeas
- Roasted pinto beans
- Roasted edamame
- Protein isolate to mix into a beverage

- Seeds—pumpkin, sunflower
- Nut butters
- Harvest snaps
- Bean chips
- Whole grain wrap with hummus

## Protecting the Supporting Structure

Runners need to be concerned about their musculoskeletal health. The wear and tear on the body coupled with food beliefs and the desire to be light and efficient can take a toll on the supporting structure. Nutrition recommendations for bone and joint health can be a valuable component of the runner's portfolio to minimize the risk of injury.

## Bone Health

Most people know that calcium is essential for bone health, but it is only one of many nutrients necessary. It is a delicate balance of emphasizing bone supporting food choices and habits and minimizing bone robbers.

| Bone Supporters | Bone Robbers |
| --- | --- |
| Optimal protein | Too little protein |
| Optimal fat intake | Minimizing dietary fat |
| Adequate sodium | Excess sodium |
| Adequate potassium | Minimal potassium |
| Optimal vitamin D | Insufficient vitamin D |
| Optimal vitamin K | Insufficient vitamin K |
| Optimal calcium | Insufficient calcium |

## Anti-inflammatory Foods

A runner's body takes a beating, especially as mileage and/or training sessions increase. Anti-inflammatory foods/supplements also offer a proactive/preventive approach to inflammation.

Some foods may increase the risk of inflammation such as fried foods, excess added sugar, sweetened beverages, and trans fat. That doesn't mean they have to be eliminated, but limited and replaced with foods that help to reduce inflammation instead. Emphasizing food as a way to reduce inflammation also provides the necessary fuel for exercising muscles.

## Anti-inflammatory Foods and Supplements

- Tart cherries/juice
- Dark green vegetables
- Deep orange fruits and vegetables
- Berries
- Tomatoes
- Fatty fish
- Ginger
- Turmeric
- Chili peppers
- Olive oil
- Nuts

### Supplements

- Sam-E
- Avocado-soybean unsaponifiables
- Curcumin
- Ginger

# Bottom Line

When it comes to fueling to go the distance, runners need to practice, fine tune, and experiment to develop a plan that is sustainable, attainable, and measurable. The sports dietitian is the nutrition coach, providing the guidance, tweaks, and suggestions to help the endurance athlete run long, and run strong.

## CHAPTER 7

# Psychology of Injury, Rehabilitation, and Recovery

## BY KEVIN N. ALSCHULER

## Key Points

1. Self-monitor across the physical, psychological, and social domains to identify opportunities for growth and barriers to success.
2. Employ strategies such as goal setting to be process-oriented during rehabilitation.
3. Use imagery, meditation, and other forms of relaxation to manage stress and embrace the power of the mind.
4. Consider unmet opportunities for growth to focus on while recovering from injury.
5. Remain active in the social side of sport despite the physical limits imposed by injury.
6. Utilize resources within the sport and medical communities for support and professional assistance in maximizing recovery.

## Introduction

Virtually every long distance runner will experience an injury. As described elsewhere in this book, some will be serious, while others will be minor. Regardless of the severity, the injury will interfere with the runner's ability to participate fully in the sport they love.

When a runner is injured, the focus is most often on the physical experience: what, exactly, is injured and what can be done to expedite a return to running. The reality, however, is that while running injuries may be physical in origin, how runners experience and respond to injuries is largely a psychological experience. Thus, understanding the role of psychology is vital to maximize recovery and minimize barriers to returning to run.

# Injury is More than a Physical Phenomenon

Sport is largely viewed as a physical phenomenon, and therefore so is injury. Yet just as sport has placed a greater emphasis on the "mental game" in recent years, sports medicine has placed greater importance on a "biopsychosocial" perspective that extends beyond a singular focus on physical functioning to also include psychological and social concepts. A successful foundation for coping with injury is rooted in understanding the breadth of this model. Consider the following:

- When a runner is injured it most often hurts; when something hurts, individuals interpret the significance of that pain and the related threat to their well-being. For most, pain—"an unpleasant sensory and emotional experience associated with actual or potential tissue damage, or described in terms of such damage" (1)—is an alarm that warns us that we may be in danger. In many cases, this serves a vital purpose: if I accidentally place my hand on a warm burner, I receive a warning that I am about to seriously harm myself; when I receive that warning, I respond by removing my hand to limit the extent of the injury. I then process the event, recognizing that stoves are dangerous, and forever remain motivated to be more cautious so I do not burn myself again. Many would argue that this virtually automatic process is a major contributor to our survival.

- Runners experience the same process. When an injury occurs, particularly one that is painful, it is alarming. To limit injury, many stop running, although the culture of sport often motivates—and even encourages—pushing through pain. However, running injuries are often significantly more complex to understand relative to accidentally burning oneself on the stove. In particular, it might be difficult to determine how the injury occurred, so the optimal response is likely infinitely more complex than "don't put your hand on a hot burner." Moreover, the recovery process is likely more complex: The "pain means stop" message does not apply fully, as recovery and return to running may involve enduring some discomfort or overcoming a fear of a recurrence of the injury. The way a runner makes meaning of the injury, the emotions they experience, and the cognitive and behavioral responses to the injury are psychological and can greatly impact the experience of and recovery from injury.

- The psychological response to pain can modify the severity of pain. Although theory has become increasingly sophisticated over time, the

Gate Control Theory (2) serves as an excellent example of what we are describing. This theory suggests that when a sensation is experienced on the periphery (e.g., at the ankle, knee, hand, etc.), the signal then travels up through the central nervous system to the brain for interpretation. It is proposed that along the way the pain signal travels through a number of "gates" that may disrupt the signal. Those gates can be controlled by any of a number of factors, including the individual's thoughts and emotions, and how the signal travels through the gates would impact the subsequent interpretation of severity and significance of the sensation. Although the entirety of the theory is nuanced and complex, an important take-home point is that this was among the first theories to suggest that factors beyond physical pathology contribute to the human experience of pain.

• The way individuals think about pain and respond to pain can dramatically impact post-injury functioning. Consistent with other aspects of health, scientists now view pain and injury through a biopsychosocial perspective that considers the physical problem in a multifaceted context that also incorporates psychological and social perspectives (3). Given that the majority of this book is focused on the physical side of injury, the rest of this chapter is devoted specifically to the psychosocial experience of the injured athlete. Today, pain psychology has grown to explore how individuals think about their pain (pain-related cognitions and beliefs), how they behave in response to pain (pain behaviors), and how this relates to meaningful outcomes, including how much pain hurts (pain intensity) and how much it gets in the way of functioning (pain-related interference). Although early research was focused primarily on what people do "wrong" in coping with this discomfort (negative or maladaptive responses to pain), an increasing amount of recent research has focused on the factors that make positive outcomes more likely (positive or adaptive responses to pain). Additionally, a parallel body of literature has focused on factors external to the individual, such as social interactions and social context that impact pain-related outcomes (e.g., a spouse's response type can be helpful or hurtful to recovery) (4). Importantly, in the past twenty years, a sport-specific integrated model of sport injury (5, 6, 7, 8) has been developed to tailor the biopsychosocial perspective to the sport setting.

- Injury may be particularly threatening to runners, given optimizing physical functioning is central to success. Runners spend a significant amount of time, energy, and resources on their physical functioning in an effort to get fitter, stronger, and—most importantly—faster. One might argue, then, that an injury carries a greater threat value to athletes because of the perceived direct interference with the ability to reach one's primary goal. More research is needed to understand whether this is the case.

- Being unable to participate in sport following an injury can impact emotional wellness and an individual's general sense of well-being. Participation in sport often serves multiple purposes for athletes. Examples include sport being a source of exercise, competition, social engagement, and stress management. Therefore, a hidden threat of injury is that its negative impact may be widespread and may leave the individual feeling inadequately prepared to manage any of a number of key aspects of daily life. It is therefore not surprising that numerous studies have now shown a higher likelihood of lower mood in injured athletes; more importantly, these studies have highlighted that this is yet another barrier to return to sport, as lower mood may be associated with poorer recovery, particularly in the immediate aftermath of an injury (6, 9, 10, 11).

- Navigating social factors—particularly social pressures—can be uniquely challenging for athletes. Culturally, athletes are urged to push themselves to their limits, enduring a level of non-injury discomfort on a regular basis that would be avoided by the average person. With this comes an expectation of toughness accompanied by encouragement to take risks. Injury does not intersect particularly well with this culture. If one is injured, they might worry that not participating will be a sign of "weakness" and that others might doubt them. They might have their own doubts, wondering whether they should push through the discomfort to save face. They might also have fears of losing ground to others by not training. Thus, the perceived social consequences of being injured are often threatening to injured athletes and can play a prominent role in how the athlete approaches the recovery process.

# Individual Recovery Should Be Built upon One's Own Strengths

Before a deep dive into all of the threats to successful recovery, it is important to remember that many—perhaps even most—athletes adapt in healthy ways to their injuries (12). Therefore, most athletes have numerous strengths that can serve as the foundation for successful outcomes post-injury.

- Psychology is not just about what people do wrong; it is also about what people do right. In recent years, psychologists have increased their focus on positive psychology. Standing in contrast to psychology's historical focus on dysfunction, positive psychology is about identifying and building upon individual strengths. Some might consider positive psychology as the underpinning of sport performance psychology: greater emphasis is now being placed on using the power of the mind to improve performance, rather than only calling on a psychologist when an athlete is facing a psychological barrier or problem.
- A particularly popular focus within this topic has been the concept of resilience: a person's ability, in the face of adversity, to maintain or restore their well-being through the use of adaptive strategies (13, 14). Although it is still open for debate, resilience likely encompasses a number of characteristics. Some factors may be inherent to the individual (e.g., some may be naturally more optimistic than others), but many are modifiable factors that can be enhanced (13, 15). For example, the resilient individual may be more likely to:
  - Put forth a full effort, despite challenges, by maintaining or regaining focus on the steps needed to achieve the desired outcome.
  - Think flexibly about challenges and solutions, resulting in the use of new or different approaches to solve a challenge, as opposed to rigidly continuing with prior strategies that may no longer be effective.
  - Attend to their thought content to frame challenges appropriately, keeping the challenge in perspective.
  - Identify a way forward after a setback, by orienting towards progress and goal attainment rather than getting derailed by negative thoughts or emotions.

It is important to recognize that strengths and weaknesses can co-occur, as they are not necessarily opposites of each other. Thus, a person may be resilient in many ways, but may demonstrate weaknesses in other ways. Enhancing one's strengths, such as by growing facets of resilience, may buffer against the negative impact of areas of difficulty (16, 17).

## Proactive Prevention of Barriers to Success

There are an infinite number of psychological challenges to injury, but a few—fear of pain and re-injury, low mood, and poor adherence to rehabilitation—have garnered the most attention from psychologists interested in sports injury:

- Pain is an undesired experience and can inspire behaviors that unintentionally slow return to sport. For many, the experience of pain is unpleasant, scary, a sign of danger, and a threat to well-being. Not surprisingly, the human instinct is to first make it stop, and then make sure it does not happen again. In the immediate aftermath of an injury, this is helpful. If our leg breaks, we need to know. If our hand is on a hot burner, we need to know. Moreover, the desire to not experience the pain again is likely central to our survival as humans: if introducing oneself to a bear results in a painful injury or death, we need to know to (a) run away (we call this "escape") and (b) never stand face to face with a bear again (we call this "avoidance"). Few would argue that this response set has been valuable to our survival.

There is little concern over the initial response of a runner to injury. But consider the impact of this line of thinking once it is time to confront the pain, threat of pain, or threat of re-injury through rehabilitation or the return to sport: If we apply the "bear" logic from above, we will have determined that (a) if we have pain from running, we should stop (escape), and (b) to avoid future pain, we should not run (avoid). The problem here is obvious—we want to return to running, but that stands in conflict with our logic. Importantly, the extent to which a runner subscribes to this line of thinking can dramatically impact recovery and return to sport.

The challenge described here has now been the focus of greater than twenty years of study in the pain psychology literature, particularly focusing on the concept of fear-avoidance (18, 19, 20, 21, 22). Many individuals respond in an appropriate way to this pain or discomfort during rehabilitation and recovery; this ideal response is shown on the right side of Figure 7-1. These individuals confront the pain and are able to pursue a return to full function without being hindered by fear. Others, however, struggle, as shown on the left side of the figure. These individuals may have more extreme worries about the meaning of the pain (catastrophizing), or may demonstrate a

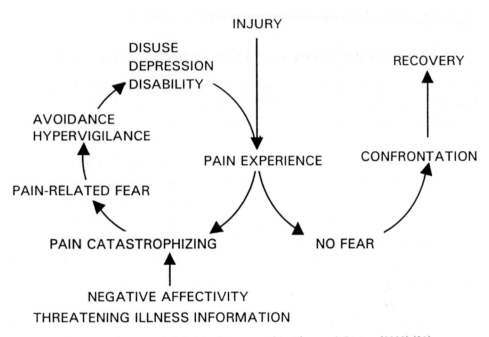

**Figure 7-1** Fear-avoidance model. Originally appeared in Vlaeyen & Linton (2000).(21) Reprinted with permission obtained from Dr. Vlaeyen.

fear response to pain or a fear of re-injury, which then causes the individual to function at a lower level than they desire.

Anecdotally, fear of pain may be somewhat lower in athlete populations relative to other populations, as the culture promotes a desire to push through pain and, generally, there is a tendency to embrace discomfort, particularly in high-level sport. In contrast, fear of re-injury is likely a more prominent issue, particularly when an injury is more significant, as the threat of repeat injury to the athlete's function is quite worrisome and problematic. For example, research on athletes returning to sport from anterior cruciate ligament repair indicates that higher levels of fear of re-injury are associated with lower quality of performance upon return to sport (23). Although the exact reasoning for this is unclear, the fear-avoidance model would suggest that individuals are more likely to engage in self-protecting behaviors that may unintentionally limit full engagement with the activity (e.g., shorten stride length, avoid fully planting foot to pivot).

- Running injuries are a bummer. They can derail training, interfere with an enjoyable activity, and alter social relationships. While disappointing for all injured runners, some may respond with greater despondence or may suffer more significantly from the consequences, which can then have a trickle-down effect on desired outcomes: poorer outcomes are associated with low mood for a variety of reasons, such as that individuals with lower mood perceive a painful stimulus as more painful than a person with higher mood who experiences the same stimulus (24); individuals with low mood may have a harder time fully engaging with tasks (25), such as rehabilitation; and individuals with low mood may be more prone to cognitive patterns that are detrimental to recovery and function, such as catastrophizing (26).

- Sticking with a rehabilitation regimen can be difficult. Much has been made of adherence to rehabilitation programs (the extent to which an individual participates in the prescribed program as designed). Although there remains debate over the relationship of adherence to the speed and quality of recovery, the difficulty of maintaining adherence is conceptually intriguing, particularly because attending rehabilitation sessions is one of the most controllable factors for the injured athlete. There is limited research on exactly why individuals have difficulty maintaining adherence to rehabilitation, but numerous theories have been offered (see Spetch & Kolt [27] for summary). Possible theories include perceived susceptibility to harm, negative emotional responses, or even a grief response. Taken together, we believe there are at least two possible areas of concern with poor adherence: first, to the extent adherence to rehabilitation relates to recovery-focused outcomes, there is the direct concern that individuals are hindering their own recovery when their adherence is low. Second, regardless of the relationship of adherence to recovery-focused outcomes, there is the clearer perspective that poor adherence may be caused by maladaptive cognitive and behavioral processes that also relate to other critical areas, such as the fears and low mood described earlier in this section.

Of the three barriers emphasized here—fears of pain and reinjury, low mood, and poor adherence—all can arise quite naturally in response to an injury. Thus, there are the final points to consider: first, these challenges can develop in an apparently benign fashion. A choice here or a choice there can add up over time to steer a person toward the "wrong" path. As will be discussed in the next section, being educated on these potential pitfalls gives the injured athlete a greater opportunity to intervene before a problem develops. Second—and equally important—the natural development of these challenges also suggests that in a high percentage of cases there is nothing "wrong" with the athlete who has these struggles. Sometimes there is a sense of shame from athletes, embarrassed that they cannot "handle" the challenge of their injury or frustrated that they are struggling in the face of this adversity. Understanding that many of these pitfalls are rooted in natural responses to threats to our well-being can provide a more comfortable starting point for intervention.

## Use of Specific Strategies to Facilitate Success

There are numerous strategies that one can employ in an effort to optimize their response to and recovery from injury. Psychologists take great pride in tailoring recommendations to the individual, but are still able to offer some strategies here that runners can employ independently:

- Be proactive when considering the opportunities and threats across the biopsychosocial spectrum. Successfully navigating the psychology of injury, recovery, and rehabilitation requires a certain level of awareness of the experience. In particular, being aware of how athletes experience injury across the biopsychosocial spectrum provides a chance for athletes to identify opportunities and threats in real time so as to be proactive in promoting a positive outcome. It is often the case that, in hindsight, problems that develop over time or missed opportunities that pass could have been recognized in real time. Injured athletes are routinely encouraged to do ongoing self-assessments, whereby the athlete takes stock in their current coping (again, across the entire spectrum) and evaluates both threats and opportunities for growth.
- Be process-oriented. Although the ultimate goal of injury recovery and rehabilitation is a specific outcome (i.e., successful return to sport), it is actually a multi-step process that adds up to the desired outcome. Thus, the injured runner is tasked with staying engaged with the steps of the process to reach the desired outcome; exclusive focus on the outcome can accidentally be a distraction. There are numerous threats to this engagement, ranging from psychological barriers (such as the fear-avoidance phenomenon described above) to other more subtle barriers, such as feeling overwhelmed by the process or simply not wanting to be forced to do rehabilitation.
  - Goal setting is an often recommended and relatively straightforward method for remaining process-oriented (7, 28). Many athletes are

actually quite good at goal setting, often through the use of training goals that are positioned as markers of progress toward a desired goal. In addition to objective markers (i.e., incremental changes in mile pace), successful athletes often also have process goals that are focused on their engagement with training. Goal setting in the context of injury recovery is similar. There are likely a series of smaller accomplishments that serve as intermediate steps from injury to recovery. Additionally, there are also engagement goals related to, for example, participation in rehabilitation or completion of an at-home rehabilitation routine.

- Appropriately set goals are effective because they keep one on track, they define specific steps to aid in moving toward the desired outcome, and they provide sources of motivation on the way to the long-term outcome. The best goals are often defined in terms of the SMART acronym—specific, measurable, action-oriented, realistic, time-based. (For example, one might have the goal of doing their physical therapy exercises once per day for two weeks.) In using this format, an injured runner can assure that the goals are reasonable, quantifiable, and within their control. Importantly, these goals may also aid in sustaining motivation and effort, helping the individual progress more quickly to their desired end result. Figure 7-2 provides a template to develop and record one's goals.

- Embrace the power of the mind. Throughout this chapter the case has been made that the way individuals view pain and injury can impact injury-related outcomes. It is therefore important for athletes to consider opportunities to shape their thought process to enhance positive outcomes.

  - One method is through the use of imagery, which is a form of mental rehearsal (7, 29). Imagery is utilized in a variety of ways across psychology. For some, imagery is a form of relaxation, such that an individual may imagine (in detail, utilizing all senses) a pleasant experience, such as sitting on a beach. This form of imagery has been shown to be an effective way to relax the body physically (e.g., decrease muscle tension, slowing heart rate), as well as to improve emotions and sense of well-being. Other imagery is more task or skill specific, such as rehearsing a specific athletic endeavor. This type of imagery is believed to improve performance above and beyond what can be achieved when an individual does physical practice without also doing imagery. Both methods can be effective for injured athletes. Relaxation-focused imagery can be utilized at regular intervals to aid in stress management and promote positive emotions in the setting of injury-related challenges. Skill-oriented imagery can provide a level of participation in sport to replace some of the loss of training, of course recognizing that it cannot replace aerobic training.

- Another popular strategy for embracing the mind's role is through meditation. In contrast to imagery, which employs active thought about an experience, meditation focuses on sitting with one's present experience. There are many forms of meditation, but most focus on sitting quietly, eyes closed, breathing calmly, with emphasis placed on following one's breath, allowing all other thoughts, smells, and sounds allowed to come and go without engagement. Akin to relaxation imagery, effectively used meditation can reduce markers of stress. An added bonus with meditation is the emphasis on allowing thoughts to pass through, a skill which can be quite valuable to athletes in the midst of a training run or race (i.e., distressing thoughts about the ability to finish a race might be best managed by simply letting them pass through, rather than trying to fight back against them).

- Imagery, meditation, and other forms of relaxation are skills. As such, they take practice. Athletes should be encouraged to engage in this practice daily, starting with shorter intervals and building up to more robust efforts.

- Capitalize on the opportunity to become a better athlete. It is the rare athlete who feels that he or she is doing everything possible to maximize performance. Most have room for growth, but have not taken the time to embrace some new facet of their training or preparation. It might be that they have not taken the time to learn mental performance strategies, or wanting to more closely examine running technique, or wanting to improve diet. In many cases these desired areas remain unaddressed out of fear of losing valuable training time to implement these new areas; in the face of not being able to train, injured runners might find that this is an ideal time to try something new without the perceived training cost. There are numerous anecdotes about athletes making great use of this time, such as football players who finally do the film study they have not previously done, or golfers who get good at putting because they cannot take full swings and spend substantially more time working on their short game.

- Remain an active participant in the social side of sport. People who are injured often end up more removed from their social supports than they need to be. Athletes should be encouraged to think about ways they can still interact with their fellow athletes, even if physical participation is

Figure 7-2 SMART goals template.

| SMART Goals | |
|---|---|
| Identify a series of goals that lead you on a path to recovery. These may be goals for small achievements, but may also be goals oriented towards specific tasks (e.g., completing therapy exercises). For each goal you develop, ensure they meet the SMART criteria | |
| Goal #1 | Specific |
| | Measurable |
| | Action-oriented |
| | Realistic |
| | Time-oriented |
| Goal #2 | Specific |
| | Measurable |
| | Action-oriented |
| | Realistic |
| | Time-oriented |
| Goal #3 | Specific |
| | Measurable |
| | Action-oriented |
| | Realistic |
| | Time-oriented |
| Goal #4 | Specific |
| | Measurable |
| | Action-oriented |
| | Realistic |
| | Time-oriented |
| Goal #5 | Specific |
| | Measurable |
| | Action-oriented |
| | Realistic |
| | Time-oriented |

limited. This could include participating in the warm-up or a portion of a workout, or attending team-related social events. Additionally, it can be as simple as taking extra steps to call, text, or email with teammates. There's no question that being injured ruins the natural flow of the social interactions, but with effort athletes can guard against some of the social isolation they might otherwise experience.

- Utilize community and resources to ease the process. Most athletes are not physicians, athletic trainers, or physical therapists. Therefore, they should not expect to have the expertise to independently guide their rehabilitation process. Surrounding oneself with a trusted team can ease this process significantly and provide an opportunity to return more quickly and with fewer barriers.

Particularly, it is important to remind athletes of the potential benefits of working with a psychologist. Most modern psychologists are interested in helping any person improve their functioning. Psychology is present throughout sports injury; therefore, there is opportunity to help athletes optimize their response to and recovery from injury through our intervention. There is no need to wait for a problem.

Taken together, these key points provide a recipe for success: be educated, be process oriented, use the power of the mind, capitalize on the opportunity to become a better athlete, remain engaged with the running community, and utilize community and professional resources to maximize return to running. Being injured will never be easy, but our hope is that fully embracing the psychological side of recovery will result in the most positive outcome possible.

# SECTION 2

# Evaluation, Treatment, and Prevention of Musculoskeletal Injuries

## CHAPTER 8

# Foot Care

## BY GRANT S. LIPMAN

## Key Points

1. Good fitting shoes that are broken in can help prevent blisters.
2. Consider application of paper tape to "pre-tape" areas that are prone to hot spots and blisters.
3. If a blister does not hurt or is not at risk for spontaneous rupture, leave it intact.
4. Treat a painful blister or hot spot as soon as possible.
5. Whenever possible, preserve a blister's "roof."
6. Try to avoid taking off blister tape once applied to minimize chances of tearing open fragile blister skin.
7. Try to avoid draining blood-filled blisters unless they are at risk of spontaneously popping open.

Any runner knows the inordinate amount of pain and suffering that can be caused by even a small blister. For some, a foot blister may be considered merely a nuisance; for others, it may ruin an outing, necessitate dropping out of a race, or even lead to medical complications from infection of the skin or the body (1, 2). Blister rates in the outdoor community range from 54 percent in wilderness area backpackers to 64 percent of long distance hikers on the Appalachian Trail (3, 4). Blister rates in marathoners range from 0.2 percent to 39 percent (5), 76 percent to 100 percent in multi-stage ultramarathon runners (6, 7, 8, 9), and were found to be the most common factor to adversely affecting race performance in elite single-stage ultramarathon finishers (10). Foot care represents the most commonly reported injury attended to by medical teams in both multi-stage ultramarathons and expedition-length adventure races, 74 percent and 33 percent, or 45 percent, respectively (11, 12, 13).

# Blisters: Where They Come From

The earliest etymology of the word friction, described from 1704, is "to rub; to crumble; they injure" (14). The mechanism of a friction blister injury is the repeated action of skin rubbing against another surface. As the external contact of either sock or footwear moves across the skin, the frictional force (Ff) opposes this movement. Frictional force increases with increasing external force. When external force exceeds the frictional force, movement occurs at the interface. In addition to magnitude of the frictional force, frequency of the cycling of the object across the skin leads to higher probability of blister development (15). There is an inverse relationship between these two variables; at higher frictional forces, it takes fewer cycles to form blisters (15, 16, 17, 18). There is wide variation in the amount of friction between the skin and various substances, with increased friction equating to increased resistance and decreased ease of movement. Also, frictional properties of the skin depend on inherent suppleness and hydration, as well as a host of external factors, including temperature and humidity (20).

Sheer forces extend horizontally between skin layers, skin and sock interface, between socks, and between socks and footwear. When the forces overcome resistance, sliding occurs. Repeated sliding at a friction point causes exfoliation of the stratum corneum and erythema in and around this zone (15, 16, 17, 18, 19). This is experienced as an initial sensation of heat, the well-known "hot spot," which represents an impending blister. Continued friction on a hot spot causes epidermal cells in the stratum spinosum to delaminate and split (1, 21). With continued rubbing, a sensation of stinging or burning occurs as a narrow pale area forms around the central reddened region. This enlarges inward (19). The skin becomes elevated as the underlying epidermis fills with fluid, and a blister is created (21). The intact superficial cells of the stratum corneum and stratum granulosum form the blister's "roof." The separated cleft in the area under the blister roof quickly fills with a low-protein fluid (22). The underlying basal skin layer and associated epidermal–dermal interface is usually unaffected and undamaged.

Healing of the blister is rapid if one can reduce further friction, cycles of rubbing, and the exacerbation of the injury. After 120 hours, a new stratum corneum will have been made (23). In the presence of continued friction and pressure when continued ambulation and activity are unavoidable, the body needs assistance to heal.

## Blister Prevention

The perpendicular directed normal force between the foot and the insole is determined by the weight of the runner and the weight being carried. Reducing the magnitude of the forces on the feet that cause a friction blister can be as simple as reducing either weight or the carried load (24), as increased body mass has been found to be a significant risk factor for number of blisters developed in multi-stage ultramarathons (8). Another way to minimize force on the feet is to use a padded insole or arch support. There are my different generic and custom mold-able insoles on the market. Although an insole or orthotic does not technically reduce the perpendicular forces on the feet, it helps to more evenly distribute pressure over the plantar surface of the foot. Greater pressure occurs when there is a high load on a smaller surface area of the foot, which may cause that area of skin to be more susceptible to blister formation.

Either increasing or decreasing the ease with which two surfaces rub against each other can reduce the chances of blister development. Making it very easy for the foot to slide, or conversely, maximizing the frictional forces through well-fitted footwear, will result in little or no movement at the skin–surface interface.

## Reduction of Movement within the Footwear System

Shoes should fit properly and comfortably. Allowing for ample time to break in a new set of footwear before use increases flexibility in the material, thereby reducing potential high-friction areas against the foot.

- Shoes that are too tight can increase contact points of pressure on the foot.
- Shoes that are too loose can allow excess movement that allows generation of frictional forces.
- Narrow shoes can cause blisters on the large and small toes.
- Loose shoes can create blisters on the tips of toes from sliding forward and getting the tips jammed into the toe box.
- A toe box that is too shallow can cause blisters on the tops of the toes from repeated contact.
- It is important to fit a shoe in the evening, because feet tend to swell throughout the day and the fit will be similar to the natural swelling that feet undergo while active.
- When trying on shoes, wear the same socks and/or insoles or orthotics that you will be using when running.

## Increasing Movement within the Footwear System

Various sock layer combinations can create a weak sheer layer and minimize the frictional forces against the skin of the foot itself. The goal of a layered sock combination is to have friction occur between the two layers of socks, not between the skin and socks. However, the double sock combination may be challenging to implement in a snug-fitted running shoe.

- A smooth, thin, snug-fitting synthetic sock worn as an inner layer against the foot will move with the foot, whereas a thicker, woven sock tends to move with the footwear and cushions against shocks.
- Socks that have a low frictional coefficient worn close to the foot have been found by computer modeling to reduce plantar shear stress.
- The thinner synthetic liner sock will also assist in humidity control by retaining less moisture and wicking moisture and perspiration away from the skin surface (28, 29).

A study was conducted to determine the effect of sock fiber on frequency and size of blisters. Two different visually identical socks were tested, one with acrylic and the other with 100 percent natural cotton fibers. Acrylic fiber socks were associated with fewer blister events and blister size when compared with cotton fiber socks (28). The take-home message on socks is a good fit and synthetic fiber.

## Minimizing Moisture

Repetitive rubbing on moist skin produces higher friction than on very wet or dry skin (1, 15, 21). Cutaneous hydration leads to increased contact area, adhesion, and maceration, resulting in more frequent blisters (Figure 8-2). Frictional forces on dry skin may exfoliate superficial cells of the stratum corneum, lubricating the feet in a manner analogous to the lubricating effects of graphite powder (19). Consider the addition of gaiters to help eliminate mud, dirt, gravel, sand, or rocks from entering the sock–shoe system. Consistently moist skin or sweaty feet may require frequent changing of socks.

## Feet Preparation

Repeated low-intensity Ff exposure results in cellular proliferation and epidermal thickening. These adaptations to underlying skin may reduce the likelihood of developing blisters. A soft and supple foot will be more adept at withstanding frictional stress than dried out and cracked feet with friable epithelium.

- Many podiatrists and ultra-endurance athletes recommend preparing feet with a moisturizer (e.g., Bag Balm, hand lotion, or other softening

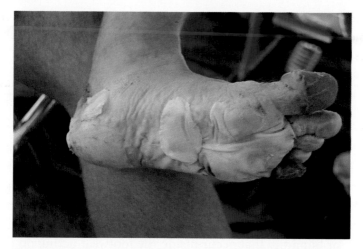

**Figure 8-2**  Moist, macerated feet. Courtesy of Mark Ellis, MD.

agent) for months before an event. Other athletes take serial footbaths in povidone-iodine to promote epidermal proliferation and thickening, which they believe will withstand sheer stress better (5).

- Calluses should be filed down with a pumice stone or emery board to prevent them from tearing off, which would leave an open wound. Blisters deep to a callus are extremely painful and difficult to drain.
- Toenails should be kept short and beveled at a 45-degree angle with an emery board to potentially reduce the incidence of a blister underneath the nail (i.e., subungual hematomas). Before a big run, consider treating yourself to a professional pedicure. Have this done at least a week before the planned outing allows time for the manipulations to the epidermis and cuticles to heal, to prevent potential bacterial entry and infection on the trail. Also, athletes may want to avoid an opaque nail color, as this could interfere with diagnosis of a subungual hematoma.

## Blister Prevention Compounds

The key to blister prevention involves decreasing sheer forces on the skin. Despite extensive studies regarding the impact of sheer forces on development of blisters, there are few studies examining the efficacy of various modalities (e.g., powders, antiperspirants, lubricants, tapes, pads). Theoretically, each of the above options offers a distinct advantage. Lubricants, tapes, and pads are proposed to decrease the friction that leads to blisters, whereas powders and antiperspirants are thought to limit perspiration and resulting skin wetness that leads to increased blister incidence. Antiperspirant mechanism of action is by the metallic salt that dissolves at the skin surface, forming an acidic solution that hydrolyzes upon contact with more alkaline sweat, precipitating and "plugging" of the sweat gland (25, 26).

## Preventive Taping and Pads

A preventive barrier between the footwear and potential point of blister formation is a proactive treatment that can prevent a blister. Barriers are best used as preventive measures before blisters form, either at the beginning of the day prior to the run or as soon as a hot spot develops. The barrier needs to be adhesive so it can remain fixed to skin, despite the action of frictional forces, heat, or humidity that occur inside the footwear acting on the barrier. The concept of prevention is to have a layer over the skin such that the shear stresses will occur between the barrier and the footwear, not the footwear and the skin. The shelves of drugstores and running stores are filled with products that can be applied to the foot. These include Micropore paper tape, cloth tape, Elastikon, Kinesio tape, Moleskin, Spenco hydrocolloid Blister Pads, Blist-O-Ban, and duct tape, to name a few (Table 8-1). Use of an adhesive-like tincture of benzoin or Pedi-Pre Tape spray can help keep the barrier fixed to the skin.

Taping is a relatively easy and cost-effective method to prevent hot spots and subsequent blister injuries at various sites on the foot. Ideally, taping products should be thin, easy to apply, adhere well, and provide limited seams that may become friction points. Paper-like surgical tape (i.e., paper tape) (Figure 8-3) can be easily placed over and around the toes, heel, plantar, dorsal aspects of the foot, or other blister-vulnerable areas (Figure 8-4). Due to its low cost, ease of use, and silky feel, it is this author's go-to product to apply on a hot spot or to historical blister-prone areas prior to a run to prevent blister formation. It is not recommended to empirically tape the entire foot, which has not been shown to pre-

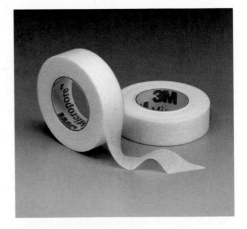

**Figure 8-3** Paper tape. Courtesy 3M.

vent blisters and may actually increase the rate of blisters on the toes when combined with Injinji single-toed socks (7). Rather, pre-taping only an area where one is predisposed to develop blisters has been found to have a robust protective

**Table 8-1** Foot care tapes and pads.

| Product | Description | Advantage |
|---------|-------------|-----------|
| Blist-O-Ban® | Ultrathin patented BursaMed dome reported to decrease the forces along the skin by deflecting forces away from the skin. Useful over hot spots or mild blisters. | Ultrathin, easy to apply, hypoallergenic, multi-day use, water resistant. |
| Compeed® | Sterile gad hypoallergenic plaster reported to protect vulnerable skin from friction damage. | Easy to apply, water resistant, flexible, multi-day use. |
| Duct Tape | Polyethylene tape with flexible shell and pressure sensitive adhesive quality. However, not very breathable and difficult to remove. May be used over any surface. | Strong, easy to apply, multi-day use. |
| Elastikon | Flexible tape made of a porous high twist, cotton elastic cloth tape with a rubber based adhesive. Useful over heels and plantar surface of foot. | Breathable, easy to apply to uneven surfaces. |
| Leukotape® | Slightly thicker tape with zinc oxide and Rayon backing. May be utilize over any part of the foot. | Breathable, easy to apply. |
| Micropore Paper Tape | Breathable pressure-sensitive adhesive tape. Useful for preventative taping and underneath thicker tape. However not well suited for wet environments. | Easy to apply and remove, hypoallergenic, multi-day use. Robust benefit in studies. |
| Moleskin | A heavy cotton fabric sheared on one side and adhesive backing on the other. Useful over relatively even surfaces to offset the direct pressure on large blisters. | Easy to apply, hypoallergenic. |
| Spenko® 2nd Skin | Series of products ranging from non-woven cotton tape to a hydrogel pad designed to assist with fluid absorption and wound healing. The pads are very useful for complicated blisters without any skin cover. | Easy to apply, hypoallergenic, multi-day use. |

effect. In a multi-site prospective randomized trial that analyzed 128 multi-stage ultramarathon runners, pre-taping was found to reduce blister incidence by 40 percent, with a success rate of over 70 percent (8). Preventive taping with paper tape appears to be an ideal method for preventing blisters in those at-risk areas, with the caveat that due to the light adhesive, paper tape will likely need to be reapplied after getting wet. For tips on preventive toe taping, see section on treatment of toe blisters (page 132).

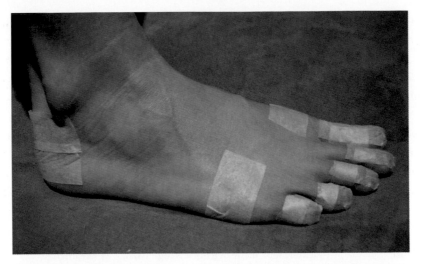

**Figure 8-4** Paper tape prophylactically applied to prevent hot spots. Courtesy Mark Ellis, MD.

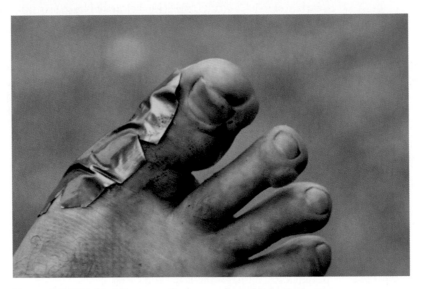

**Figure 8-5** Wrinkled duct tape that can promote blister formation.

Sturdier and wider tape (i.e., Elastikon) may be used over the soles of the feet, heels, and top (or dorsum) of the feet. Because of the rough feel of this tape, it should not be used on the toes as it may induce blisters on the neighboring toes. Duct tape has been used with variable success in areas such as the heel of a foot. However, there are innate qualities that make this product less than ideal for blister prevention. Duct tape is non-porous, causing increased moisture content and maceration of skin beneath the tape; it wrinkles easily, leading to pressure points (Figure 8-5); and the adhesive backing often sticks too well, which can lead to ripping off of skin along with the tape. Detailed descriptions on taping techniques for prevention are discussed in the blister treatment section of this chapter.

Like taping, pads (which are a combination of adhesive dressing with a central thicker composite pad) are relatively easy to apply to prevent or treat developing blisters. Pads can be extremely easy to apply over relatively smooth surfaces such as the Achilles region or ball of the foot. However, these products are usually bulkier than tape, making them more difficult to apply on uneven surfaces or in small areas, such as between the toes. Improper application can lead to excessive friction around the product and further epidermal injury. Also, pads are exponentially more expensive than tape, which may limit their use. Caution should be used when applying and removing pads with strong adhesive qualities (i.e., Compeed), as friable blister skin layers are pulled off along with the bandage (Figure 8-6).

The adhesive bandage Blist-O-Ban is uniquely suited for wet environments. The product decreases the incidence of new blisters in treated feet compared with untreated feet, and adheres well in humid conditions. However, these studies did not address blister formation in common areas, such as between the toes, and these can be difficult to treat with a bulkier bandage (27, 28).

Any discussion on foot care would be remiss without mentioning Moleskin, the ubiquitous product that has been a fixture for blister care for generations.

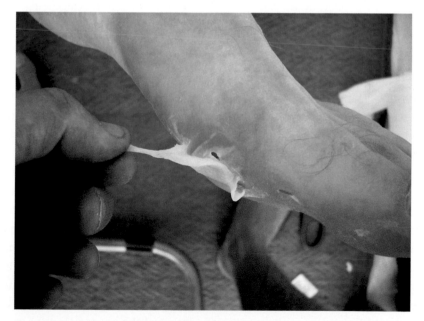

**Figure 8-6** Removing a Compeed bandage that had been placed over a blister, showing strong adhesive qualities and tearing of the blister's roof. Courtesy Grant S. Lipman, MD.

The technique of using Moleskin is to affix a doughnut-shaped patch around a hot spot or blister, securing the material with the irritated skin in the opening, in the hope that friction will act on the perimeter of felt-like material rather than the original spot. Although large or open heel blisters may benefit from being surrounded by Moleskin or the thicker Molefoam (Figure 8-7), this intervention is not recommended for treatment or prevention of hot spots or blister treatment. Anecdotally, it has a high failure rate, is difficult to anchor, and the volume of the product in a well-fitted shoe box may cause a "contrecoup" blister on the toes or even under the Moleskin product itself because of its high coefficient of friction (29).

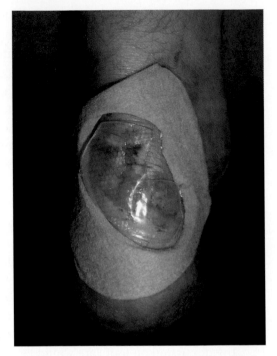

**Figure 8-7** Moleskin doughnut with hydrocolloid pad in the center. Courtesy Paul Langer, DPM.

## Antiperspirants and Powders

Antiperspirants and powders (Table 8-2) have been proposed as preventive measures to decrease the amount of moisture at the foot–sock interface. Limited studies provide conflicting findings in regard to blister prevention and the impact on foot perspiration. A small study assessed the effectiveness of two different aluminum-based antiperspirants in reducing sweat accumulation and preventing blisters. Each of the subjects applied one of the antiperspirants and then completed a one-hour treadmill march in a warm environment. Overall, both groups experienced a significant decrease (greater than 50 percent) in foot-sweat accumulation, but not in number of blisters. However, there was an increase in the incidence of skin irritation (irritant dermatitis) (30). The largest of these antiperspirant studies was a double-blind trial of 667 US military cadets randomized to either a 20 percent aluminum-based antiperspirant or placebo for five days before a short hike. For compliant subjects who used the preparation for at least three nights, the incidence of blister formation was 27 percent lower in the antiperspirant group. However, these results were tempered by a 51 percent greater

**Table 8-2** Foot antiperspirants and powders.

| Product | Description | Advantages | Ingredients |
|---|---|---|---|
| Pedifix Neat Feat® Antiperspirant Spray | Antiperspirant foot spray designed to eliminate odor, prevent irritation, and cool feet. | Spray makes application extremely easy. | Aluminum, oils. |
| Dr Scholl's® Foot Powder | Powder utilized to control foot odor, cool and soothe irritated skin, absorb wetness. | It absorbs moisture, controls foot odor and odor-causing bacteria. | "Special cooling product." |
| Gold Bond® Powder | Medicated body powder used to prevent skin irritation and relieve itching. | It absorbs moisture, controls foot odor and odor-causing bacteria, provides itch relief, and cools and soothes irritated skin. | Zinc oxide and menthol. |
| Odor-Eater's® Foot Powder | Powder combing special ingredients with baking soda to control odor and protect against wetness. | Odor and wetness protection. | Unique combination of odor-destroying ingredients and baking soda. |

incidence of skin irritation in the antiperspirant group then placebo (31). The gained benefit in blister prevention from antiperspirant may not be worth the risk for resulting irritation, and should not be considered as a first-line blister prophylactic unless runners have excessively sweaty feet (hyperhidrosis). If the decision is made to use an antiperspirant, a trial should be attempted at least a week before the planned outing to avoid having skin irritation in an outdoor setting.

A variety of powders are designed to help with foot odor and perspiration. These powders are typically composed of an astringent to ease itching and an inorganic compound (e.g., talc or sodium bicarbonate) to assist with wetness. Despite widespread marketing of these compounds, there is no published scientific evidence to suggest that these products prevent foot blisters (32). In addition, it has been suggested that powders may increase the risk for blisters because of their tendency to clump with perspiration. Despite anecdotal support for use of powders, they are likely best used to dry out feet in the evening, rather than being used on the trail.

## Lubricants

Lubricants allegedly prevent blister formation by decreasing friction at the foot-contact material interface. Lubricants have been developed that are more

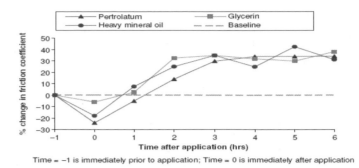

**Figure 8-8** Effect of lubricant cosmetic ingredient on skin friction coefficient. Reproduced with permission from Sivamani RK, Goodman J, Gitis NV, et al. Skin Res Technol 9:227, 2003.

advanced than traditional Vaseline, which is greasy and tends to attract grit particles that irritate and may increase friction and blister production (Table 8-3). Lubricating agents that have a subjective "greasiness" leave skin with a higher coefficient of friction than those with a sensation of "slipperiness" (33). Advanced lubricants use silicone and petrolatum mixes that have a silky feel and are thought to work by altering skin smoothness and moisture content of the skin. Several studies have shown that after applying lubricating substances to skin, there is an initial decrease of the coefficient of friction, but that within an hour, it returns to baseline with a subsequent increase in friction 35 percent over baseline over the next three to six hours (Figure 8-8) (18, 33). These studies suggest that with prolonged exercise the use of lubricants might contribute to blister formation, so if used, they need to be reapplied frequently.

## Blister Treatment

Treating a blister as soon as possible improves healing rates (34), reduces pain, and minimizes complications from either subsequent tissue damage or infection. In the early stages of blister formation, the initial sensation of warmth from the hot spot is the warning sign. Heed it. Prompt attention and rapid treatment can stop the abrasive process that prevents progressive blister formation. Options for hot spot treatment include the blister-preventive taping/lubricating measures mentioned earlier in the chapter.

Proper blister care is not complicated, yet may be time-intensive depending on the extent of damage to the feet. Individuals should become familiar with techniques before heading outside and facing a blister predicament. This author's medical experiences with multi-stage ultramarathons around the world have shown that implementation of mandatory personal foot care kits for competitors and the expectation of self-care takes a huge burden off the

**Table 8-3** Foot care lubricants.

| Product | Description | Advantages | Application | Ingredients |
|---|---|---|---|---|
| Bodyglide® | Hypoallergenic, non-petroleum based moisturizer that helps prevention against friction, rubbing from footwear, and blister formation. | Non-greasy, non-fragrant, sweat and water-resistant. | It is packaged as an applicator (i.e., deodorant stick) that can make it slightly awkward for application to the foot. | Allantoin 0.5; Aloe-barba-densis (aloe vera) leaf extract, C18-36 acid triglycerides, caprylic/capric triglycerides, tocopheryl acetate, tribehenin. |
| Hydropel® | Silicone-based skin lubricant used to prevent blisters, chafing, and chapping of skin in extreme environments. | Non-greasy, non-fragrant, sweat and water-resistant. | Ointment allows easy application to any body part. | Dimethicone 30%, petrolatum, aluminum starch, octenylsuccinate. |
| Sportslick® | Skin gel comprised of antifungal and antibacterial ingredients used to prevent blisters, chafing, and chapping of skin in dry and water environments. | Skin gel comprised of antifungal and antibacterial ingredients used to prevent blisters, chafing, and chapping of skin in dry and water environments. | Non-greasy, sweat and water-resistant. | Tolnaftate 1%, triclosan, silicone, petrolatum, aloe, vitamin E, soybean oil, and oil fragrance. |
| Sportshield® | Silicon-based liquid roll-on or towelette used to minimize friction that causes blisters, chafing, and irritation. | Non-greasy, water-resistant, odorless. | Relative easy of application to any body part depending upon product used. | Dimethicone, aloe vera extract, vitamin E. |
| Vaseline® | Petroleum-based product used to minimize friction that causes blisters, chafing, and irritation. | Water-resistant, odorless. | Easy to apply to any body part. However, the product is greasy. | 100% pure petroleum jelly. |

**Table 8-4** Personal foot care kit.

| |
| --- |
| Safety pins |
| Alcohol swabs squares |
| Benzoin swabs squares |
| Spenco® 2nd Skin burn pads (in re-sealable bag) |
| Lubricant (i.e., Hydropel®) |
| Paper tape |
| 4" Elastikon roll |
| Small roll duct tape |
| Small scissors |
| 18-gauge needle |

medical team (Table 8-4). The blister treatment techniques discussed in this chapter have been easily taught and mastered by numerous ultra-endurance race participants.

There is no one correct way to care for feet. For every technique and product mentioned, there are multiple different options. The goals of blister treatment are to optimize comfort for continued activity, maximize prevention of infection, assist with recovery, and prevent further blister enlargement when staying off your feet is not an option.

## General Taping Rules

Any tape used for blister treatment or prevention should be applied as smoothly as possible. The tape ideally acts as a second layer of skin, so that friction, abrasion, and rubbing acts on the tape, not on the underlying skin. Any folds or wrinkles in the tape should be avoided because they may lead to high-pressure and friction areas. Cut the tape corners to round them and to avoid "dog-ears" that have a tendency to roll off under a sock. All tape should be cut long enough to extend well beyond the border of the blister and any blister pads underneath the tape. Try to not overlap tape, and avoid circumferential wrapping of the feet that may lead to blood vessel constriction and swelling.

Before taping, ensure that the skin is clean of dirt and grit and as dry as possible, which will enhance natural adhesion of tape. Consider using an adhesive substance such as benzoin to ensure security of the applied dressing. Extra care must be given to securing the tape, possibly using duct tape (which should be applied cautiously as it can rip off the underlying skin when removed) or extra tape as an anchor at high friction areas. As a general rule, try not to remove blister tape unless it is peeling off or there is increasing discomfort at the tape site. Leaving tape on as long as possible during repetitive activity minimizes the risk for "deroofing" the blister upon tape removal. When tape is to be removed (ideally after the activity is finished and feet will not be subjected to further abuse), soaking the bandages before removal will loosen adhesion and minimize chances of ripping open intact blisters.

## Basic Blister Treatment

The pain from a blister is due to pressure on an incompressible fluid between skin layers. As abrasion and pressure build, there is further pain and separation of skin layers, increasing the potential for rupturing the blister, which would leave exposed raw and sensitive skin. The best protection for a blister is its own "roof," so efforts should be taken to maintain this natural skin protection.

The best method for treating a symptomatic blister is to drain the fluid. The seminal prospective blister treatment trial found that blister drainage in the first twenty-four hours led to the quickest healing rate versus no drainage (75 percent versus 16 percent) (34). Small blisters that are not causing significant discomfort can be left intact. If the blister is punctured with a needle and drained, it will often refill within a few hours. If a large hole is made that allows continuous fluid drainage, there is the risk for losing integrity of the blister and having the blister's roof tear off, and leaving a large damaged area. It is best to use a safety pin or similar-sized needle to create the optimum-sized hole. Blisters that recur under intact tape can be drained with an alcohol pad prepared safety pin through the tape.

- Prepare the blister skin and safety pin with an alcohol pad. Alcohol pads commonly have two hinged sheets; one sheet can be used to clean the blister-draining implement and the other to clean the skin.
- Puncture the blister with the prepared pin at a point further away from the center to allow natural foot pressure to continually squeeze out fluid. If more drainage is required, use several small holes rather than one large hole, limiting risk for deroofing the blister.
- Gently blot out the expressed fluid (Figure 8-9).
- Cover the now-flattened blister with paper tape that is cut or torn to overlap the edge of the blister (Figure 8-10). This very important step protects the roof of the blister from being ripped off when the overlying tape is removed.

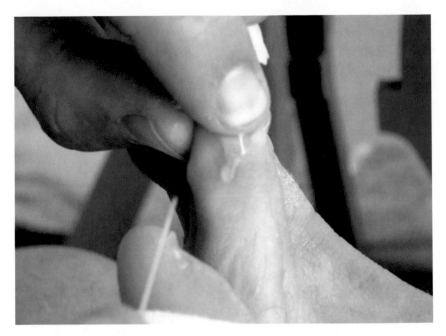

**Figure 8-9** Expressing fluid from a toe blister. Courtesy Grant S. Lipman, MD.

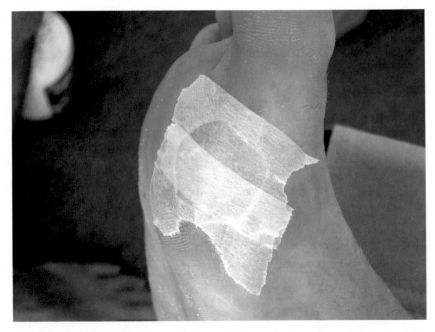

**Figure 8-10** Paper tape covering of a drained blister. Courtesy Grant S. Lipman, MD.

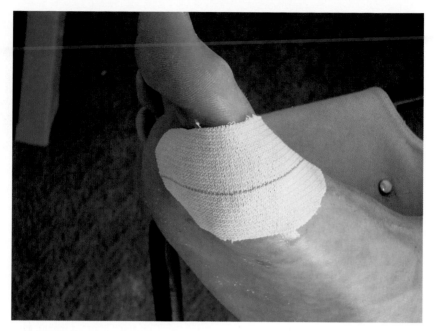

**Figure 8-11** Rounding off the corners of the overlying adhesive tape will prevent it from peeling off. Elastikon tape layer over paper-taped blister. The elastic quality of the tape allows smooth application and contours to the foot. Note the rounded corners to prevent peeling. Courtesy Grant S. Lipman, MD.

- Cover paper tape with benzoin adhesive to optimize that stickiness of the final layer of tape.
- Apply shaped Elastikon adhesive tape over the paper-taped blister (Figure 8-11).

## Open Blister Treatment

Caring for ripped-open blisters builds on the preceding basic blister treatment.

- Carefully unroof the blister (Figure 8-12), completely trimming off the dead skin. Devitalized skin is insensate and not painful to remove. The open blister may appear like a raw wound (Figure 8-13).
- Place a hydrocolloid pad (i.e., Spenco 2nd Skin burn pad) over the exposed base of the blister, extending slightly beyond the external margins (Figure 8-14). The moisture content of these hydrocolloid pads absorbs moisture and promotes collagen production and healing while providing cooling relief and padding. They should be stored in a ziplock bag to keep them moist.

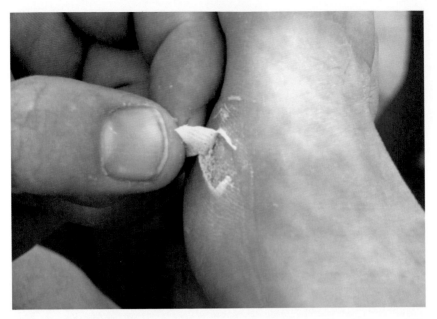

**Figure 8-12** Removal of the torn roof of an open blister. Courtesy Grant S. Lipman, MD.

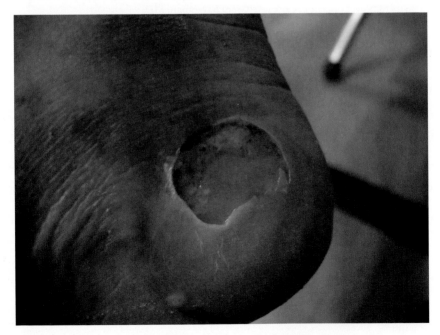

**Figure 8-13** Large open heel blister. Courtesy Grant S. Lipman, MD.

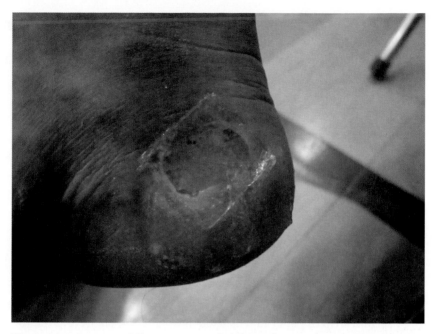

**Figure 8-14** Spenco 2nd Skin cut to size, slightly overlapping the open blister circumference. Courtesy Grant S. Lipman, MD.

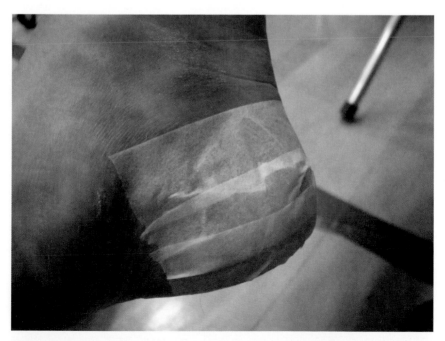

**Figure 8-15** Paper tape over the Spenco 2nd Skin covered open blister. Courtesy Grant S. Lipman, MD.

- Finish dressing the blister by covering the moist pad as you would a basic blister with paper tape (Figure 8-15), a benzoin adhesive layer, and finishing with shaped Elastikon tape or other tape product of choice.

## Toe Blisters

This technique of treating toe blisters is the same as preventing toe blisters with paper tape. Only paper tape should be used on toe blisters, because tape with rough texture can cause irritation, abrasion, and blisters on neighboring toes.

- Drain a clean blister with a prepared safety pin.
- If a blister is at the end of a toe (Figure 8-16), apply a piece of paper tape longitudinally covering the distal toe from the top to the bottom (sole) aspect (Figure 8-17).
- A second strip of paper tape is used as an anchor, encircling the toe circumferentially (Figure 8-18), which will also work to cover and treat blisters between the toes.

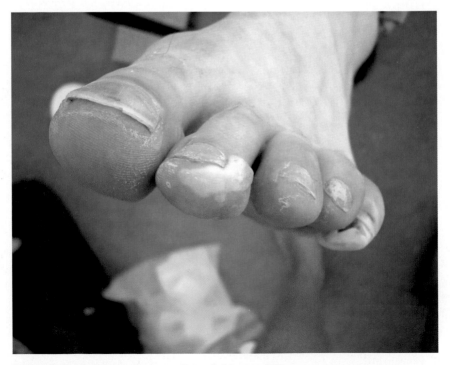

**Figure 8-16** Toe blister. Courtesy Grant S. Lipman, MD.

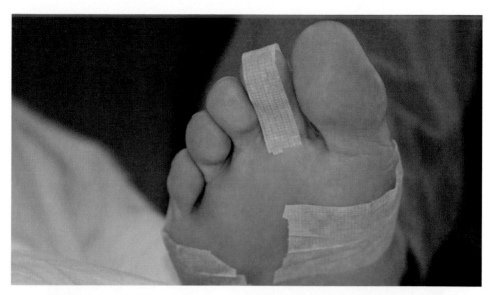

**Figure 8-18** Circumferential strip of paper tape over a toe, which both anchors the long strip and treats between-the-toe blisters. This technique can be used for preventive pre-taping. Courtesy Grant S. Lipman, MD.

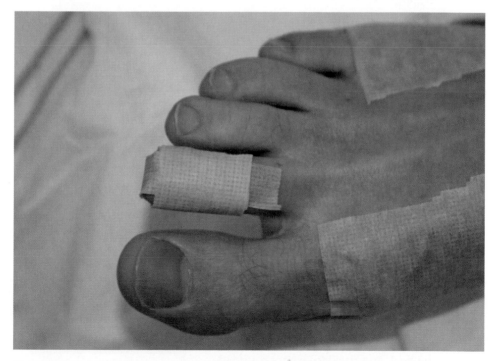

**Figure 8-17** Longitudinal strip of paper tape over a toe. This technique can be used for treatment of toe blisters, or for prophylactic pre-taping. Courtesy Grant S. Lipman, MD.

- If there is an isolated blister in the web space, just applying the circumferential wrap should be sufficient. Care should be taken to not overlap the tape multiple times, constricting the toe, and to leave the tape end on the top of the foot, to avoid irritating neighboring toes.
- Pinch the tape closed, and trim any dog-ears or wrinkles.
- Blisters that occur at the base of the nail (Figure 8-19) can be treated the same way as the tip, which will provide significant pain relief when drained.

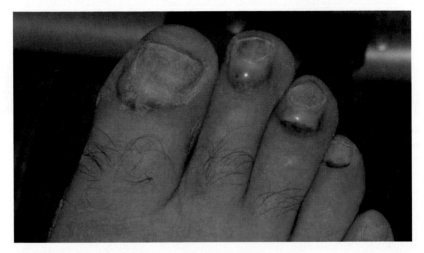

**Figure 8-19**  Base of toe blisters. Courtesy Mark Ellis, MD.

## Heel Blisters

Heel blisters are notorious for the size and potential for pain and disability (Figure 8-20). This author has witnessed exasperated people cut out the heel of a shoe to remove the instigating point of friction. A "heel cup" is a useful technique to provide a large surface area over the blister, while providing a large anchoring surface to compensate for the large shear stresses.

- A large 10-cm (4-inch) piece of thick tape (i.e., Elastikon) is cut to cover the heel, and the corners are rounded off. A horizontal incision is cut almost

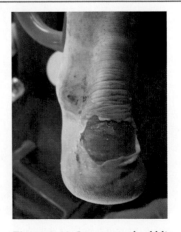

**Figure 8-20**  Large open heel blister. Courtesy Grant S. Lipman, MD.

completely through the tape, leaving an anchoring piece in the middle like a large sideways "H" (Figure 8-21).

- The upper portion is wrapped around the upper heel and the lower "wings" are wrapped over the heel and up over the ends of the upper portion, anchoring them down (Figure 8-22).

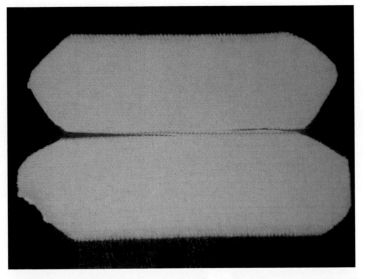

**Figure 8-21** A 10-cm (4-inch) Elastikon tape is prepared for heel cup application; the tape is cut longitudinally with a central connected piece. Note the rounded edges of the tape to minimize the edges peeling off. Courtesy Grant S. Lipman, MD.

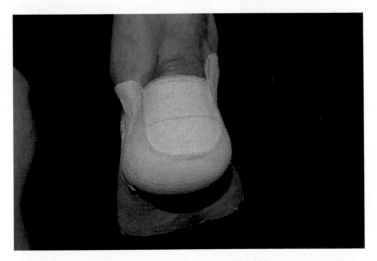

**Figure 8-22** A completed heel cup covering a heel blister. Courtesy D. J. Kennedy, MD.

- A strip of anchoring tape can be placed perpendicular to the Achilles tendon at the top of the heel cup, to prevent bandage slippage and abrasion (Figure 8-23 and Figure 8-23).
- Overlapping "dog-ears" of tape should be trimmed off to results in a smooth surface that will minimize underlying pressure points (Figure 8-25 and Figure 8-26).

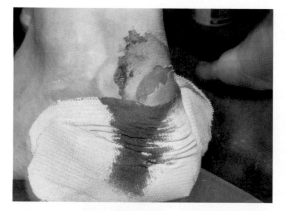

Figure 8-23 Abraded heel cup and open blister. Courtesy Grant S. Lipman, MD.

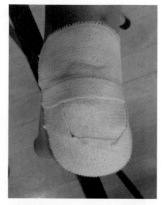

Figure 8-24 The top border of a heel cup stabilized with a perpendicular piece of Elastikon tape. Courtesy Grant S. Lipman, MD.

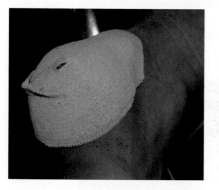

Figure 8-25 Completed heel cup with "dog ears." Courtesy Mark Ellis, MD.

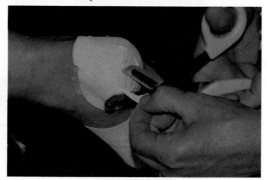

Figure 8-26 Trimming the edges and "dog ears." Courtesy Mark Ellis, MD.

## Ball-of-Foot Blisters

Blisters occurring on the ball of the foot may be very painful because this is a large weight-bearing surface (Figure 8-27). These blisters are often difficult to reach. Taping across the ball and up the sides of the foot is an option, but because the tape is running perpendicular to the mechanical movement of the foot in the

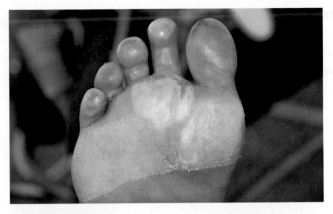

**Figure 8-27** Ball-of-foot blister. Courtesy Mark Ellis, MD.

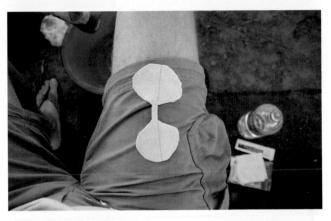

**Figure 8-28** "Blister origami." Courtesy Mark Ellis, MD.

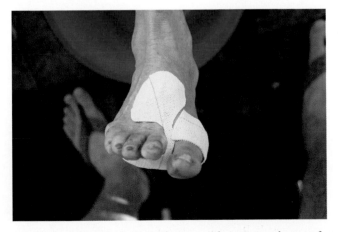

**Figure 8-29** Note the large anchoring surface area on the top of the foot of the blister origami. Courtesy Mark Ellis, MD.

shoe, it has a tendency to pull off. The author prefers a method dubbed "blister origami." During this process, the blister is drained and treated using either the open or closed method described earlier. Figure 8-29 shows a dumbbell or butterfly shape cut out of Elastikon tape with a thin connector piece. This provides three important functions. The tape has a large surface area to cover and protect the blister; it has a large surface area to be anchored on the top of the foot; and the thin strip of material connecting the two halves of tape passes between the web space of the toes, causing minimal irritation and avoiding further web-space blisters (Figure 8-29). If needed, a piece of paper tape can be laid between the toes first to minimize the abrasion of the overlying Elastikon tape. An anchoring strip of Elastikon may be placed perpendicular over the top of the foot to secure the blister origami (Figure 8-30).

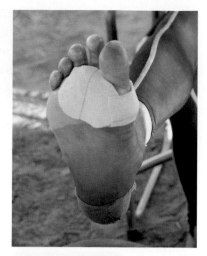

**Figure 8-30** A ball-of-foot blister treated with blister origami and stabilized with a perpendicular piece of Elastikon tape. Courtesy Mark Ellis, MD.

## Subungual Hematomas

A subungual hematoma is a collection of blood that develops underneath the nail bed. The mounting pressure makes this very painful. It is common to acquire a

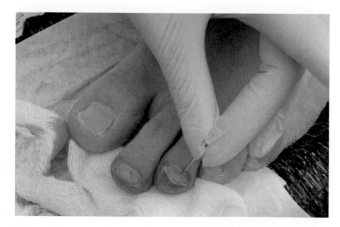

**Figure 8-31a** A subungual hematoma about to be drained with an 18-gauge hypodermic needle. Courtesy Brandee L. Waite, MD.

subungual hematoma on downhill runs when the toes are repetitively jammed into the toe box. A toenail that has been beveled downward at a 45-degree angle may disperse the pressures upward rather than straight back into the nail base. Some people find silicone toecaps are useful to prevent these injuries. Other athletes have gone so far as to have all their nails removed prophylactically. This is a drastic measure.

Subungual hematomas are easily treated. This is an exception to the rule to avoid draining bloody blisters. The release of blood under pressure through the 18-gauge hole may be dramatic, causing it to squirt, so one should use appropriate universal precautions (i.e., surgical gloves). The 18-gauge needle should be cleaned, recapped, and likely will need to be reused for the same patient, because these blisters have a tendency to recur.

- An 18-gauge hypodermic needle is held perpendicular to the proximal nail bed over the area of greatest fullness (Figure 8-32a).
- With gentle downward pressure, hold the needle between the thumb and first finger (Figure 8-31b).
- Gently twirl the needle back and forth between the thumb and finger and it easily drills into and through the nail, releasing the hematoma and resulting in significant relief (Figure 8-31c). Be careful not to hit the nailbed.

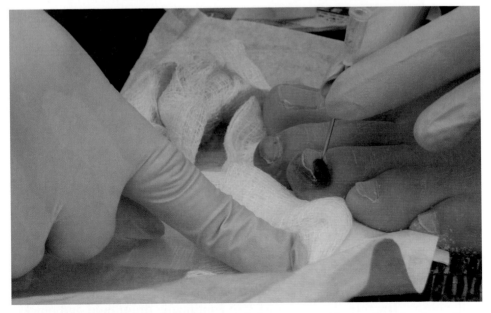

**Figure 8-31b** Moderate downward pressure applied to a rotating 18-gauge hypodermic needle will drill a hole and release the blood under a toenail. Courtesy Brandee L. Waite, MD.

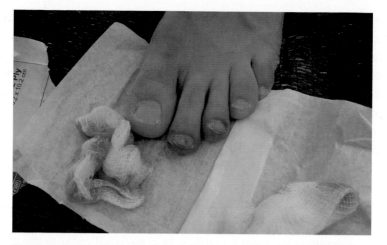

**Figure 8-31c** The drained subungual hematoma. This should then be wrapped with paper tape as a regular toe blister. Courtesy Brandee L. Waite, MD.

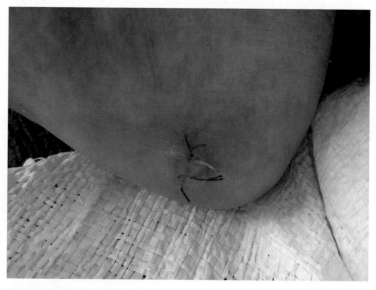

**Figure 8-32** Needle-and-thread blister technique. Courtesy Brian J. Krabak, MD.

## Alternative Blister Care Treatments

In the needle-and-thread technique (Figure 8-33), a needle is cleaned with alcohol and passed through the blister, leaving thread hanging out on either side of the blister. The thread acts as a wick to continually drain fluid and quickly dry the blister. Although this method seems to work well, it is only cautiously mentioned, since any route for fluid out of a blister is a potential entry point for bacteria.

Techniques to chemically treat blisters have variable rates of success, yet consistently high levels of procedural pain. One method to seal a blister's roof uses benzoin. After the blister has been drained, benzoin or "liquid bandage" is directly injected into the blister cavity, and then pressure is applied to the roof of the blister. This seals or "glues" the blister together. A similar technique has been attempted (cutting off the blister roof, blotting away the blister fluid, and then gluing the blister's roof down) in a study with tissue glue. There was no significant difference in blister size or time to return to normal activity versus no gluing; however, the glue arm was associated with significant procedural discomfort (35). As such, using glue on your blisters (medical grade or the "super" variety) is not recommended.

A particularly uncomfortable technique is the application of merbromin antiseptic (i.e., mercurochrome) to a manually deroofed blister. This mercury salt compound effectively dries out the blister base by a type of chemical cautery, which is quite painful. But by causing an instant dry and callus-like base to the

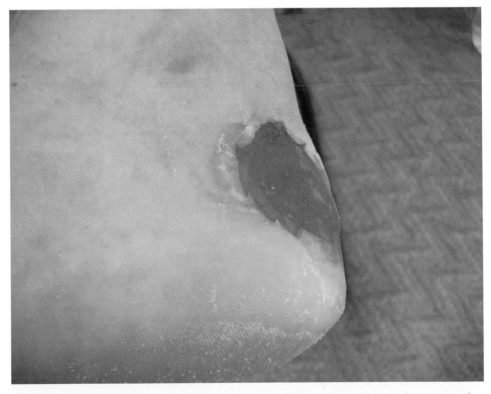

**Figure 8-33** Mercurochrome applied to a large open heel blister with resulting red staining and desiccated skin. Courtesy Grant S. Lipman, MD.

blister, this technique allows further activity with little discomfort (Figure 8-34). Of note, this product was moved from the "generally recognized as safe" into the "untested" classification by the US Food and Drug Administration in 1998 over concerns about mercury toxicity (36), effectively stopping its US distribution. It is widely available internationally.

## Blood-Filled Blisters

Blood-filled blisters represent injury to the dermal blood vessels, which run deep to the superficial epidermis (Figure 8-34). If unroofed and open to the environment, this blister represents a potential route for bacteria to enter the wound and bloodstream, which can lead to a skin infection called cellulitis, or systemic infection called sepsis. Blood blisters should be left intact unless they are large, fluctuant, and at risk for spontaneous rupture. To drain a blood blister, cover the area with a povidone-iodine solution (Figure 8-35), wear medical gloves, and follow the basic blister techniques described previously. Consider applying antiseptic ointment to the drained blister before taping. Recheck the blister site frequently for redness, streaking, or purulent drainage in which case any infection should be treated promptly with a systemic antibiotic.

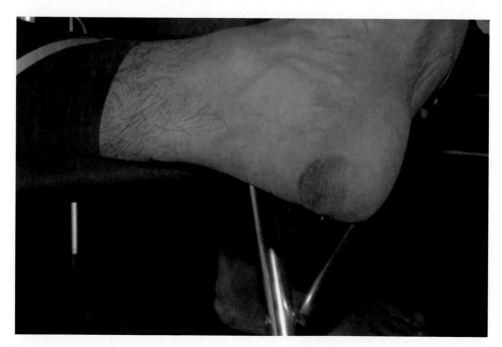

**Figure 8-34**  Large fluctuant blood blister. Courtesy Mark Ellis, MD.

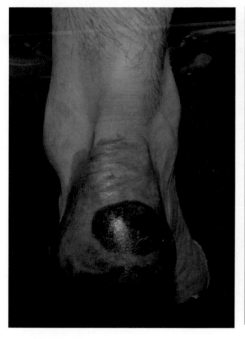

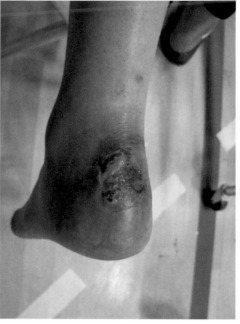

**Figure 8-35** Povidone-iodine swabbed blood blister about to be drained. Courtesy Mark Ellis, MD.

**Figure 8-36** Infected open heel blister with surrounding redness and swelling (cellulitis). Courtesy Grant S. Lipman, MD.

## Infected Blisters

A blister with murky, hazy fluid or pus may be infected. The blister should be opened (deroofed), irrigated with povidone-iodine, and then have antiseptic or antibiotic ointment applied to the cavity before being covered with the "open blister" technique. This blister's roof is more sensitive than most devitalized blister skin. An infected blister surrounded by tender and warm red skin or streaking may represent cellulitis (Figure 8-36). This blister should be opened and managed as described, with the addition of a systemic antibiotic. If the patient begins to show signs of worsening local infection or systemic symptoms, such as chills, fevers, nausea, or weakness, definitive care should be sought as soon as possible.

## Sub-callus Blisters

Blisters deep to a callus should not be drained. These blisters are difficult to access, yield little blister fluid, and quickly refill after drainage. Drainage can introduce infection to the deep space. These blisters are painful, but there is no other good treatment option beyond taping as for a basic blister and allowing the fluid to be absorbed by the body. These painful and difficult-to-manage blisters are examples of why it is beneficial to minimize blisters with a pumice stone or emery board before an outing.

CHAPTER **9**

# Musculoskeletal Injuries: Muscle, Tendon, Ligament, and Joint

BY BRANDEE L. WAITE AND BRIAN TOEDEBUSCH

## Key Points

1. Many long distance runners will experience a muscle, tendon, or joint injury while training for an event, which can decrease performance or prevent competition.
2. Risk factors for injury in the long distance runner include a previous history of injury, increasing training mileage to quickly, inexperience with long distance running, and poor running form.
3. Muscle and tendon injuries can occur anywhere in the lower extremity but are most common in the knee, followed by foot/ankle, and then hip.
4. Patellofemoral pain is the most common cause of pain in the front of the knee.
5. Iliotibial band syndrome is the most common cause of pain in the outer knee.
6. Achilles tendon problems and plantar fasciitis are the two most common causes of heel pain.
7. Pain in the front of the hip is most often due to osteoarthritis, cartilage injury, or muscle strain.
8. Pain in the outer hip is most often due to tendon injury.
9. Conservative treatment starts with rest, ice, and over-the-counter pain medications.
10. Therapeutic exercises, various injections, and improved training can help most injuries without requiring surgery.

## Introduction

As participation in long distance running events increases, so does our knowledge of common injuries that occur as a result. The term "musculoskeletal injury" refers to an injury to the muscle, tendon, ligament, or skeletal bone, usually presenting in or around a joint. Previous analysis has shown that among all ultramarathon race day injuries and illness, musculoskeletal injuries account for approximately 18 percent of all medical-treated encounters (1). In addition, nearly two-thirds of all individuals training for a long running event will have their program interrupted because of injury (2). For those training for a marathon, the reported yearly incidence of a running related injury is as high as 90 percent. Because these types of injuries are such a common occurrence with long distance running, it is important for participants to have a basic understanding of the most frequent injuries.

Musculoskeletal injury rates vary depending on the length of the run. They range from 19 percent to 75 percent in marathons, 2 percent to 18 percent in continuous single-staged ultramarathons and 19 percent to 22 percent in multi-stage, multiday ultramarathons (3, 4, 5). For all runners, the most commonly affected joint is the knee, followed by foot and ankle, then hip and pelvis, and finally the lower back (6). Shoulder, arm, elbow, and hand injuries are rare in runners, unless associated with a fall. The most frequent injuries in all runners are medial tibial stress syndrome (see Chapter 10), Achilles tendinopathy, and plantar fasciitis (3). In ultramarathon runners, Achilles tendinopathy and patellofemoral syndrome are the most common injuries. The majority of race day injuries are considered minor, and runners are therefore able to continue training. However, up to 22 percent of major injury/illness encounters during multi-stage ultramarathons are due to musculoskeletal injuries, which prevent an athlete from finishing a race. Injuries in runners may decrease performance, and result in decreased training, if not withdrawal from a race. The purpose of this chapter is to explain the common musculoskeletal injuries, specifically detailing proper evaluation and management.

## Risk Factors

There are many factors that may lead to increased risk of injury in long distance runners. The three most common risk factors are an increase in weekly mileage too quickly, a history of previous injury, and a competitive training regimen (7). Longer running distance has been attributed to increased risk as well. This is demonstrated by a sharp increase in injury risk when training crosses a threshold of forty miles per week (8). A common recommendation for increasing mileage is no more than 10 percent increase per week or 30 percent increase over a two-week period (9). Previous injury within the past twelve months is also a strong predictor of recurrent musculoskeletal injuries. This may be due to incomplete recovery from earlier injury and/or change in biomechanics causing a new injury (8). Also, novice runners with less than five years of experience and runners who did not perform interval training on a regular basis demonstrated higher injury rates (10). Experienced runners were found to be at a decreased risk of injury because they were able to recognize initial symptoms and compensate with appropriate modifications to running (11).

# General Injuries

**Table 9-1** An overview of basic musculoskeletal injuries and treatment.

| Basic Injury Type | Symptoms | Initial Treatment | Injection Options |
|---|---|---|---|
| Muscle Strains<br>1. Hamstring<br>2. Calf<br>3. Groin | - Sudden tear or pop in muscle<br>- Pain with contraction or stretch<br>- Muscle weakness | - Rest, ice, gentle stretch<br>- Acetaminophen then anti-inflammatories (oral or topical)<br>- Physical therapy with gradual strengthening | - Limited, no steroid<br>- Platelet Rich Plasma or Autologous Blood options<br>- Saline or sugar water (Prolotherapy) |
| Tendon Injuries<br>1. Achilles<br>2. Hamstring<br>3. Patellar tendon<br>4. Inner/outer ankle | - Initial pain at site of tendon attachment<br>- Initially improves after warm up<br>- Long standing pain of tendon at all times<br>- Pain with stretching tendon | - Rest, ice, gentle stretch<br>- Acetaminophen then anti-inflammatory (oral or topical)<br>- Physical therapy with gradual strengthening<br>- Massage<br>- Bracing<br>- Extracorporeal shockwave therapy | - Steroid injection around (not into) the tendon<br>- Platelet Rich Plasma or Autologous Blood into the tendon<br>- Saline or sugar water (Prolotherapy) |
| Back Pain<br>1. Muscle strain<br>2. Degenerative disc or joint disease<br>3. Pinched nerve/ radiculopathy<br>4. Sacroiliac pain | - Centralized low back pain<br>- Radiating pain into legs in pinched nerve<br>- Numbness or tingling in legs with pinched nerve<br>- Numbness in groin or change in bowel/ bladder = seek emergent care | - Rest, heat, gentle stretch<br>- Acetaminophen or anti-inflammatory (oral or topical)<br>- Physical therapy with gradual strengthening<br>- Massage therapy<br>- Consider acupuncture or chiropractic treatment | - Trigger point injection to muscle<br>- Steroid injection to degenerative joint<br>- Steroid injection for pinched nerve<br>- Steroid injection for sacroiliac pain |
| Osteoarthritis<br>1. Knee<br>2. Hip<br>3. Ankle | - Joint ache early in the morning<br>- Improves with mild activity<br>- Limited swelling, but may swell with bad flare up | - Rest, ice, gentle stretch<br>- Acetaminophen or anti-inflammatory (oral or topical)<br>- Glucosamine or chondroitin<br>- Physical therapy with gradual strengthening<br>- Bracing | - Steroid injection into the joint<br>- Platelet Rich Plasma into the joint<br>- Hyaluronic acid into the joint |

## Muscle Strains

Muscle strains are a common injury in long distance runners and have been reported as the most common reason of premature race termination in 250,000 off-road ultramarathons (12). The most common locations for muscle strains are the calf (gastrocnemius) and hamstring. Injury occurs during eccentric contraction, when the muscle fires while it is lengthening/stretching at the same time. Pain occurs immediately after muscle strain and there may be involuntary spasms. The runner may even feel a pop in the muscle at the time of injury. Typical hamstring strains occur in the gluteal/buttock region where the tendon originates at the sits bone (ischial tuberosity), but may also occur anywhere throughout the length of the muscle in back of the thigh and knee. Hamstring pain may be described as deep pain that is aggravated when accelerating or running uphill. Of note, chronic hamstring strain may be confused as low back pain.

In the initial stage of muscle strain, runners should be treated with ice, rest, and compression. If the injury occurs during a race, the runner with a mild strain may continue to race, as tolerated. However, if gait/stride is altered or if full tear occurs the runner should be withheld from competition. Following adequate rest, return to running begins with range of motion exercise with passive stretching (someone helps you stretch). Strength training and running are cautiously advanced after injury when range of motion is pain free. A severe strain or high-degree tear may require relative rest for several weeks, advanced imaging such as an MRI or ultrasound, local injection or surgery.

## Tendonitis/Tendinopathy

Tendons are dense connective tissues, which attach the end of a muscle to bone and function to transmit muscular force to produce movement of a joint. The site where the tendon attaches to bone is most prone to injury due to relatively decreased blood supply compared to the muscle itself (13). Injury may occur with repetitive overuse of a tendon. This is extremely common in the lower extremity of a runner and can be a cause of hip, knee, or ankle pain. More specific tendon injuries are discussed in detail throughout this chapter.

While there are several terms that may be used to describe tendon injury, the essential terms are tendonitis, tendinosis, and tendinopathy. Tendonitis is the initial stage of injury to the tendon and refers to early inflammation in the tendon. If tendon pain continues after several weeks, this is known as tendinosis or tendinopathy. During this stage microscopic examination would show decreased inflammation but increased collagen degeneration, like scar tissue in the tendon. Often the term tendinopathy is used as a clinical description of prolonged tendon pain.

With early tendon injury pain is present at the beginning of a run but usually improves as the run goes on. But without rest or treatment of tendinopathy, the intensity of pain may increase and last throughout the entire run. In the prolonged injury stage, pain may be constant throughout the day. There may also be swelling at the site of injury. Initially, reduced activity and ice will be beneficial for pain control. Oral or topical non-steroidal anti-inflammatory (NSAIDs) drugs are effective in the early stage, though currently there is some discussion that this may actually stunt the body's natural healing process. Strengthening and stretching are beneficial for recovery once pain is decreased. Steroid/cortisone injection around the tendon can be effective to decrease inflammatory pain but will not heal the tendon. Other types of injections (platelet rich plasma, stem cells, prolotherapy) are currently being investigated by researchers as treatments for tendinopathy. Various bracing or orthotics can be used depending on the location. Lastly, surgery for chronic pain lasting more than six months may be considered if conservative treatment fails.

## Back Pain

The incidence of back pain in long distance running (marathons and ultramarathons) is 12.4 percent (14). Various causes include muscle strain, spasm, disk injury, or chronic degenerative changes in structures of the lower back. Initial treatment should include rest, heat, and gentle stretching of core muscles. If there are symptoms of radiating pain into the lower leg, or numbness or tingling in the legs, this raises suspicion for a pinched nerve (radiculopathy). If a radiculopathy is suspected, the runner should be removed from training/racing and referred for medical evaluation. Urgent evaluation is required for back pain with significant weakness in the leg, numbness or tingling in the groin, or loss of control of bladder or bowel function. These symptoms may indicate spinal cord injury. The natural course of lower back pain is to improve with time. Oral pain medication, topical muscles creams, physical therapy, massage, acupuncture, chiropractic treatment, improved running, and workplace ergonomics (science of designing workspace) are all things that may help back pain in active people. If symptoms do not improve within several weeks, then evaluation by a spine specialist is recommended.

## Osteoarthritis

Osteoarthritis (OA) is chronic wear and tear of cartilage in joints, which leads to abnormal bone growth with joint narrowing. It is the most common cause of joint pain and affects 80 percent of the population age sixty-five or older. Risk factors for OA include age, obesity, history of joint injury, and occupational or environmental repetitive joint stress (15). Many studies have attempted to determine if running increases the risk of OA development. A review of previous research concluded that there is no link between low and moderate distance running leading to OA (16). However, there is currently inconclusive evidence regarding high-volume running (more than sixty-five miles per week) and the development of OA.

OA can occur in any joint but is most common in the knee and hip. Knee OA is described as pain that is located along the joint line. Hip OA is recognized most frequently as groin pain. Pain from OA is typically at its worst early in the morning and with standing. The pain subsides during the day or with rest. Treatment is conservative and includes oral medications, physical therapy, braces or mobility aids, and lifestyle modifications including weight loss, if applicable. Common medications used to treat pain associated with OA include oral anti-inflammatory medications, also known as NSAIDs (like ibuprofen, naprosyn), acetaminophen, glucosamine, chondroitin, and joint injections with steroids or hyaluronic acid. Ultimately joint replacement surgery may be required if pain is not controlled with conservative treatment and ideal function is lost.

# Specific Regions of Pain

## Hip Pain

### *Outer Hip: Bursitis/Tendonitis*

Greater trochanteric pain syndrome (GTPS) refers to pain originating from the structures on the outside of the hip. In the past, the pain was thought by specialists to be from inflammation of the fluid sacks between tendons (bursa) and was called hip bursitis. Additional research has shown that majority of this pain is due to a buttock muscle (gluteus medius) tendinopathy at its site of attachment on the side of the hip (17). This condition is most commonly found in females over the age of forty and in long distance runners. It can often be confused with radiating lower back pain. Pain is reproduced with directly pressing on the side of the hip and often is increased at night when lying on the affected side. There is also weakness with muscles that rotate the hip outward (external rotation) and push the leg away from the body (abductor). The treatment is the same as for tendon injury as described above. Physical therapy for this specific problem should focus

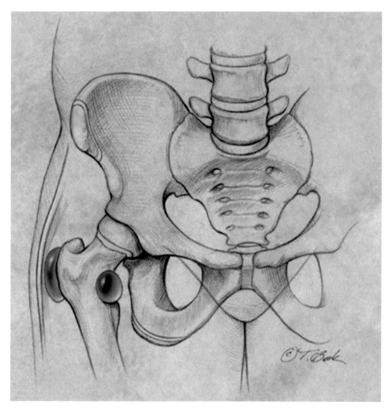

**Figure 9-1** Hip Bones and Bursa. © Todd Buck Illustration, Inc.

on strengthening of the gluteal muscles that pull leg away from the body and muscles that rotate the leg out. Injection with steroids, saline, or blood products, like platelet rich plasma, may be used for pain that does not improve with initial treatment. An ultrasound or MRI may be required to diagnosis significant tearing in pain that does not respond to therapy and injections, which may ultimately need a surgery to repair the tendon.

## Inner Hip

For hip arthritis, see section on OA above.

### Groin (Adductor) Strain

The adductor muscles are located on the inside of thigh and bring the legs together. These muscles usually are injured with a sudden change of direction. Often the individual will feel a "pull" in the groin when the injury occurs. At first, pain is localized to either the muscle belly or near the origin in the groin. There will be tenderness to pressing on the muscle and increased pain with stretching of the groin. Treatment follows the guidelines described above for muscle strains. Injections or surgery may be considered in certain cases but is rarely necessary.

## Hip Impingement/Labrum Tear

The labrum is a cartilage ring in the socket of the hip, which provides additional stability to the hip joint. Tears of the labrum commonly cause groin pain and occasionally cause buttock region pain. Runners with an abnormal bony structure of the hip, known as femoral acetabular impingement (FAI), have increased risk of labrum tears. Repetitive twisting and pivoting on the hip will make the labrum more prone to tear. Despite persistent hip pain with a labrum tear, it may be difficult to distinguish this from other causes of groin or hip pain. The runner may notice locking, clicking, or catching in the hip with a labrum tear. An MRI with dye injection to the joint is the most reliable test to diagnosis this condition. Initial treatment is with conservative care. Often pain will improve with strengthening of hip muscles and avoiding repetitive motion at the end of range of motion like deep squatting. Ultimately, various injections or hip surgery may be necessary to fix the labrum if it does not heal by itself.

## Knee Pain

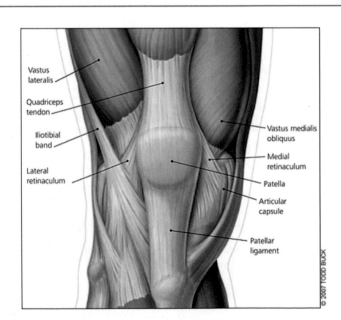

**Figure 9-2** Knee anatomy. © Todd Buck Illustration, Inc.

---

## Front of Knee

---

### *Patellofemoral Syndrome "Runner's Knee"*

Patellofemoral syndrome (PFS) is one of the most commonly reported running injuries, especially in long distance runners. It is pain between the kneecap (patella) and the underlying end of the thigh bone (femur), commonly known as "runner's knee." The prevalence in ultramarathon runners is 7.4 percent to 15.6 percent (3, 14). Females are two to three times more likely than men to have PFS (18, 19, 20, 21). This is believed to be associated with anatomic and biomechanical variations in women compared to men. Anatomic risk factors include kneecap maltracking (abnormal motion), increased mobility of the kneecap, quadriceps weakness, abnormal quadriceps activation, and decreased flexibility of soft tissue around the knee joint (22). Biomechanical risk factors include hip abductor and external rotator muscle weakness, impaired hip muscle endurance, and overpronation of the foot. Lastly, training errors such as abrupt escalation in exercise intensity or frequency, excessive downhill running, and inadequate recovery time may contribute to PFS.

In PFS, the runner will often notice vague frontal knee pain. There may be popping or grinding of the kneecap. Symptoms usually arise without any specific trauma or injury. Pain may be increased by prolonged sitting with bent knee, walking down stairs, running, or squatting. There may be tenderness to the touch along the deep borders of the kneecap. Pain can be reproduced with single leg squats, and there tends to be exaggerated inward rotation/thrust of the knee when squatting. See Figure 9-3 for abnormal single leg squat often seen in PFS. Outward deviation of the kneecap occurs when the knee is straightened from a bent position (23).

Initial treatment of PFS is conservative and includes activity modifications, ice, and oral medications. Physical therapy focuses on strengthening of quadriceps, hip abductors, and hip external rotators. In addition to strengthening, stretching protocols for the quadriceps, hamstring, gastrocnemius, and iliotibial band should be included in physical therapy (24). Patellar taping with McConnell tape has been shown to control maltracking and hypermobility (25). Also, short-term use of a patellar stabilizing brace has been reported to immediately reduce pain (22). Knee injections or surgery are rarely necessary for PFS.

### *Patellar Tendinopathy/"Jumper's Knee"*

The patellar tendon attaches the kneecap to the lower leg bone (tibia). It functions to transmit the muscular force of the quadriceps to straighten the knee joint.

Figure 9-3: Single Leg Squat

- A & B Correct form: the trunk remains upright, knee well aligned over the ankle and pelvis is level.
- C & D. Incorrect form: With poor control seen in patellofemoral single leg squat, the trunk leans forward, pelvis tilts, and knee may deviate inward and move forward over the toes due to abnormalities in strength and alignment.

**A. Correct Form**

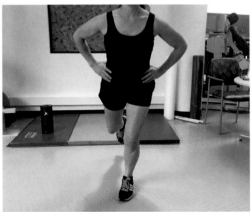

**B. Correct Form**

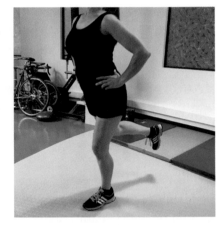

**C. Incorrect Form**

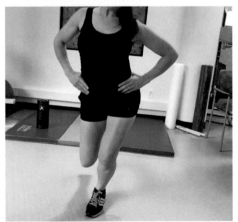

**D. Incorrect Form**

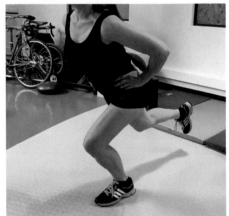

**Figure 9-3**

When the tendon becomes overused a painful tendinopathy occurs just below the kneecap. Traditionally, this has been referred to as "jumper's knee" because of its high prevalence in sports such as basketball and volleyball. However, it is also a common cause of knee pain in long distance runners. The most tender spot is found just below the kneecap when pressing on the tendon. Pain will increase with squatting, running downhill, or decelerating. There typically is no knee swelling or change in range of motion of the knee.

Ultrasound can be used to diagnose patellar tendinopathy, and may show swelling of the tendon and increased blood flow around the tendon. Treatment is similar to other tendinopathy. Bracing with a Cho-Pat strap may help decrease pain. Physical therapy will focus on strengthening and stretching the quadriceps, particular with eccentric exercises like single-leg squats and lunges. Injections with blood products like platelet rich plasma may be useful for pain that does not improve with physical therapy. Finally, surgical debridement can be used for recurrent pain does that does not improve after several months of treatment.

## Outer Knee: Iliotibial Band Syndrome

This is the second most common running injury, and the most common reason for outer knee pain in runners (11). The prevalence for men has been reported as 6.8 percent and females as 9.8 percent (11). The iliotibial band (ITB) is a large ligamentous structure that spans from the upper outer hip to below the outer knee (26). Theories to explain ITB syndrome is compression of local blood vessels and nerves versus friction of the fibers over the outer thigh bone/femur as the knee bends, resulting in increased pressure at that area (27, 28). Biomechanical factors that can contribute to ITB syndrome include increased inward swing of the leg (hip adduction) and inward rotation of knee when running. Pain is usually described as longstanding outer knee pain in runners with a history of over training. The outer portion of the thigh around the knee can be very tender to the touch. Pain is most severe with compression of this area as the knee is moved from straight to slightly bent. See Figure 9-4 for an ITB stretch.

Treatment for ITB syndrome can be separated into various phases (29). During the initial phase, ice and topical NSAIDs can be used to help pain while the running is stopped. Physical therapy should begin immediately with treatments to localized trigger points (tender areas) with massage techniques such as soft-tissue mobilization or use of a foam roller. After one to two weeks of initial treatment pain should begin to subside. With advancement of treatment, the primary focus becomes ITB and lateral hamstring stretching. The final phase of recovery focuses on strengthening of the outer buttock muscles (gluteus medius and external hip rotators) (30). Common exercises that may be used include a single-leg step down, single-leg wall squat, and single-leg dead lift (31). However, if pain continues an ultrasound-guided injection around the ITB can be performed (32). Pain lasting longer than three to six months may respond better to

Figure 9-4: Iliotibial band stretch

- Lie on your back, lift the leg about half way up and loop a long strap around the foot.
- Keep the knee straight, toe pointed away and slightly inward.
- While keeping your hip and back firmly anchored to the ground, use strap to pull the straight leg across the midline.
- Adjust intensity of stretch by using strap to pull leg further up or further across the body. Once the desired level of stretching is achieved, hold stretch (do not bounce).
- Do not pull the leg up so much that you feel a hamstring stretch- the hamstring should be relaxed in order to best stretch the ITB.

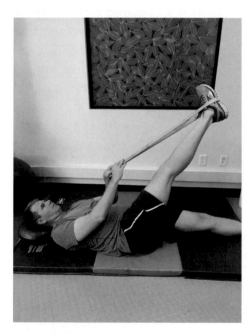

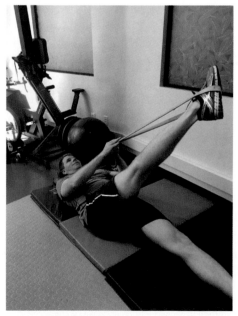

**Figure 9-4**

prolotherapy (irritant solution such as high concentration dextrose) or platelet rich plasma injections rather than steroid/cortisone injections. Return to running begins when pain is gone. Start with every other day training and on a level surface. If pain does not return after two weeks of running, then downhill running can be incorporated in the routine. Surgical treatment is rarely required for ITB syndrome but may be considered in severe cases that do not respond to medications, therapy, or injections.

## Inner or Outer Knee: Meniscus Injury

Five percent of running injuries presenting to a large sports medicine center were reported as meniscus injuries (11). The meniscus is a C-shaped cartilage shock absorber and motion stabilizer in the knee joint. See Figure 9-5 for a diagram of the meniscus. There are two in each knee and pain can be on the inner or outer portion of the knee depending on which meniscus is injured. The meniscus can be injured from wear and tear over time, or from a twisting injury while bending the knee. Acute injuries often cause noticeable knee swelling. Locking and catching of the knee are often reported. An MRI may be needed to confirm the diagnosis.

Initial treatment for meniscus injury is non-surgical unless the knee is giving out or getting stuck in a bent or position. A short course of non-weight-bearing

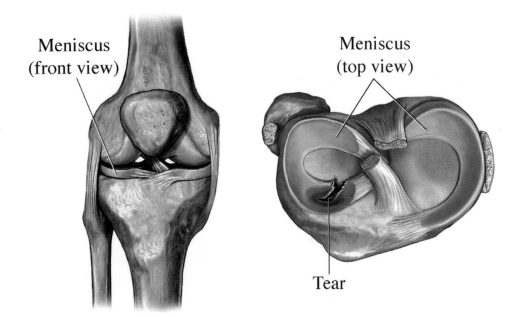

**Figure 9-5**  Meniscus anatomy. © 2017 Nucleus Medical Media.  All rights reserved. www.nucleusinc.com

may help pain. If pain does not improve with rest, it may improve with physical therapy. Sometimes a steroid injection is needed to decrease pain and swelling. Currently, there is some consideration of platelet rich plasma injections as a treatment for meniscus injury, but it is still investigatory. If surgical intervention is required, the meniscus may be repaired or partially removed depending on the type of tear present. Once part of the meniscus is removed, it does not grow back, and this may lead to increased risk of developing knee arthritis.

## Foot and Ankle Pain

### Back of Ankle: Achilles Tendonitis/Tendinopathy

The Achilles tendon attaches the calf muscles (gastrocnemius and soleus) to the back of the heel. Its main job is pushing off the ground or raising the heel (ankle plantarflexion). It is the most common cause of heel pain in runners with a prevalence of 2 percent to 18.5 percent in ultramarathon runners (3, 14). Typically the runner will complain of pain at the back of the heel or ankle. There are two common sites of pain on the tendon: the midportion of the tendon and the insertion site where it attaches to the heel bone (33). Visible swelling or redness may occur in the Achilles region. A lump on the back of the heel may be present, known as a Haglund's deformity. Pressing on the tendon may increase pain. There may be limited ability to bring toes upward (ankle dorsiflexion). See Figure 9-6 for Achilles tendon stretching technique to stretch both gastrocnemius and soleus portions of the tendon.

Initial treatment is as described for other tendons. If pain is present with standing, immobilization of the foot with a boot can provide relief. However, long term use of a boot can lead to loss of flexibility and muscle wasting. Topical nitroglycerin (which may improve local blood flow to the tendon) has been tried but does not have clear evidence to support its use (34). Physical therapy should focus on eccentric strengthening of calf muscles (35). If pain does not improve following physical therapy, then chronic Achilles pain can treated with ultrasound guided injections around the tendon. Previously, injection of steroids in to the Achilles tendon had been used to provide pain relief. This practice has been discouraged due to increased association with tendon rupture following injection within the tendon (36). If symptoms are not improved with several months of treatment then blood product or saline injections or surgery may be considered.

Figure 9-6: Achilles Tendon Stretches

- Place the heel on the ground, toes up on a step or wall, and push body weight forward over the ankle/toes.
- For gastrocnemius stretching, keep the knee straight (A).
- For soleus stretching, let the knee bend slightly and stay bent (B).

**A.**

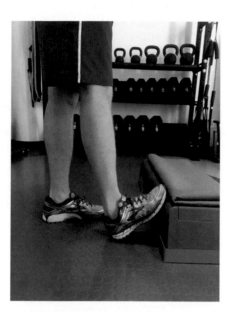

**B.**

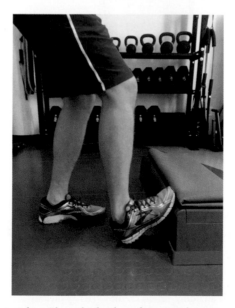

**Figure 9-6**  Achilles tendon stretches. Place the heel on the ground, toes up on a step or wall, and push body weight forward over the ankle/toes. For gastrocnemius stretching, keep the knee straight (A). For soleus stretching, let the knee bend slightly and stay bent (B).

## Inner Ankle: Posterior Tibialis Tendonitis/Tendinopathy

The posterior tibialis muscle is located deep in relation to the calf muscles on the inner portion of the lower leg, and travels behind the inner portion of the ankle to attach to multiple bones on the bottom of the foot. See Figure 9-7 for inner ankle anatomy. The primary function of the posterior tibialis is to assist the ankle with push off (plantarflexion) and inward turning (inversion) of the ankle. It also helps with stabilization of the foot and arch during standing. In one study, only 0.55 percent of runners reporting to a large sports medicine clinic had this injury (18). Pain is primarily located behind the inside of the ankle and may be confused with the less common flexor hallucis longus tendinopathy, which occurs more often in dancers. There is weakness and pain with turning the ankle inward. Management is similar to other tendinopathies. The use of a foot orthotic for arch support and correction of over pronation may be helpful (37).

Strengthening exercises should focus on high repetition plantar flexion exercises and stretching of the calf muscles. If initial treatment does not improve pain, various injections around (steroid) or into (saline, blood products) the tendon can be considered. As was mentioned previously, steroid injections may reduce pain but increase risk of tendon rupture (36). Surgery may also be considered if symptoms last more than several months.

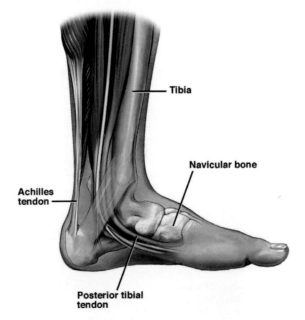

**Figure 9-7**  Inner ankle anatomy. Photo credit © 2017 Nucleus Medical Media.  All rights reserved. www.nucleusinc.com

## Outer Ankle: Peroneal Tendonitis/Tendinopathy

Peroneal tendinopathy occurs from the peroneus longus and/or brevis tendon. These two muscles comprise the outer compartment of the leg and travel together behind the outside portion of the ankle. The brevis and longus tendons function together as the primary muscles that turn the foot/ankle outward (eversion). Peroneal tendinopathy has a similar occurrence rate as posterior tibialis tendinopathy (18). With this problem, a runner will develop outer ankle pain. This may be associated with snapping sensation due to the tendon sliding over the outer ankle. Runners with increased outward bending of the ankle, known as hind foot varus, are at increased risk for injury to the peroneal tendons. Pain may be reproduced with resisted turning out of the foot. Due to the risk factor of increased hind foot varus, custom foot orthotic may be helpful including a lateral heel wedge (38). Treatment follows the same course as outlined for other tendon problems above.

## Front of Ankle: Anterior Tibialis Tendonitis/Tendinopathy

The anterior tibialis is located in the anterior compartment (front) of the lower leg. It is the primary muscle of ankle dorsiflexion, or the act of pulling up the foot at the ankle joint. With this tendinopathy pain is located in front of the ankle. This injury is more common with prolonged steep hills or inclines during running. Physical exam may show swelling or fullness in the lower anterior leg. Pressing or stretching the tendon may be painful. Treatment follows the same course as outlined for other tendon problems above.

## Plantar Fasciitis

The plantar fascia is a broad sheath of tough, fibrous tissue on the bottom of the foot that helps stabilize the inner arch. It is composed of three bands: lateral, medial, and central (39). Incidence of plantar fasciitis is 10.6 percent in long distance runners, and is slightly more common in males. Injury occurs with repeated high impact absorption in the foot and often is associated with improper arch support. The runner may notice pain located on the bottom of the foot close to the heel. Classically, pain is worse in the morning and improves during the day. Pressing on the mid-arch and inside heal is painful. Pain can be exacerbated with ankle dorsiflexion combined with great toe extension.

Initial treatment includes conservative options similar to those used for other tendon problems and stretching the plantar/bottom aspect of the foot. A rolling massage with ice, cold bottle, or golf ball underneath the arch is especially effective. Manual stretch of the plantar fascia with extension of the toes should be performed several times throughout the day (40, 41). Physical therapy with emphasis on strengthening of the foot muscles, running gait evaluation, and high load strength training with single leg calf raises, may provide pain relief. Other options include calcaneal/heel taping, various arch supports or customized foot orthotics, nighttime dorsiflexion splinting, extracorporeal shockwave therapy, acupuncture, and iontophoresis. For pain that does not improve with therapy, injections with steroids, autologous blood products, or saline may be tried to provide pain relief. In persistent cases, a surgical referral can be obtained.

## Ankle Sprain

This is a very common injury, especially with trail running or uneven terrain. The reported incidence is 10.8 percent (14). The typical mechanism of this injury occurs with inward rolling of the ankle, and results in damage to one or more of the three ligaments of the outer ankle. If the runner has an outward turning or external rotation injury of the ankle, then a more severe high ankle sprain can occur with injury to the ligament between the lower leg bones (tibia and fibula).

The runner has pain primarily located on the front and outside surface of the ankle. Shortly after the injury there is prominent swelling and occasionally bruising in the same location as the pain. Pain increases with pressing on the site of the injury. Pressing the surrounding bony structures will help determine if there is also a fracture. The Ottawa Ankle Rules are used to help determine if an X-ray should be completed (42). These rules state that if there is bone tenderness along the lower 6 cm of the back edge of the tibia or fibula, tip of the inside or outside of the ankle, bone tenderness at the outer or mid-foot, or an inability to bear weight for four steps then x-ray should be completed to make sure there is not a broken bone.

Treatment begins with PRICE—protection, rest, ice, compression, and elevation—to help control swelling and further injury. A brace or a walking boot can be used for protection and stability in the initial stages of healing. If there is suspicion of fracture, the patient should remain non-weight-bearing until this has been excluded. Some current studies suggest that oral anti-inflammatory medications should be avoided for the first few days after injury to allow the body's inflammatory response occur (43). Rehabilitation should occur early in the recovery process with emphasis on reducing swelling and restoring ankle movement. With progression in physical therapy, the focus will transition to strengthening the foot and ankle muscles, and functional balance and postural control exercises (44). The runner should return to pain-free running within a few weeks of the injury; however in more severe sprains, it can take several months for full recovery. In cases of recurrent ankle sprains or chronic instability, certain injections or evaluation by an orthopedic surgeon should be considered for repair of damaged ligaments.

## Conclusion

While musculoskeletal injuries are a relatively common problem for long distance runners, most are minor and heal with conservative measures. Runners can avoid many injuries by sticking to a training schedule that has a slow progression of distance, incorporates some interval and cross-training, and by taking time to appropriately stretch and recover after training/racing. Proper-fitting gear and timely replacement of running shoes can also help prevent problems. Injuries that do not resolve with conservative measures should be evaluated by a sports medicine physician who is familiar with the specific needs of distance runners.

## CHAPTER 10

# Bone Stress Injuries

## BY MICHAEL FREDERICSON AND EMILY KRAUSS

## Key Points

1.  A stress fracture occurs when a bone fails to withstand repetitive impact forces over time.
2.  The female athlete triad is another notable risk factor for bone stress injuries and is defined as low energy availability with or without disordered eating, menstrual irregularities (meaning absent or infrequent menstrual cycle or delayed onset of first period), and low bone mineral density.
3.  Bone stress injuries may present as a vague, nonspecific ache or pain of a body part, often making early diagnosis challenging.
4.  Magnetic resonance imaging is the diagnostic modality of choice. Most bone stress injuries are missed on routine X-rays.
5.  If the bone stress injury is located in selected high risk anatomical sites or trabecular bone (such as femoral neck or pelvis), further studies to evaluate bone health are often warranted, which may include a bone density scan, nutrition assessment, and additional lab work-up.
6.  Prevention strategies include maintaining adequate energy intake to ensure optimal energy balance and adequate calcium and vitamin D levels.
7.  Strength training can complement running by improving performance and correcting muscle imbalances, which may predispose runners to excessive stress to the skeletal framework and resultant bone stress injuries.
8.  Keep an eye on excessive or abnormal wear patterns on footwear, as this may be an early indicator of increased load on particular bones.
9.  For runners who struggle with chronic injuries, either of the bone or other soft tissue, a gait analysis may be helpful in identifying faulty biomechanics that may predispose the runners to injury.
10. A proper recovery after long runs or intense workouts is important to allow bones to repair and remodel before the next run.

# Background

Distance runners put hours of pounding on their skeletal framework day after day. When that framework fails under those forces, a bone stress injury (BSI) develops. These bony injuries are quite common in the running population with 20 percent of elite collegiate runners sustaining a BSI per year (1). This can be a frustrating setback for any runner and the injury often occurs in the heat of training, just when the runner is finding his or her rhythm. This chapter will explain what one needs to know about bone stress injuries and ways in which to avoid them in one's own running career.

# Defining Bone Stress Injury

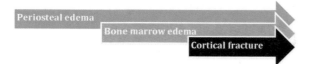

**Figure 10-1** Spectrum of bone stress injuries.

A stress fracture occurs when a bone fails to withstand repetitive impact forces over time (2). The term bone stress injury (BSI) is used to encompass the spectrum that can be seen, starting with subtle swelling (edema) or inflammation of the bone surface (periosteum), progressing to bone marrow edema, and then advancing to an overt fracture line in the outer layer of bone (cortex) (Table 10-1).

Not all BSIs are treated equally. Certain anatomic locations are considered "high risk" or "low risk" based on recovery time and increased risk of complication, such as progression to a complete fracture or delayed union of bone (i.e., delayed healing) (3). Our skeletons consist of trabecular, or spongy, bone and a denser cortical bone. Certain trabecular bone sites, such as in the femoral neck, sacrum, and pubic bones, are considered high risk due to the associated delay in return to sport (4). That said, not all trabecular bone is defined as high risk. Table 10-1 breaks down low, moderate, and high risk BSIs by anatomical location.

Along this same thought process, BSIs can be divided even further into insufficiency fractures and fatigue fractures. Insufficiency fractures usually occur when an elderly patient (usually with osteoporosis) sustains a normal stress on a weak bone, such as during a fall. A fatigue fracture is when abnormal stress is placed on a normal, healthy bone. Interestingly, some runners

**Table 10-1** High risk and low risk bone stress injuries. Pelvis stress fractures are a controversial location but recent research by Nattiv et al. showed that time to full return to play is longer in trabecular bone stress injuries, thus could be considered higher risk. *From Tenforde A S, Kraus E, Fredericson M. 2016. Bone Stress Injuries in Runners. Physical medicine and rehabilitation clinics of North America 27 (1): 139-149; with permission.*

| Low Risk and High Risk Bone Stress Injuries in Runners | | |
|---|---|---|
| **Low Risk** | **Medium Risk** | **High Risk** |
| Posteromedial tibia | Pelvis (Sacrum and pubic rami) | Femoral neck |
| Fibula/lateral malleolus | Femoral shaft | Patella (knee cap) |
| Calcaneus | Proximal tibia | Anterior tibial diaphysis |
| Diaphysis of second to fourth metatarsals | Cuboid | Medial malleolus |
| | Cuneiform | Talus (lateral process) |
| | | Tarsal navicular |
| | | Proximal diaphysis of the fifth metatarsal |
| | | Base of second metatarsal |
| | | Great-toe sesamoids |

demonstrate qualities of insufficiency and fatigue fractures, highlighting the importance of addressing both in the clinical setting.

## Who's at Risk?

Which runners are at greatest risk for sustaining a BSI? Table 10-2 provides a comprehensive list, but several deserve more discussion. Female runners are at greater risk than males, especially those who demonstrate one or more characteristics of the Female Athlete Triad (5, 6). The Female Athlete Triad (Figure 10–2) consists of low energy availability with or without disordered eating, menstrual irregularities (meaning absent or infrequent menstrual cycle or delayed onset of first period), and low bone mineral density (6). The more components of the triad that the female demonstrates, the greater the risk (7).

### Is There a Male Equivalent to the Female Athlete Triad?

A pattern similar to the Female Athlete Triad is beginning to be recognized in the male population, with males experiencing a reduction or imbalance in sex hormones, also called hypogonadotropic hypogonadism, instead of menstrual irregularities (8). The challenge clinicians encounter in the male population is

# Female Athlete Triad

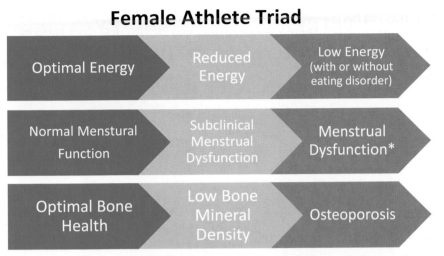

**Figure 10-2** Female Athlete Triad *Menstrual dysfunction defined as absent or infrequent menstrual cycle or delayed onset of first period.

Data from: De Souza M J, Nattiv A, Joy E, Misra M, Williams N I, Mallinson R J, Gibbs J C, Olmsted M, Goolsby M, Matheson G. 2014. 2014 Female Athlete Triad Coalition consensus statement on treatment and return to play of the female athlete triad: 1st International Conference held in San Francisco, CA, May 2012, and 2nd International Conference held in Indianapolis, IN, May 2013. Clinical journal of sport medicine 24 (2): 96-119.

**Table 10-2** Risk Factors for Bone Stress Injury. *From Tenforde A S, Kraus E, Fredericson M. 2016. Bone Stress Injuries in Runners. Physical medicine and rehabilitation clinics of North America 27 (1): 139-149; with permission.*

| Risk Factors for Bone Stress Injury | |
|---|---|
| **Biological Factors** | **Biomechanical Factors** |
| Female sex | Training patterns, including volume or changes in intensity |
| Genetics | Bone characteristics (thinner cortex, lower bone mineral density) |
| Medications (including anticonvulsants, steroids, antidepressants, antacids) | Anatomical considerations (leg length discrepancy, lean mass, foot type, smaller calf cross-sectional area) |
| Female Athlete Triad (low energy availability, menstrual dysfunction, and low bone mineral density) | History of a fracture |
| Other dietary contributors (insufficient calcium and vitamin D) | |

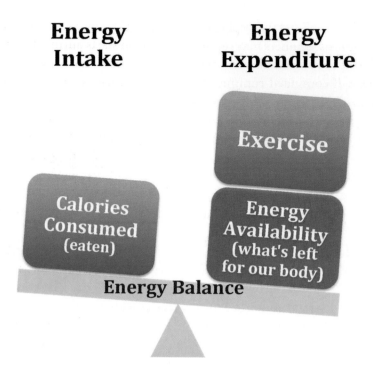

**Figure 10-3** Energy Balance and Energy Availability: Energy availability is the amount of energy left over and available for your body's functions after exercise is subtracted from the calories you take in from food.

the difficulty in finding a reliable way to test for this condition, although lower testosterone levels are seen in endurance athletes compared to their sedentary counterparts (9).

Other risk factors include insufficient calcium and Vitamin D in the diet or even certain medications, such as anticonvulsants, antidepressants, and antacids, which can impair calcium absorption (10, 11, 12). In addition to the biological risk factors, intrinsic structural abnormalities can predispose to BSIs, such as the shape of the foot (flat feet versus high arches) or a leg length discrepancy. Further, extrinsic risk factors for BSI include changes in training volume, intensity, or terrain (13, 14, 15, 16, 17). For additional information on female athlete triad, see the chapter on Injury Prevention.

## Signs and Symptoms

The challenge with early diagnosis of bone stress injuries is the often vague, non-specific presentation of symptoms. For example, a runner with a pelvic stress fracture may initially complain of a "dull ache" in the back or buttocks, which could easily be confused for a spine or sacroiliac (SI) joint problem and lead to a delay in diagnosis. Runners may report that the pain starts during the run, usually toward the latter half and becomes more noticeable over a course of days, sometimes weeks. If continued running, the pain may increase in intensity, become more localized, and occur with walking or at rest (2).

On physical examination, the runner is often very tender at a focal point on the injured bone. Depending on the location of the injury, this bony tenderness may be easy (tibia, fibula, foot bones) or difficult (sacrum, femoral neck) to pinpoint. The site of injury may be warm, or mildly swollen, due to the associated inflammatory reaction (2). Pain may also be elicited when the physician taps on the injured bone or in more severe cases, on an indirect area away from the bone stress injury.

In addition, a thorough history should be taken when evaluating a runner for a BSI. Relevant questions include a menstrual history in females, dietary habits (including any food restricting behaviors), a complete running history (i.e., changes in running volume, shoe type, duration of use, frequency of racing, change in foot strike pattern and a change in running biomechanics), any history of fractures and a personal or family history of low bone mineral density (18). Further, it's important to ask if the runner is supplementing or eating enough foods rich in calcium and vitamin D and if taking any medications such as hormones (oral contraceptive pills, estrogen, progesterone) or any other medications which may influence bone health, such as steroids or antacids.

## Diagnosis

Another challenge encountered with diagnosing BSIs is that a plain X-ray may not show abnormalities for up to three weeks and in some cases will remain negative (so don't assume a runner is in the clear with a normal X-ray). Magnetic resonance imaging (MRI) is the modality of choice for diagnosis with grading systems to aid in assessing severity of injury (19, 20). Other diagnostic modalities include bone scans or computed tomography, although both have the unwanted drawback of exposure to radiation.

## Management

Because of the many factors which can lead to these frustrating injuries, the timeline for return to running should be individualized for each athlete, under the guidance of a physician. Depending on the location of the BSI, a period of non-weight-bearing may be necessary to ensure an adequate healing response.

For example, at high risk anatomic sites runners should be non-weight-bearing (Table 10-1), and may require the use of crutches and/or a walking boot. For low risk sites, runners can often walk on the injured bone, but should avoid running (2). Repeat imaging is needed for high risk anatomic locations to ensure interval bony healing prior to progressing activity status. Pain should guide progression, as the presence of pain during or after an activity is a sign that the site of injury is being excessively loaded and the activity should be scaled back. Once able to walk without pain, runners may then transition to nonimpact training, such as with a stationary bike or underwater running. Throughout this time, strength training exercises are essential to help support and optimize running mechanics.

Although the timeline is quite variable based on site, for high risk BSIs, it may take six to twelve weeks from initial injury before initiation of a return to run protocol. An anti-gravity treadmill is one option to ensure a safe transition back to sport, because it allows the athlete to run at higher intensities while using similar muscles to land running earlier in the recovery without an excessive degree of bone-loading. One case study evaluated a return-to-run protocol using an anti-gravity treadmill in a twenty-one-year-old elite, collegiate female runner with a pelvic stress reaction (21). Ten weeks after initial injury, she successfully returned to running and competed in a 10K at the NCAA championships.

Studies show athletes may not return to pre-injury training level for three to six months from initial injury. Much of this variability is dependent on severity of injury, underlying risk factors (female athlete triad, etc.) and the type of return-to-run-protocol. Those initial weeks are a great time to address potential underlying biomechanical deficits which may have contributed to the injury so the runner can return activity with improved strength and form. Runners should also be counseled to maintain good caloric intake to meet the metabolic demands of cross-training and not inadvertently restrict caloric intake that may risk delayed healing response.

Another key player in management of BSIs is trying to address the difficult but important question runners have. First, it's important to factor in the anatomical location. If the injury is located at a high risk anatomical site (Table 10-1) or a trabecular bone site, this may warrant additional clinical investigation. For example, a DEXA bone scan will provide information on whether the runner has low bone mineral density. Lab workup may include a serum 25-OH vitamin D level, calcium (ideally measured through a twenty-four-hour urine test), and thyroid function. Female athletes should be screened for female athlete triad and both sexes should have a nutrition screen to ensure adequate energy availability

(18). In some cases, runners may need a referral to a dietitian specializing in sports nutrition who can factor in sports participation demands, caloric intake, and energy availability or a referral to an endocrinologist who specializes in bone health.

Runners may also benefit from a more formal gait assessment to address potential biomechanical factors which may be predisposing the runner to increased load on a particular bone, especially for stress fractures in the lower leg bones (tibia, fibula, foot/ankle). This should include a gait analysis, strength and flexibility assessment, and evaluation of foot structure and current foot-wear (2).

## Prevention

How can runners avoid a bone stress injury in the first place? Prevention goes beyond just thinking about the bone and requires a "whole body" approach. The following key points are a helpful guide.

## Keep the Tank Full

Adequate energy intake is essential not just for optimal running performance (or avoiding the "bonk"), but also to maintain regular menstrual function in females and a normal hormone balance in males (6, 7, 8). The timing of energy intake, such as before and after long runs or intense workouts, is important to replace energy deficits to allow for optimal repair and recovery. Restricting calories leads to low energy availability (EA), defined as the amount of energy leftover and available for your body's functions after the energy expended for training is subtracted from the energy you take in from food (Figure 10-3). Low EA can lead to hormonal deficits which disrupt the body's endocrine system. This disruption can wreak havoc on bone health, affecting bone turnover and bone mineral accrual with the consequence of early bone loss (22). If EA can be reliably estimated, the target should be at or greater than 45 kcal/kg of fat free mass (6). A sports dietitian is a valuable resource to help with calculating EA and formulating a plan to ensure optimal energy balance.

## Keep Your Bones Healthy

Runners should be taking in around 1,200 mg to 1,500 mg of calcium per day through their diet and, if needed, through the use of supplements. Vitamin D intake is recommended at 600 IU per day via diet, moderate sun exposure, and

**Table 10-3**  Dietary Reference Intakes for Calcium and Vitamin D.

| Life Stage Group | Calcium | | Vitamin D | |
|---|---|---|---|---|
| | Recommended Dietary Allowance (mg/day) | Upper Level Intake (mg/day) | Recommended Dietary Allowance (IU/day) | Upper Level Intake (IU/day) |
| 9–13 years old | 1,300 | 3,000 | 600 | 4,000 |
| 14–18 years old | 1,300 | 3,000 | 600 | 4,000 |
| 19–30 years old | 1,000 | 2,500 | 600 | 4,000 |
| 31–50 years old | 1,000 | 2,500 | 600 | 4,000 |
| 51–70-year-old males | 1,000 | 2,000 | 600 | 4,000 |
| 51–70-year-old females | 1,200 | 2,000 | 600 | 4,000 |
| >70 years old | 1,200 | 2,000 | 800 | 4,000 |

Data from: Institute of Medicine (2010). Dietary reference intakes for calcium and vitamin D. National Academy of Sciences; November 2010, Report Brief. https://www.nationalacademies.org/hmd/~/media/Files/Report%20Files/2010/Dietary-Reference-Intakes-for-Calcium-and-Vitamin-D/Vitamin%20D%20and%20Calcium%202010%20Report%20Brief.pdf. Accessed August 1, 2016.

again, when needed, the use of supplements. Table 10-3 breaks down calcium and vitamin D intake levels based on the Institute of Medicine's recommendations (23).

## Train Smarter

Once runners become fitter, there is a tendency to increase mileage and intensity too quickly during training, which can lead to a breakdown in running form, excessive loading of the bones, and an unwanted bone stress injury. As a general rule, runners should aim to increase mileage or intensity by approximately 10 percent each week; however, depending on the experience of the runner he or she may be able to tolerate more or less (24). Runners should also avoid any drastic or abrupt changes in running terrain, such as transitioning from hard (concrete, sidewalk) to medium (asphalt, road, track, treadmill), or soft (grass, gravel, trail) surfaces.

## Know Your Shoes

A full discussion on how to choose the right shoe for your foot type, gait pattern, terrain, and distance is beyond the scope of this chapter. However, there is research which states selecting a shoe using an athlete's own "comfort filter" may be a natural way to prevent running injuries, with the rationale being athletes preferentially avoid selecting footwear that is uncomfortable and potentially harmful (25). In addition, radical shoe changes should be avoided, and a new shoe should be trialed in a gradual manner. Many shoe stores will allow the runner to test out the shoe on a treadmill or around the store to ensure a proper fit.

Shoes should also be monitored for excessive and abnormal wear pattern on the treads of the soles which could indicate excessive loading at particular area of the foot, making those bones more vulnerable to injury. If possible, runners should cycle through two or three pairs of shoes at a time to allow the shoe to fully recover its cushion before the next run.

## Run Stronger

Many runners have a tendency of under-appreciating the role of strength training as a regular part of their running routine and strengthening exercises are recommended both during the training season and in the off-season. Focus should be placed on muscle control, endurance, and strength from the core to the intrinsic foot muscles (2).

Although the impact of running helps load the bone to some extent, other activities which generate higher impact and multidirectional impact-loading have been shown to have an even greater influence on bone geometry and bone density. These activities include ball sports, such as basketball, soccer, gymnastics, and jump aerobic classes (26). Although the greatest benefits are seen during childhood and adolescence when the skeleton is still rapidly growing and building bone, adults can still benefit from complementing their running with some form of higher impact activity. In addition to the aforementioned sports, routine plyometrics or box jumps are both relatively easy methods to load the bone and help preserve bone health. Conversely, cessation of sports activities, such as running, during adulthood may result in bone loss, which emphasizes the importance of consistent impact-loading activities to maintain the benefits on bone health (27, 28, 29). It is worth noting that the addition of impact-loading activities on an already high mileage training plan is not recommended, and should ideally be trialed during the off-season.

## Consider a Gait Assessment

For runners who struggle with chronic injuries either of the bone or other soft tissue (inflammation of the muscles or tendon, hip, knee, or ankle joints), a gait analysis may be helpful in identifying faulty biomechanics that may predispose the runner to injury. Gait assessments usually involve an experienced professional evaluating running form through video analysis. Gait retraining may be recommended to make subtle adjustments to stride rate (cadence) and stride length (30). Changing foot strike pattern is another consideration, transitioning from rearfoot strike to forefoot strike (31). However, to avoid excessive stress and loading of the foot bones, the transition should be done slowly and involve strengthening of the calf and foot muscles (32). In addition, barefoot running (on a soft surface) encourages a forefoot strike pattern and can also naturally encourage shorter stride length and higher stride rate compared to rearfoot strike (33).

## Respect the Recovery

Including days of rest or active recovery with cross-training (swimming, biking, yoga class) allows time for bones to repair and remodel before your next run. Runners should also keep the "easy" training days "easy" and avoid the mistake of making "easy" days harder, even if they're feeling great and want to run fast. This will allow for less stress on the body and ensure a full recovery for the next big workout or long run.

## Conclusion

Bone stress injuries are common in high level runners, but an educated runner can take steps to prevent this unwanted diagnosis. A strategy that includes adequate nutrition, hormonal balance, strength training, and sound biomechanics will help set a runner up for many fulfilling years on the road and trails.

# SECTION 3
# Common Medical Illnesses

## CHAPTER 11

# Exercise-Associated Hyponatremia

## BY TAMARA HEW-BUTLER

## Key Points

1. Hyponatremia is sometimes called "water intoxication" because in most cases too much fluid is ingested and retained by the body, diluting blood sodium levels.

2. Low blood sodium levels cause water to flow down an osmotic gradient (from low solute concentration to high solute concentration) which causes all the cells in the body to swell. Runners who die from hyponatremia, die from complications associated with brain swelling.

3. Hyponatremia is difficult to diagnose from signs and symptoms alone, because lightheadedness, nausea, vomiting, and confusion can be seen with many different medical conditions. A blood test is needed to rule out low sodium levels in a runner with a history of: drinking large quantities of fluids above thirst, body weight gain, puffiness, nausea, vomiting, and confusion.

4. The most appropriate treatment for a runner diagnosed with hyponatremia is administration of a small amount (100 mL) of a highly concentrated salt solution (hypertonic saline, or saline above the concentration normally found in blood). Reversing brain swelling with a small amount of hypertonic saline can be life-saving.

5. Hyponatremia can be prevented by drinking only when thirsty, a beverage that is most appealing at the time. Despite the somewhat misleading definition (low blood sodium), hyponatremia is more about the water and less about the salt.

## Introduction

Exercise-associated hyponatremia (or, EAH, as it is commonly referred) is a life-threatening electrolyte imbalance. Although severe symptomatic (life-threatening) EAH is rare (occurs in less than 1 percent of all runners completing marathons), asymptomatic hyponatremia (low blood sodium concentration without symptoms) can be quite common (30 to 50 percent of finishers), especially after long races held in hot climates. As such, a lot of research has been performed on this topic—specifically in long distance runners—with respect to understanding the causes, signs and symptoms, treatment options, and prevention of EAH. This chapter will highlight what we currently know about EAH, from the perspective of this research.

What is hyponatremia? Hyponatremia is defined as any blood sodium concentration ([Na+]) that is below the normal range for the laboratory instrument analyzing the blood sample. Quite literally, "hypo" refers to "low" while "natremia" means "sodium in the blood." For most laboratories, the threshold blood sodium concentration which defines hyponatremia is 135 mmol/L (sodium content in millimoles in relationship to a liter of plasma water). Hyponatremia that occurs during exercise is called "exercise-associated hyponatremia" or "EAH" for short (1). Therefore, any runner with a blood sodium concentration below 135 mmol/L is, by definition, hyponatremic.

Why is hyponatremia bad? The dire consequence of a low blood sodium concentration is cellular swelling. In simplistic terms, the body strives to maintain "tonicity balance" which means that water is in equilibrium with the solute particles that are both inside and outside of the cells. This is important because water will freely (passively) flow in and out of cells across an osmotic gradient. Sodium (Na+) ions (as a solute) are primarily found outside of the cells (i.e., in the extracellular fluid, or ECF, space) while potassium (K+) ions (as a solute) are primarily found inside of the cells (i.e., in the intracellular fluid, or ICF, space). Since neither sodium nor potassium ions can passively cross the cell membrane barrier, each functions as an effective "osmole" attracting water molecules across cell membranes. So, in the case of hyponatremia, water molecules will flow from areas of low solute concentration (outside the cell) to areas of high solute concentration (inside the cell) through the process of osmosis (water flowing down an osmotic gradient). Thus, when a runner becomes hyponatremic, the low sodium concentration will cause all of the cells in the body to rapidly swell. If the brain swells (encephalopathy) more than roughly 8 percent of its original size, than it will run out of space within the confines of the skull. The pressure of the swollen brain can force the brainstem out of the base of the skull (brainstem herniation through the foramen magnum), which is how runners die from hyponatremia (2). Cell swelling from hyponatremia can also lead to whole body edema (puffy hands and fingers), pulmonary edema (water inside the lungs), and rhabdomyolysis (increased muscle damage due to fragility of swollen muscle cells). Figure 11-1 represents changes in cell size with changes in sodium concentration (natremia). Thus, severe hyponatremia is a life-threatening medical emergency and an increasingly common cause of death during exercise.

How widespread is hyponatremia? From a historical perspective, the first case of hyponatremia was reported in 1935 and involved a fifty-year-old woman administered approximately nine liters of tap water via proctoclysis (water enema) following gallbladder surgery (3). This patient subsequently died from what was called "water intoxication" (3). In modern times, the incidence of hyponatremia ranges between 30 and 40 percent in critical care (4) and post-operative patients (5) and is the most common electrolyte imbalance seen in hospitalized patients. Outside of the hospital, life-threatening hyponatremia (with brain swelling) has been seen in otherwise healthy individuals who ingest exuberant amounts of fluid that far exceed excretion rates. Such "non-compensated" fluid intake characteristically occurs when any hypotonic fluid (i.e., less sodium than that is found in blood or below a concentration of 140 mmol/L) is ingested well beyond the physiological dictates of thirst. This means that almost all beverages, such as tea, diet cola, sports drinks, and beer, can cause hyponatremia if ingested beyond excretion rates (1, 6, 7, 8). Typical scenarios in which hyponatremia develops from drinking too much fluid include: when competing homeostatic mechanisms supersede the suppression of thirst (hungry infants fed water instead of formula), individuals believe that excess water is good for heath (athletes fearful of dehydration), cognitive abilities are impaired (schizophrenics), or when superfluous fluid intake is not recognized as potentially toxic (college hazing).

In 1985, the first cases of exercise-associated hyponatremia (EAH) were described in detail in four 90K Comrades Marathon runners (9). By 2000, EAH

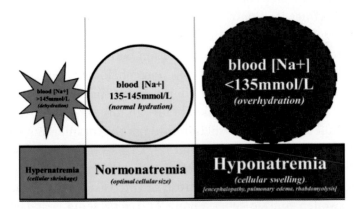

**Figure 11-1** Change in cell size with changes in sodium concentration (natremia).

was reported in clusters of marathon runners, with five deaths confirmed in marathon runners from EAH-associated brain swelling. Severe symptomatic cases of EAH have now been reported in athletes following half marathons, cycling, trekking, canoeing, swimming, yoga, weightlifting, and American football practice sessions. Additionally, multiple blood samples taken from ultramarathon runners, rugby players, and elite junior rowers reveal that over half of athletes tested were hyponatremic at one point during training. The medical relevance of these transient low sodium values during training and racing without apparent symptomatology is unknown. Thus, reports of EAH continue to increase with low sodium levels being detected with increasing frequency across a wider variety of sports.

How is hyponatremia diagnosed and classified? Hyponatremia that is detected through routine blood testing (e.g., for research purposes), and without any apparent symptoms (aside from long distance running), is called "asymptomatic" hyponatremia. Conversely, we refer to "symptomatic" hyponatremia as any blood sodium concentration below 135 mmol/L plus significant clinical signs and symptoms which would prompt runners to seek medical attention. Symptomatic EAH can be further classified into categories along a continuum of mild through severe, depending on the presence or absence of neurological signs and symptoms.

Mild symptomatic EAH is characterized by somewhat vague signs and symptoms, which include dizziness, lightheadedness, bloating, and nausea. Unfortunately, these non-descript symptoms overlap with many other causes of exercise-associated collapse (e.g., hypoglycemia, hypernatremia, heat illness, postural hypotension), which makes the diagnosis of EAH especially difficult without a blood test. There is little evidence for neurological involvement with "mild" symptomatic EAH. However, clinicians argue that the neurological impairment associated with asymptomatic or mild hyponatremia is often very subtle, manifesting as an unsteady gait or balance disturbance (10). When hypothetically translated to running, even a minor impairment in gait or balance could have disastrous musculoskeletal consequences in longer races over rough terrain. Thus, even asymptomatic or mild hyponatremia may have deleterious effects on a runner's health and performance.

Severe symptomatic EAH is diagnosed when neurological signs and symptoms associated with acute brain swelling become apparent. The signs and symptoms of cerebral edema (encephalopathy) include vomiting, confusion, altered mental status, combativeness, seizures, and coma. Unfortunately, these signs and symptoms often overlap with the other common causes of exercise-associated collapse which cause encephalopathy (e.g., hypoglycemia, hypernatremia, heat stroke). Severe EAH may also induce respiratory symptoms (non-cardiogenic pulmonary edema) such as wheezing and pink frothy sputum. Hyponatremic encephalopathy is an urgent, life-threatening emergency requiring immediate treatment. Thus, if any of the above-mentioned symptoms are present in a runner, especially when associated with body weight gain and a history of high fluid intake, a blood sodium test is highly recommended to rule out hyponatremia.

What causes hyponatremia? The primary cause of both symptomatic and asymptomatic EAH is excess fluid consumption during or immediately following long distance running combined with an inability to pee out, or excrete, the excess fluid. In a gross simplification of what is clearly a complex overlapping process, hyponatremia occurs when: 1) too much water is forced into the body (over-hydration/hypervolemia) which dilutes sodium levels; or 2) water is abnormally retained by the body (fluid retention/euvolemia) which dilutes sodium levels; or 3) overt sodium is lost from the body without adequate replacement (volume depletion/hypovolemia). These three main causes (mechanisms) of EAH are briefly summarized in Figure 11-2.

1.  Over-hydration (hypervolemic mechanism): When excess fluid is ingested (or administered intravenously) far beyond excretion rates, fluid overload hyponatremia may develop. This is sometimes called "water intoxication" (3) and occurs when fluids are consumed compulsively and well beyond the sensation of thirst. Prompt urinary excretion of any excess water is the main defense mechanism which usually protects against fluid overload, with maximal kidney excretion rates somewhere between 778 to 1043 mL/hr when the body's main anti-diuretic hormone (ADH), called arginine vasopressin (AVP), is maximally suppressed (11, 12). Maximum sweat rates in elite athletes, working at high exercise intensities for short periods of time, often reach 2 L/hr (13). However, long distance runners must exercise at far

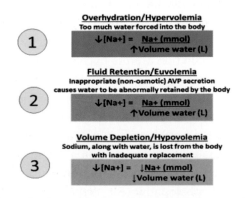

**Figure 11-2** Three main mechanisms of Exercise Associated Hyponatremia.

lower intensities and thereby have much lower sweat rates (<500 mL/hr). Thus, runners moving at slower speeds are able to drink exuberant amounts of water (beyond need) and are at greater risk for developing EAH if they compulsively drink beyond thirst.

2. Fluid retention (euvolemic mechanism): As stated above, the maximum amount of water that the kidneys can pee out ranges between 778 to 1043 mL/hr when AVP is maximally suppressed (i.e., there is no AVP within the circulation) (11, 12). However, exercise above the intensity of a brisk walk is a stimulus to AVP secretion which causes immediate water retention (14). This "exercise-induced AVP secretion" makes evolutionary sense, because moderate to vigorous physical activity induces sweating, which is necessary for evaporative cooling. In order to preserve total body water, the body instinctively "shuts off" urinary water losses to compensate for additional sweat water losses. So, if humans drink too much fluid at rest, the excess water is immediately pee'd out to protect blood sodium levels from becoming overly diluted. If a runner drinks too much during exercise (above sweat water losses), however, urinary water excretion is impaired due to exercise-associated anti-diuretic hormone (AVP) secretion. Additionally, there are many other stimuli to AVP secretion which occur during long distance running, such as nausea with or without vomiting, plasma volume contraction, heat, pain, hypoglycemia, and other hormones stimulated during exercise which will also facilitate water retention (14). Thus, sustained fluid intake above sweat water losses, combined with the inability to pee out any fluid excess during exercise, is the main cause of dilutional EAH in runners.

3. Volume depletion (hypovolemic mechanism): It is impossible to completely deplete total body sodium stores. However, significant sodium losses can occur from vomiting or diarrhea as well as from sweating during prolonged (greater than eigtheen hours) running in the heat, especially when under-acclimatized (15) or when a genetic defect is present that increases sweat sodium output (i.e., cystic fibrosis) (16). Sustained, under-replaced, sweat and/or gastrointestinal sodium losses may cause the circulating plasma volume to shrink (i.e., less sodium in the vascular space will attract less water into the circulation), which will activate AVP as well as the renin angiotensin-aldosterone (RAAS) system (17, 18). The hormone, angiotensin, will directly stimulate thirst within the brain while AVP serves to retain all fluids ingested during running. This combination of water retention plus volume-driven (baroreceptor-mediated) thirst may facilitate the development of the "volume-depletion" (not "sodium depletion") form of hyponatremia, which is far less common than the dilutional mechanisms mentioned above. The hypovolemic variant

of hyponatremia is often associated with body weight loss from relative over-drinking with respect to sustained, under-replaced sweat sodium and water losses. The typical sodium content of diarrhea (30 to 90 mmol/L) (19) and sweat (10 to 70 mmol/L) (20) is significantly less than that of blood (normal range of 135 to 145 mmol/L). So in the absence of fluid intake with gastro-intestinal losses and/or prolonged sweating, more water is actually lost than sodium which would actually trigger hypernatremia (the opposite of hypona-tremia). Thus, runners participating in long (greater than eighteen hours) races in the heat—while not fully heat-acclimatized and/or with vomiting and/or diarrhea—are at increased risk for developing the hypovolemic form of hyponatremia if they do not replace both sodium and water.

How is hyponatremia treated? Once EAH is confirmed with a blood test (sodium concentration reading below 135 mmol/L or below the normal reference range for the laboratory running the test), then treatment is guided by the runner's signs and symptoms. Although it would seem intuitive that the lower the numerical value for blood [Na+], the more dire the signs and symptoms, this is not always the case for EAH. The rate (i.e., how fast blood [Na+] falls over time) of sodium decline is just as important as the actual numerical value for sodium because EAH is (in most cases) an "acute" hyponatremia (1). Any hyponatremia which develops "acutely" (less than forty-eight hours) can be more damaging to the brain, as brain cells do not have enough time to counteract osmotic swelling (like in chronic hyponatremia, whereas brain cells can adapt and limit cellular swell-ing). For example, a marathon runner who starts a race with a blood [Na+] at 144 mmol/L and then finishes the race with a blood [Na+] of 130 mmol/L may have more severe signs and symptoms compared with a runner starting the race at 136 mmol/L (and then drops to 130 mmol/L during the same time frame) because the "drop" in sodium over time was greater in the first runner. Therefore, the treat-ment of EAH is always tailored toward reversing the symptoms first—especially those symptoms associated with severe EAH with encephalopathy—and not nec-essarily completely reversing the actual blood sodium value (i.e., greater than 135 mmol/L). The return to normal blood sodium levels will occur once the runner starts urinating again (with AVP suppression).

When asymptomatic EAH is encountered, fluid should be restricted until the runner starts to urinate freely. Alternatively, highly concentrated salt solutions can be given, making sure that the sodium concentration of these broths is well above blood sodium concentrations (greater than 140 mmol/L; a "hypertonic" saline solution). One study showed that four bouillon cubes dissolved in four ounces (half a cup) of water improved blood sodium levels within thirty minutes of ingestion

(21). Another showed an increase in blood [Na+] regardless of whether or not the salty solution (approximately three ounces of 3 percent saline, or the salinity of seawater) was given by mouth or through an arm vein (intravenously) (15).

When mild EAH is diagnosed, fluids should be restricted until the onset of urination occurs or, more practically, runners may be given small amounts of salty solution (see above) until the symptoms resolve. If runners with mild EAH cannot tolerate oral fluids, than a small amount (100 mL or approximately three ounces) of hypertonic saline should be administered intravenously by a trained professional until he or she feels better and/or starts to urinate freely. Since the condition of athletes diagnosed with asymptomatic or mild EAH has been shown to deteriorate within a few hours of race finish (as fluids are absorbed into the blood from the gut with the cessation of exercise), hypertonic salty broths and close monitoring of signs and symptoms are encouraged over the next twenty-four hours.

Last but not least, severe EAH is a life-threatening medical emergency. Runners with signs and symptoms of severe EAH should be promptly treated with intravenous hypertonic saline until his or her condition improves (or at least stabilizes) before immediate transport to the nearest hospital. Oral hypertonic saline broth (i.e., four bouillon cubes dissolved in four ounces of water) has also been shown to reverse severe EAH in marathon runners able to ingest fluids by mouth (21). The aim of this life-saving hypertonic saline treatment is to reduce fatal brain swelling (the sodium will attract water out of the brain cells and into the vascular space) rather than restore blood sodium levels back into the normal range. Thus, brain swelling from water intoxication can be quickly reversed with prompt administration of hypertonic saline. If EAH-associated brain swelling exceeds 5 to 8 percent, then a runner will likely die from brainstem herniation.

As detailed above, hypertonic saline is the most appropriate treatment choice for all three mechanisms of hyponatremia. Isotonic, or normal (0.9 percent), saline should only be administered intravenously when there are clear signs of hypovolemia (hypovolemic hyponatremia) such as low or unstable blood pressure, orthostatic hypotension (fainting when standing), thirst, decreased body weight, and/or elevated blood urea nitrogen. If the runner's condition begins to deteriorate with isotonic saline treatment, then blood [Na+] measurement should be repeated (if possible) and normal saline replaced with hypertonic saline. In extremely rare occasions, hyponatremia may be seen in combination with significant and symptomatic rhabdomyolysis (muscle breakdown—detected by a marker called creatine kinase of "CK" for short). This scenario may occur in longer races over difficult terrain. Our treatment of choice is to administer a small amount (100 mL) of hypertonic saline first (to remove the plasma volume stimulus to AVP and limit brain swelling) and then follow up with isotonic saline (to help "flush" the kidneys) (22). This rare combination of medical maladies should be monitored closely by medical personnel, with both electrolyte status and kidney function re-assessed at regular intervals to guide subsequent treatment.

How can hyponatremia be prevented? Individualized hydration guidelines (drinking to thirst or using body weight and urine specific gravity as a rough estimation) in order to prevent the extremes of both dehydration and over-hydration, will be covered in greater detail in a separate chapter. Broadly speaking, drinking according to the dictates of thirst will prevent most (if not all) cases of EAH in runners across a variety of distances. Thirst is an evolutionary protective mechanism against the development of dehydration in all mammals, including humans (23, 24). Drinking above the physiological dictates of thirst has been associated with most severe cases of EAH documented in the literature (1). Overzealous fluid consumption before, during, or immediately following running will not prevent heat stroke, muscle cramps, nor enhance performance. Drinking to thirst will satisfy the body's water requirements to maintain both osmolality (cellular size) and circulating plasma volume.

Additionally, thirst (and AVP secretion) respond to perturbations in fluid homeostasis in real-time (seconds to minutes) by the activation and suppression of nerve impulses, hormones, and aquaporin water channels. There are sensors located in the brain, called osmosensors, that continuously monitor blood osmolality (for which blood [Na+] is the biggest contributor). There are also sensors located in the great vessels in the heart that continuously monitor circulating plasma volume, called baroreceptors, which send nerve signals to the brain when plasma volume decreases beyond 8 to 10 percent. Thus, because long distance running is a dynamic activity in an ever-changing environment, listening to the body's internal signals is a far better approach than strict adherence to a hypothetical hydration plan. A fluid intake plan that may have worked well in the past may cause hyponatremia when both environmental temperature and AVP secretion are abnormally high.

When fluids are replaced to maintain body weight, during exercise, sodium replacement in the form of sports drinks may keep blood [Na+] higher when compared with the ingestion of plain water (25, 26). However, because sports drinks contain such a small amount of sodium (10 to 50 mmol/L) when compared with the concentration of sodium in the blood (approximately 140 mmol/L), a sports drink will not prevent the development of hyponatremia if consumed in excess. If fluids are ingested in response to thirst during competitions, then extra sodium ingestion does not appear to influence post-race blood sodium concentrations in temperate climates (27, 28). However, sodium supplementation may be necessary to maintain plasma volume during prolonged (greater than eighteen hours) exercise, performed in the heat, when not properly heat-acclimatized. In these extreme environmental conditions (or when sweat sodium is particularly high), ingestion of 40 to 50 mmol (460 to 920 mg) of sodium per liter of water may prevent the development of hypovolemic hyponatremia (20).

In general, a wide variety of fluids should be available during races, at refueling stations spaced 5 km apart, with instructions to drink whatever beverage is most appealing and only when thirsty. For athletes who desire a (very) rough estimate of fluid replacement needs (to match losses), weighing before and after sixty minutes of running—at expected race pace and ambient temperature—is a good starting guide. However, the best hydration, fueling and racing strategy is to start with a plan and then adjust according to thirst and sodium palatability.

## Conclusion

Exercise-associated hyponatremia is an electrolyte imbalance in which there is too much water in relationship to sodium ions circulating within the blood. Hyponatremia causes all of the cells within the body to swell, which can be fatal if brain swelling exceeds the confines of the skull. Although death is rare, 30 to 50 percent of race finishers in long, hot races may have hyponatremia without knowing it. Drinking only when thirsty will prevent most cases of EAH in runners. Runners participating in long (greater than eighteen hours), hot races while unacclimitized to the heat will need to replace sodium (according to palatability) to maintain circulating plasma volume and prevent the (less common) volume depletion form of EAH.

## CHAPTER 12

# Running in the Heat

## BY WILLIAM M. ADAMS, YURI HOSOKAWA, AND REBECCA L. STEARNS

## Key Points

1.  Exercise in the heat places added stress from a cardiovascular and thermoregulatory perspective on the exercising individual. This has been shown to have adverse effects on exercise performance and increases the risk of exertional heat illness.
2.  Implementing strategies such as individualized hydration plans, heat acclimatization, and optimizing recovery from daily stress via sleep during endurance training can enhance training and performance.
3.  Exertional heat illness is a broad term describing the medical conditions that can arise during exercise in the heat; heat syncope, exercise-associated muscle cramps, and heat exhaustion are conditions that may impede exercise performance.
4.  Exertional heat stroke is a medical emergency that may lead to death or long term illness if not treated appropriately.
5.  Exertional heat stroke is caused by a failure of the body's thermoregulatory system to balance heat loss and heat gain.
6.  Recognition of exertional heat stroke signs and symptoms and appropriate treatment using cold water immersion within thirty minutes of collapse maximizes the chance of survival with no long term complications.
7.  Returning to activity following exertional heat stroke requires coordinated efforts with one's primary care physician or other medical personnel to closely monitor the athlete from immediately post-incident to full return to activity.

## Introduction

During exercise, particularly in the heat, the body is subjected to various stressors that can increase the risk of suffering from exertional heat illness (EHI) and have adverse effects on performance. While the incidence of EHI is not 100 percent preventable, steps can be made during training and competition to mitigate the risk. In the event of EHI during endurance running events, appropriate steps in the recognition and the treatment is vital in optimizing the outcome. The purpose of this chapter is to address the topic of heat-related illness in the context of long distance running; a particular focus will be centered on strategies to maximize performance and optimize safety during exercise in the heat and provide the readers with an in-depth background on the prevention, recognition, treatment, and return to activity following EHI.

## Temperature Regulation

During exercise in the heat, the body undergoes a series of normal physiological responses in an attempt to maintain exercise performance. These whole body responses result from the increased level of stress placed on the body by the coupling of exercise and increased environmental temperatures. Without these responses during exercise, body temperature would continuously rise to levels that would adversely affect performance or put an individual at a high risk for potential life-threatening medical conditions like exertional heat stroke.

During rest, body temperature is tightly controlled and regulated by the hypothalamus in the brain to maintain a temperature of 37 degrees C (98.6 degrees F) (1, 2, 3). During exercise, metabolic rates increases by a factor of fifteen to twenty times that of resting values, where 80 percent of the energy produced is given off in the form of heat (4, 5). The increase in body temperature attempts to dissipate the metabolically produced heat via mechanisms of conduction, convection, radiation, and evaporation (Table 12-1) (6, 7). Table 12-2 defines each of these mechanisms to provide an understanding of how heat can be lost or gained

**Table 12-1** Physiological responses for dissipating metabolically produced heat during exercise in the heat.

| Physiological responses | Method of heat dissipation |
| --- | --- |
| Evaporation of sweat from the skin<br>Cardiovascular responses | •Evaporative heat loss<br>•Dry heat losses: Conduction, Convection, and Radiation |
|   - Increased cardiac output (↑Heart Rate, Stroke Volume) | |
|   - Peripheral vasodilation and visceral vasoconstriction | |

**Table 12-2**   Mechanisms of heat gain or loss.

| Mechanism | Definition | Factors Impeding Heat Dissipation during Exercise in the Heat |
|---|---|---|
| Radiation | Transfer of heat via electromagnetic waves | When environmental temperatures are greater than skin temperature heat is gained within the body |
| Conduction | Movement of heat between two objects in direct contact | During exercise, this process involves contact of feet with the ground. Heat transfer is negligible (~1 percent) |
| Convection | Movement of heat down its thermal gradient via circulating air/water | When environmental temperatures are greater than skin temperature heat is gained within the body |
| Evaporation | Loss of heat through the latent vaporization of water (process of sweat going from liquid to gas) | When relative humidity increases (increased water vapor in the air), evaporative capacity is reduced |

within the body and the limitations of these mechanisms of heat dissipation (4, 6). Evaporation of sweat becomes the primary means of heat dissipation during exercise, especially when ambient temperatures exceed skin temperature. When environmental conditions are hot and humid the ability of the body to effectively dissipate stored body heat is markedly reduced due to the decreased water vapor gradient, which elevates the risk of exertional heat illness as well as degradation of exercise performance.

## Strategies to Maximize Performance and Safety

While performance and safety can be compromised during exercise in the heat, there are multiple strategies that can be utilized to mitigate these risks. Hydration, heat acclimatization, and sleep can be strategically implemented into daily training regimen to optimize long distance running performance.

## Hydration

Hydration plays a vital role in optimizing performance and safety during exercise in the heat. Research has shown that dehydration as small as 2 percent loss of body mass, can degrade endurance performance by as much as 7 to 29 percent (8, 9, 10) and exacerbate physiologic strain from both a cardiovascular (11, 12, 13) and thermoregulatory (14, 15, 16) perspective. Additionally, for every 1 percent dehydration while exercising heart rate increases by a magnitude of three beats/

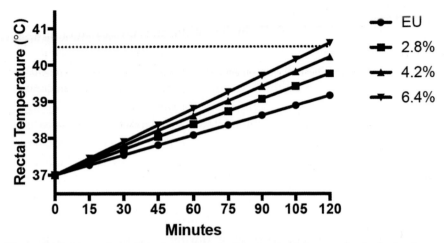

Theoretical change in body temperature during steady state exercise in the heat with progressive dehydration compared to a euhydrated state. It is assumed that the individual is a 70kg runner with running at a set intensity with a metabolic increase in body temp of 0.18°C•min$^{-1}$ when euhydrated. Thermoregulatory strain is assumed to be 0.22°C for every 1%BML (Huggins, 2012). EU=minimized fluid losses during exercise; 2.8%=runner with 1.0 L•hr$^{-1}$ sweat rate; 4.2%= runner with 1.5 L•hr$^{-1}$ sweat rate; 6.4= runner with 2.0 L•hr$^{-1}$ sweat rate. Dotted line depicts threshold for EHS.

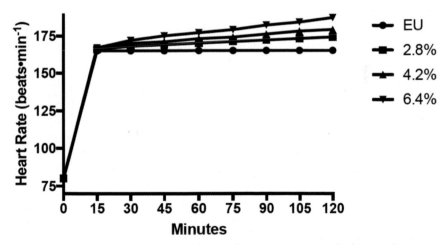

Theoretical change in heart rate during steady state exercise in the heat with progressive dehydration compared to a euhydrated state. It is assumed that the individual is a 70kg runner with running at a set intensity with a metabolic increase in body temp of 0.18°C•min$^{-1}$ when euhydrated. Cardiovascular strain is assumed to be 3 beats•min$^{-1}$ for every 1%BML (Adams, 2014). EU=minimized fluid losses during exercise; 2.8%=runner with 1.0 L•hr$^{-1}$ sweat rate; 4.2%= runner with 1.5 L•hr$^{-1}$ sweat rate; 6.4= runner with 2.0 L•hr$^{-1}$ sweat rate.

**Figures 12-1 and 12-2**

min (17) and body temperature increases 0.22 degrees C (0.5 degrees F). Figures 12-1 and 12-2 depict a theoretical model of the thermoregulatory and cardio-vascular strain that may occur with progressive dehydration during prolonged exercise. While the model assumes steady state exercise, as the magnitude of dehydration increases throughout exercise, exercise intensity will decrease with self-adjustment of the pace to accommodate for the increased stress on the body.

During exercise in the heat, the blood flow needed to provide oxygen and nutrients to the working muscles competes with the need for blood flow to reach the skin and extremities to aid in heat dissipation. Dehydration causes a reduction in plasma volume, which further increases the competition for blood flow in the body leading to an impairment of performance by means of a reduced central venous pressure and cardiac output regardless of acclimatization status (Table 12-3) (19, 20).

Minimizing the extent of dehydration during endurance running in the heat will minimize physiologic strain and assist in optimizing performance and safety. Fluid needs are highly variable and are dependent upon a multitude of factors such as individual sweat rate, fitness and acclimatization status, exercise intensity, and environmental conditions (21). Developing an individualized hydration strategy based on one's sweat rate is essential for minimizing fluid losses during exercise (Table 12-4).

It may not be possible to fully replace fluids according to the sweat rate during exercise. Those with high sweat rates may not be able to tolerate large amounts of fluids during exercise, as the stomach is only able to absorb roughly 1 liter of fluid per hour. Additionally, water availability may be limited increasing the risk of dehydration. To optimize hydration needs during exercise, prevent performance deficits, and mitigate safety risks runners should begin exercise euhydrated (in a normal state of hydration). This is typically well regulated by the brain via a sensation of thirst. Then, minimize fluid losses during exercise based on one's individual sweat rate and replace remaining fluid deficits following exercise.

**Table 12-3** Effects of hydration on exercise in the heat.

| | Exercise in the Heat | Exercise in the Heat (Heat Acclimatized) | Exercise in the Heat (Hypohydrated) |
|---|---|---|---|
| Exercising Heart Rate | ↑ | ↓ | ↑↑ |
| Sweat Rate | ↑ | ↑↑ | ↓ |
| Rise of Core Temperature | ↑ | ↓ | ↑↑ |
| Skin Blood Flow | ↑ | ↑ | ↓ |
| Plasma Volume | ↓ | ↑ | ↓↓ |
| Cardiac Output | ↓ | ↑ | ↓↓ |
| Overall Exercise Performance | ↓ | ↑ | ↓↓ |

←→: Negligible Change,   ↑: Small Change   ↑↑: Moderate Change,   ↑↑↑: Large Change

**Table 12-4** Steps to determine fluid needs (measuring sweat rate) during exercise.

| | |
|---|---|
| 1 | Prior to the start of exercise, empty your bladder and obtain a nude body mass. *Example: A runner takes a nude body mass before exercise and weighs 70kg (154lbs).* |
| 2 | Go outside and exercise for 60 minutes at an intensity that is normal for your training. Note: During this time do not consume any fluids or use the bathroom to minimize the variables in the following calculation. |
| 3 | Following exercise, dry yourself off with a towel and re-weigh yourself in the nude. *Example: Runner completes exercise and weighs in at 68.5kg (151lbs).* |
| 4 | Calculate your sweat rate using the equation: Sweat rate=(Pre body mass-Post body mass) + (volume of fluid consumed and/or urine if applicable)*(Time[min]/60). Assume that 1kg=1L. *Example: 70kg-68.5kg=1.5kg•hr$^{-1}$=1.5L•h$^{-}$1.* |
| 5 | Once your sweat rate is measured, you will know how much fluid you are losing per hour and you can plan your hydration strategy based on this. Note: The stomach may only be able to handle 1–1.2L of fluid per hour so those with a higher sweat rate should aim to minimize fluid losses during exercise. |
| 6 | It is advantageous to measure your sweat rate numerous times throughout training as this will change depending on fitness status, acclimatization status, environmental conditions, and exercise intensity. Measuring sweat rate numerous times will refine your individual sweat rate over time and allow you to optimize your fluid replacement strategy. |

## Heat Acclimatization

Heat acclimatization is a term used to describe the physiological adaptations that occur during exercise in the heat that reduces cardiovascular and thermoregulatory strain and improves heat tolerance (22). This process takes approximately ten to fourteen days and requires repeated bouts of heat exposure (exercise in hot conditions) at an intensity sufficient enough to elicit the elevation of skin and body temperature and a sweating response (23). These adaptations include a reduction in exercising heart rate, expansion of plasma volume, reduction in exercising body temperature, increased sweat rate with an earlier onset of sweating, and an increased retention of sodium within the body (Figure 12-3) (22, 23).

A shortened period of heat acclimatization (four to seven days) can be achieved as 75 to 80 percent of the adaptations occur during this time period (24, 25). Particularly, highly trained athletes or sports teams that are traveling to warm environments for competition may benefit from short term heat acclimatization, as cardiovascular adaptations occur during this time frame (26, 27, 28).

In order to obtain the full benefits of heat acclimatization, a sufficient number of days exposed to heat stress while exercising is necessary. Furthermore, heat acclimatization is dependent upon exercise intensity and exercise duration. The goal of exercising heat stress should focus on a progressive overload model,

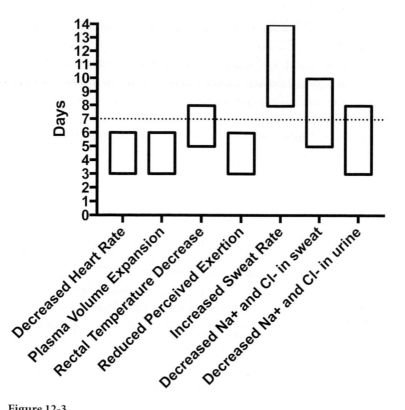

**Figure 12-3**

where overall workload is increased throughout the duration of the acclimatization period while achieving controlled hyperthermia (exercising body temperature should be at or above 38.5 degrees C) (29).

For the long distance runner training for a competition in warm environmental conditions, it is advantageous to undergo a period of heat acclimatization prior to the competition. This can be done in a natural environment (if living in a warm-weather location) or artificially, which can be done in a climate-controlled facility. If it is not feasible to undergo a period of heat acclimatization prior to competition, arrival to the location a few days prior to the event allows an individual the opportunity to train in those conditions to acquire some of the benefits of heat acclimatization in an effort to improve performance.

## Sleep

Sleep is an essential component of life, and during times of bodily stress, such as exercise, it is said to be the "gold standard" for whole body recovery and restoration (30, 31, 32). Maintenance of energy metabolism (33), neural plastic-ity, hormonal responses (34), and immune function (35) requires that individuals achieve an adequate amount of sleep on a nightly basis. Also, the amount of time spent in slow-wave (deep) sleep is directly proportional to improved sleep quality and whole body recovery (32). For example, in a cohort of elite swimmers, the amount of time spent in deep sleep was directly related to their training volume; the higher peaks in training volume showed that the percentage of time spent in deep sleep the following night was increased (36).

Sleep and exercise have been shown to work in synergy with each other; evi-dence shows that sleep optimizes and enhances exercise performance (37, 38, 39), and exercise has been shown to enhance the duration and quality of sleep (37, 40, 41). Overall sleep quality has been shown to improve when regular, moder-ate intensity exercise is performed, especially when done later in the day such as during evening hours (41, 42, 43, 44). Conversely, as sleep and exercise can be complementary to one another, changes in one can adversely affect one another. Loss of sleep has been shown to have adverse effects on both exercise perfor-mance and overall health (45, 46, 47). Specifically, sleep loss has been shown to impair cognitive function (48, 49, 50), exacerbate thermoregulatory strain (51, 52, 53), and impair exercise performance (38, 47, 54). Similarly, high-intensity or exhaustive exercise may disrupt overall sleep quality (55, 56). Establishing a regular sleep regimen of adequate length (six to eight hours) optimizes the body's ability to recover from daily stressors such as exercise and prime the body for the next day's training regimen.

Dehydration, lack of heat acclimatization, and sleep deprivation can place an individual at risk for exertional heat illness and can impair exercise perfor-mance. It must also be acknowledged that these factors can have compounding effects on one's ability to perform optimally, especially during hot environmen-tal conditions. For example, while lack on heat acclimatization and dehydration both increase the risk of exertional heat illness and impairs exercise performance independently, exercising in the heat in a state of hypohydration negates any ben-efits associated with heat acclimatization, which may elevate an individual's risk profile (15). While less is known about the interrelationships between sleep and hydration, researchers are beginning to investigate the influence that these fac-tors have on heat stress and risk of EHI (57).

## Exertional Heat Illness

Exertional heat illness is a broad term describing the medical disorders that involve environmental heat. It has been identified as the disorders that have environmental heat as one of its etiological factors (58). During exercise in the heat, the risk of EHI is increased due to the added stress placed on the body from the environment. The exertional heat illnesses that are most commonly seen during exercise in hot conditions include exercise-associated muscle cramps (EAMC), heat syncope, heat exhaustion, and exertional heat stroke. While most of these conditions (heat syncope, EAMC, and heat exhaustion) are not life-threatening and treatment leads to rapid revival, exertional heat stroke is a life-threatening emergency, and without immediate treatment can lead to death or life-long complications.

While the etiology of each of these disorders often involves environmental heat, there are other identifiable causes that are used to differentiate these conditions from one another. Knowledge of effective ways to prevent, recognize, and treat these disorders provide the long distance runner the ability to optimize both safety and performance.

## Exercise-Associated Muscle Cramps

Exercise-associated muscle cramps is a broad term that has recently been differentiated from the traditional classification of heat cramps, as a secondary type of cramping. While both involve painful, involuntary muscle spasms or muscle cramps (usually in the legs but also in other large muscles) during or after fatiguing exercise performed in the heat (59, 60, 61), heat cramps are usually associated with exercise in the heat when athletes have been sweating profusely and may have had large electrolyte loss (59, 60). Exercise-associated muscle cramps (EAMC) has been described as a result of cramping during exercise due to muscular fatigue and possibly overload, which could occur in any environment but is common in the heat (61). The mechanism behind the cramping is ultimately what differentiates these two terms, however they are both common within athletes exercising intensely in the heat.

In the classical view of heat cramps, the cause is usually due to electrolyte loss. Excessive salt loss can be problematic due to its diverse functions throughout the body. Sodium plays a large factor in the regulation of fluids between cells and compartments. Sodium also contributes to retention of fluids in the kidneys (59). Therefore, athletes that are exercising for extended durations in the heat or those that are "salty sweaters" are at particular risk for large salt losses, especially if no attempt is made to replace the salt during exercise (59). Sweat losses may be increased by exercise lasting longer than a few hours, intense exercise, adequate fluid intake (to maintain sweat function), exercise with protective equipment and exercise in hot environments. Additional considerations that could increase an individual's risk include:

- Athletes who are not acclimatized to the heat (and therefore may not retain sweat sodium losses as effectively).
- Athletes that wear additional protective equipment or clothing that can interfere with heat loss.
- Athletes who have multiple practice sessions in a day, consecutive days of strenuous exercise, or both (thus increasing total sweat loss potential).

When cramping can be attributed to EAMC, it suggests that the muscles have become fatigued and the exercise session is greater (either in intensity, duration, or both) than what the muscle could handle, resulting in cramping. This theory was first introduced in 1997 as a result of observations in cramping cases that did not have the classical signs/history consistent with electrolyte losses or because the cramping did not occur in a hot environment (61). It was suggested that local muscle fatigue was responsible for cramping (61). In such cases, cramping would be more localized to the specific fatigued muscle.

Though no clear mechanism has been defined, there is evidence to support both theories (62, 63). In some cases, the consumption of a carbohydrate beverage with sodium allowed athletes to exercise longer before cramping occurred (62), whereas other literature has demonstrated that when athletes completed faster race times they were more likely to cramp, regardless of hydration or electrolyte balance (63). Based on current literature, the best recommendations to prevent muscle cramping for athletes are:

- Train for the anticipated race/competition demands to avoid unique stressors on that day.
- Acclimatize to warm/hot environments (which will assist in retaining sweat sodium losses).
- Educate athletes to replace fluids and electrolytes appropriately. Athletes should minimize body mass losses to 2 percent when exercising intensely in the heat and replace fluids according to their individual fluid needs and sweat rate.
- Athletes who experience recurrent issues with cramping may benefit from a full diet and sweat electrolyte analysis to determine if electrolytes are being appropriately replaced.
- Supplement workouts with electrolyte drinks if you anticipate the session to last more than one hour, multiple bouts of exercise in the same day, athletes have not yet acclimatized to a warm environment, the

athletes have a history of cramping, or know they are considered a "salty sweater."

Cramping from either heat cramps or EAMC is generally self-resolving by resting and gentle stretching, though the cramps can be incredibly painful and result in soreness on subsequent days. The critical step for those who experience or suffer from cramping is to identify the cause and work toward reducing the factors that place them at risk for cramping. Athletes with heat cramps or EAMC may follow the same return to play guidelines as heat syncope (7).

## Heat Syncope

Heat syncope is a fainting episode that spontaneously resolves and occurs when an individual is exposed to environmental conditions, particularly with prolonged standing, a sudden change to an upright posture from sitting, or sudden cessation of exercise (64). This can be commonly seen at the end of a prolonged endurance event where a runner suddenly stops once crossing the finish line. The cause of heat syncope is a combination of dilation of blood vessels in the periphery of the body, with pooling of blood, decreased blood flow return to the heart, and subsequent decreased blood outflow from the heart and resulting decrease in oxygenated blood flow to the brain (cerebral hypoperfusion) (64). With exercise there is a shunting of blood flow from the internal organs to the periphery, where the blood provides the working muscles with nutrients and oxygen to perform work. With a sudden stop in running, the combination of increased blood flow to the muscles in the legs with a diminished venous return leads to pooling of blood in the lower extremities and diminished oxygen to the brain, resulting in the fainting episode. Exercise in the heat exacerbates the risk of heat syncope due to the added stress on the body requiring blood flow to compete with the working muscles and the skin for heat dissipation.

The prevention of heat syncope can largely be done through a proper heat acclimatization by inducing desirable cardiovascular adaptation to expand the cardiac output capacity (65). Athletes are also encouraged to minimize the amount of dehydration to prevent large reduction in plasma volume, which may also pose athletes at risk for heat syncope (7, 66). Incorporating a proper cool down following activity may also protect the athlete from heat syncope by preventing the cardiovascular system from experiencing the rapid change in blood pressure. During a competition, race organizers can set up the finish line area in ways to promote a constant flow of people to allow constant movement to prevent the pooling of blood in the lower extremities.

Athletes with heat syncope may have an elevated body temperature (hyper-pyrexia) due to the metabolic heat produced from the physical activity, however, it should be within the normal range for exercising individual (usually about 39 degrees C) (66). Athletes may experience weakness, lightheadedness, and dizziness. They may also complain of tunnel vision prior to the collapse. Other common signs include decreased blood pressure, dehydration, profuse sweating, and pale skin. Nonetheless, differential diagnoses with more serious conditions are warranted since many of the signs and symptoms overlap (7, 66).

Heat syncope is typically self-resolving with rest and often rehydration. Athletes with heat syncope should be moved to a cool area and lay supine with their legs elevated above the heart to facilitate the venous return. Return to play following heat syncope should generally be delayed until the following day or at least until the individuals sign's symptoms are no longer present (indicating that the contributing factors have been sufficiently addressed). Generally this can easily be done within a twenty-four-hour period assuming no other conditions or medical issues are present (7).

## Heat Exhaustion

Heat exhaustion is defined by the inability to continue exercise in the heat (67, 68). The cause is primarily attributed to dehydration, large sodium losses, or energy depletion. Literature supports that there are two types of heat exhaustion: water depletion and salt depletion heat exhaustion—both due to the inadequate replacement of water or sodium to sustain exercise (69, 70). Independent of the root cause of heat exhaustion (water or salt depletion), this condition arises due to a reduction in extracellular volume leading to cardiovascular insufficiency, which limits the ability to perform exercise (67).

The prevention of heat exhaustion can be largely done with the implementation of a proper heat acclimatization period during exercise in the heat. Athletes should be cognizant of their physical fitness and exercise capacity, especially during the first few workouts in the heat (66).

Heat exhaustion is a self-limiting condition where the athlete can no longer continue the exercise. Common signs and symptoms include weakness, fainting, lightheadedness, dizziness, heavy sweating, decreased blood pressure, and decreased muscle coordination (7, 66, 71). Individuals with heat exhaustion may have a normal or elevated temperature, but do not have an altered level of consciousness. As temperature measurements may not be available, the absence (or presence) of an altered sensorium can differentiate this condition from exertional heat stroke (72).

Athletes with heat exhaustion should be moved to a cool area and body cooling should be initiated. Excess clothes should be removed to expedite the cooling, and if dizzy the athlete's legs should be elevated to facilitate venous return to reduce the cardiovascular strain (7). When dehydration is suspected, the athlete should be encouraged to rehydrate orally. Intravenous fluid replacement should only be considered when the athlete cannot safely ingest the fluid (7).

For athletes with heat exhaustion, same day return is not recommended (7). The athlete should be provided time to rest followed by gradual reintroduction of exercise in the heat. This can take place over the few days following their heat exhaustion. Lastly, it will allow the athlete to gauge his or her recovery and report any symptoms that could arise with the re-introduction of exercise in the heat.

## Exertional Heat Stroke

Exertional heat stroke is a medical emergency that occurs when the body's thermoregulatory system is unable to balance heat gain with heat loss during physical activity. This may be due to excessive heat gain derived from exercise intensity and/or environmental heat stress or the inhibition of heat dissipation mechanisms (7). The uncontrolled rise in body temperature (uncompensable heat stress) elicits a cascade of physiologic events causing increased gut permeability, the release of toxins into circulation, decreased oxygen to cells, and if left untreated may lead to multi-organ failure, abnormalities in the body's ability to control blood clotting and bleeding, and death (73, 74, 75).

The cause of exertional heat stroke is often multi-factorial and individualized (76). Intrinsic risk factors include items that are internal to one's body such as sleep loss, dehydration, and lack of physical fitness/heat acclimatization, whereas, extrinsic factors include items such as extreme environmental conditions, clothing/protective equipment, and inappropriate work-to-rest ratios. While many risk factors are modifiable if appropriate steps are taken to implement strategies to mitigate risk, other factors may not be modifiable within the context of a particular bout of physical activity in the heat (Table 12-5).

Similar to the prevention of heat syncope and heat exhaustion, proper heat acclimatization will provide a protective advantage in allowing the body to cope with thermal strain while exercising in the heat. Athletes should also modify the activity and attire accordingly to the environmental stress (66). Anyone with history of heat-related illness should consult their primary physician to identify extrinsic and intrinsic factors that may have led to the previous heat-related illness episode.

**Table 12-5** Exertional Heat Stroke Risk Factors

| Modifiable | Non-modifiable |
| --- | --- |
| • Work-to-rest ratio | • Previous history of heat-related illness |
| • Clothing | • Climate |
| • Hydration status | • Recent illness |
| • Heat acclimatization status | • Race distance and technicality |
| • Cardiovascular fitness | |
| • Pacing appropriate to physical fitness | |
| • Sleep | |

Two hallmark signs of exertional heat stroke are: temperature greater than 40 degrees C (104 degrees F) and central nervous system dysfunction (7, 66, 72). Central nervous system dysfunction may present as altered mental status, change in personality, aggression, irritability, hysteria, delirium, or even seizures or unconsciousness. Athletes may also experience weakness, fainting, lightheadedness, dizziness, heavy sweating, lack of sweating, diarrhea, and dehydration.

Exertional heat stroke is a time-critical emergency. The goal of exertional heat stroke treatment is to cool the core temperature below 39 degrees C (102 degrees F) within thirty minutes after collapse (77). The gold standard for cooling is whole-body water immersion using cold water with ice and a cooling tub. This is the only method that has demonstrated an acceptable cooling rate to rapidly reduce the body temperature and minimize the risk of adverse events following prolonged hyperthermia (e.g., kidney failure, liver failure, death) (78). When a cold water immersion tub is unavailable, utilizing a tarp as a basin to contain water has demonstrated cooling rates that are comparable to traditional cold water immersion tub method (79, 80). If the only immersion option is a natural body of water, submerge the victim to the nipples, but ensure to support the upper body to prevent water aspiration and drowning.

Return to play from exertional heat stroke will largely be determined by the severity and duration that the athlete is exposed to a dangerously hyperthermic state. Therefore, immediate and aggressive cooling that lowers body temperature within thirty minutes from the onset of the exertional heat stroke will ultimately provide not only the best chance of survival, but an improved recovery and ability to return to physical activity. Generally with this treatment, athletes with no other complicating factors may begin to return to exercise within one month. During this time, athletes should refrain from exercise and be monitored by a physician to ensure that normal blood work results (for liver and kidney panels, electrolytes, and muscle enzyme levels) are obtained prior to the gradual re-introduction of exercise. Once normal blood work and seven to twenty-one days of rest have been obtained, the runner may begin to exercise again with physician clearance. Generally this gradual return should be supervised by a medical professional who is familiar with sport injuries and progress from low-intensity exercise to high-intensity exercise in a temperate environment. If this progression goes smoothly, without the athlete reporting any new or increased symptoms, then a graded progression of heat acclimatization should take place. Ideally and to ensure the athlete's safety, rectal temperature and heart rate should be monitored. If the individual experiences any side effects or negative symptoms the progression of exercise should be slowed, delayed, or stopped completely. Return to play will be highly individualized and in the most optimal cases may take two to three months, but in cases where there are complications or where adequate onsite treatment was not provided this process could be extended to up to a year or more. In rare cases where treatment was largely lacking, athletes may not be able to return to activity (7). Complicated cases of exertional heat stroke or those that struggle with returning to activity should seek expert consultation and consider further tests such as a heat tolerance test, to evaluate an individual's potential for return to activity (7, 81).

## CHAPTER 13

# Running in the Cold

## BY JESSIE R. FUDGE

## Key Points

1. Be prepared for and respond to changing weather conditions. Cold injury prevention is more effective than treatment.
2. The combination of cold, wet, and wind increases the risk of frostbite and hypothermia.
3. Understand windchill and how it relates to frostbite and hypothermia risk.
4. A layered approach to clothing can prevent injury and allow rapid response to changing weather conditions.
5. Avoid the use of facial emollients while running as this can increase frostbite risk.
6. If prolonged running in cold and wet conditions, dry socks should be changed into regularly.
7. Protect exposed skin and eyes from exposure to cold and windy conditions.

## Introduction

Cold-related injuries can easily occur in the running athlete, although the incidence is not well-documented in the literature. Running in cold weather increases the risk of hypothermia, frostbite, non-freezing skin and eye conditions, and exacerbation of underlying medical conditions. Most cold-weather-related injuries can be prevented through preparation and proper dress. A layered system of clothing and a rapid response to symptoms and changing weather conditions allows for safe participation in most temperatures.

## Physiology of Cold Exposure

Each individual athlete has a different risk of cold injury during the same weather conditions. Runners with a higher percent body fat and higher muscle mass can maintain their core temperature better than individuals with less muscle and fat (1). Women, and runners who are younger than twenty years old or older than sixty years old may have a higher risk of cold-related injuries due to these differences (2).

A balance of heat production to heat loss is required to maintain a normal core body temperature and protect the extremities from cold injury. Temperature alone cannot be used to determine the full risk of injury. The weather combination of cold, wet, and wind is most likely to predispose a runner to both freezing and non-freezing cold injuries through evaporation, conduction, and convection (1, 2, 3). Convection results in heat loss through the direct transfer of heat from the body to moving currents, like wind or water (4). Wind decreases the effective insulation of clothing if there is no vapor barrier (1, 2). The windchill temperature index (Figure 13-1) reflects convective heat loss rates and is a better indicator of frostbite risk than discrete environmental temperatures (5). The windchill temperature estimates the temperature felt on the average human face that would result in the same heat loss rate in calm wind conditions. For example, with wind speeds of twenty miles per hour, frostbite can occur after thirty minutes of exposure to an ambient temperature of -18 degrees C (0 degrees F), ten minutes at temperatures below -26 degrees C (-15 degrees F), and five minutes below approximately -37 degrees C (-35 degrees F) (2, 5). The time to frostbite is reduced as wind speeds increase. The risk of frostbite is less than 5 percent when the ambient temperature is greater than -15 degrees C (5 degrees F) (1).

## Wind Chill Chart

| Wind (mph) | \ Temperature (°F) | | | | | | | | | | | | | | | | | |
|---|---|---|---|---|---|---|---|---|---|---|---|---|---|---|---|---|---|---|
| Calm | 40 | 35 | 30 | 25 | 20 | 15 | 10 | 5 | 0 | -5 | -10 | -15 | -20 | -25 | -30 | -35 | -40 | -45 |
| 5 | 36 | 31 | 25 | 19 | 13 | 7 | 1 | -5 | -11 | -16 | -22 | -28 | -34 | -40 | -46 | -52 | -57 | -63 |
| 10 | 34 | 27 | 21 | 15 | 9 | 3 | -4 | -10 | -16 | -22 | -28 | -35 | -41 | -47 | -53 | -59 | -66 | -72 |
| 15 | 32 | 25 | 19 | 13 | 6 | 0 | -7 | -13 | -19 | -26 | -32 | -39 | -45 | -51 | -58 | -64 | -71 | -77 |
| 20 | 30 | 24 | 17 | 11 | 4 | -2 | -9 | -15 | -22 | -29 | -35 | -42 | -48 | -55 | -61 | -68 | -74 | -81 |
| 25 | 29 | 23 | 16 | 9 | 3 | -4 | -11 | -17 | -24 | -31 | -37 | -44 | -51 | -58 | -64 | -71 | -78 | -84 |
| 30 | 28 | 22 | 15 | 8 | 1 | -5 | -12 | -19 | -26 | -33 | -39 | -46 | -53 | -60 | -67 | -73 | -80 | -87 |
| 35 | 28 | 21 | 14 | 7 | 0 | -7 | -14 | -21 | -27 | -34 | -41 | -48 | -55 | -62 | -69 | -76 | -82 | -89 |
| 40 | 27 | 20 | 13 | 6 | -1 | -8 | -15 | -22 | -29 | -36 | -43 | -50 | -57 | -64 | -71 | -78 | -84 | -91 |
| 45 | 26 | 19 | 12 | 5 | -2 | -9 | -16 | -23 | -30 | -37 | -44 | -51 | -58 | -65 | -72 | -79 | -86 | -93 |
| 50 | 26 | 19 | 12 | 4 | -3 | -10 | -17 | -24 | -31 | -38 | -45 | -52 | -60 | -67 | -74 | -81 | -88 | -95 |
| 55 | 25 | 18 | 11 | 4 | -3 | -11 | -18 | -25 | -32 | -39 | -46 | -54 | -61 | -68 | -75 | -82 | -89 | -97 |
| 60 | 25 | 17 | 10 | 3 | -4 | -11 | -19 | -26 | -33 | -40 | -48 | -55 | -62 | -69 | -76 | -84 | -91 | -98 |

Frostbite Times    ▢ 30 minutes    ▢ 10 minutes    ▢ 5 minutes

$$\text{Wind Chill (°F)} = 35.74 + 0.6215T - 35.75(V^{0.16}) + 0.4275T(V^{0.16})$$

Where, T = Air Temperature (°F)    V = Wind Speed (mph)    *Effective 11/01/01*

**Figure 13-1** Wind-chill temperature index with corresponding expected time to frostbite injury. (Courtesy of The National Weather Service. http://www.nws.noaa. gov/om/winter/windchill).

Conduction results in heat loss to an object in direct contact with the skin, like wet clothing. Runners exposed to rain are at risk for greater heat loss at higher temperatures than would be expected in dry weather (1). The American College of Sports Medicine's (ACSM) consensus statement on the prevention of cold weather injuries suggests that the ambient temperature used when assessing windchill equivalent temperatures for frostbite risk should be 10 degrees C lower than the actual ambient temperature if the skin is wet and exposed to the wind (1). Evaporation of water directly from the body (wet skin or clothing) also increases the rate of heat lost to the environment (2, 4). Through a combination of conduction and evaporation, wet clothes may double the heat loss seen in dry conditions at an air temperature of 5 degrees C (41 degrees F), highlighting the importance of proper clothing (1). Wet, windy conditions also increase the risk of frostbite. Skin cools faster, reaches a lower temperature, and freezes at a higher threshold than dry skin (1, 6, 7).

Underlying medical conditions can change the body's response to cold exposure. Runners should review any medical conditions that can alter thermoregulation with their doctor. These can include endocrine conditions (e.g., hypothyroidism, diabetes) and chronic skin conditions (e.g., psoriasis, eczema). Medications for blood pressure and anxiety can also change the body's response to cold (1, 2, 3).

## Food and Fluid Intake for Cold Weather Running

If the body's core temperature remains elevated above resting values during exercise, then increased cold weather caloric requirements are not expected to be above normal (1). However, runners often expend more energy in cold weather if they increase their effort by running in snow or keeping warm through shivering. Proper dress can help prevent increased caloric needs. If calorie expenditure is higher for an individual runner, then increased calories can be obtained through frequent snacks. For runners who maintain adequate core and muscle temperatures, fatigue may be related to carbohydrate availability rather than increased caloric expenditure related to the cold (1). Since carbohydrate availability is important for cold weather running, carbohydrate loading to maximize muscle glycogen stores may be beneficial (1). Similar to temperate environments, marathon runners in the cold can maintain performance by eating carbohydrate-rich foods (1).

Dehydration does not appear to increase the risk of cold injuries, but can decrease performance (1). Dehydration is more common in cold weather exercise due to a combination of cold-induced increased urination, reduction in voluntary fluid intake, and sweat loss. Cold exposure decreases the release of hormones that trigger thirst. This is likely due to cold-induced vasoconstriction increasing core and brain blood volume, which in turn stimulates central volume receptors and results in decreased thirst sensation at rest and with exercise in the cold (8). Since thirst is less noticeable in cold compared to hot weather, runners should focus on adequate hydration before and during their activity (1).

## Prevention of Cold-Weather-Related Injuries

Preparation for environmental exposures is the most important intervention a runner can do to prevent frostbite, hypothermia, and other cold-related injuries. Injuries in cold temperatures occur when tissue heat loss exceeds heat production, which can result in the freezing of tissues and a drop in core body temperatures. Understanding the weather conditions will help to determine your risk of cold injury and allow proper preparation.

Layering of clothing and rapid response to changing weather conditions can help maintain adequate core temperature and decrease heat loss in cold weather. Runners need different clothing layers depending on their planned running distance, individual heat production, and the weather conditions. Layering should be individualized based on past cold weather experience and training (1, 2). The risk of cold injury increases in wet conditions, so clothing layers must maintain heat while limiting internal wetness (1, 2, 3). The innermost layer, which is in direct contact with the skin, should wick moisture away from the body to maintain an insulating air layer next to the skin and transfer water to outer layers of clothing (1, 2, 3, 4). The middle layer or layers are primarily for insulation and the number of layers is dictated by the temperature and exertion level. As exercise intensity increases, the amount of clothing insulation needed to maintain body heat at a given temperature decreases. The outer vapor layer must allow moisture transfer from inside to outside, allow ventilation, and protect against wind and rain (1, 2, 3, 4). Avoid exercising in the outer protective vapor layer unless it is wet or windy, and instead use it for changes in weather conditions or during rest periods to prevent overheating, increased sweat production, and subsequent wetting of the inner layers (1, 2, 3). It is important for athletes to realize that exercise sweat rates can easily exceed the breathability of many waterproof or water resistant materials. These outer layers may become a vapor barrier that traps moisture next to athletes' bodies. It is safe to assume that the more waterproof clothing is, the less it will breathe (2, 3).

Loose clothing is also important to minimize restrictions in hand and foot blood flow to help maintain adequate digit temperature. Clothing or footwear that is too tight can constrict peripheral blood flow and increase the risk of frostbite injury (1, 2, 3). If more than one pair of socks is needed, then an athlete should go up one shoe size. Adding an extra pair of socks for increased insulation may inadvertently constrict blood flow to the feet and increase the risk of frostbite.

Chemical hand and foot warmers can be used to maintain peripheral warmth as long as they do not constrict blood flow (2, 3). The use of skin protecting emollients increases the risk of frostbite and should not be used (1, 2, 3, 9, 10). It has been found that study subjects who used skin emollients doubled the incidence of facial frostbite in the areas where emollients were applied (9). This may have been due to subjective skin warmth, a false sense of protection, and neglect of other protective measures (9, 10). Eyeglasses should be used to protect the eyes from snow blindness (if snow running) and cold injury.

Running increases core body temperatures, but core temperature can drop rapidly when the exercise is decreased or stopped while the runner is still exposed to the elements. It is critical to ensure that the exercise can be stopped in a warm, dry, and safe environment. Adequate training, nutrition, and hydration for a cold weather running event is necessary to complete the activity safely. More specific prevention and treatment strategies will be reviewed for each individual diagnosis below.

# Hypothermia

Hypothermia is best prevented through layered clothing and early recognition of changing weather conditions. Hypothermia is defined as a core body temperature below 35 degrees C (95 degrees F) and occurs when total body heat loss exceeds heat production (1, 4, 11, 12). Hypothermia is often characterized as mild, moderate, or severe depending on the presenting symptoms and signs. Mild hypothermia can be recognized by increased shivering, social withdrawal, and other behavior changes, with preservation of the mental state (1, 4). As blood is shunted from the periphery to the core to maintain warmth of the body's vital organs, athletes may develop pale, cool skin and extremities (4). Rapid response to these symptoms is critical. Symptoms worsen if the early hypothermia changes are not recognized and core body temperature drops even further. Symptoms of worsening hypothermia to "moderate" include confusion, sleepiness, slurred speech, and behavior change. People may appear as if intoxicated, and the confusion can lead to runners inadvertently leaving the course and getting lost in cold conditions. As hypothermia worsens, athletes will eventually lose the ability to shiver, and ultimately lose consciousness (1, 12). The risk of cardiac arrest from a fatal heart rhythm increases as the core temperatures drop below 30 degrees C

(86 degrees F) and is even more likely below the temperature threshold for severe hypothermia, 28 degrees C (82.4 degrees F) (11).

The symptoms of hypothermia vary between runners, even at the same core body temperature, and early recognition is important for long-term recovery and survival (1). Runners should suspect hypothermia if the conditions are fitting and empirically treat based on symptom recognition. The field treatment of hypothermia relies primarily on passive external rewarming. Runners should be removed from the environment as soon as possible, change into dry clothes, and allow shivering to continue (4). Warm drinks, high calorie drinks and food, and active movement can also increase core temperature (11). The athlete should be protected from wind, moisture, and further cold exposure. Treatment in a hospital may be required if the individual has lost their shivering response or their altered mental state cannot be reversed.

For unresponsive runners in cold environments, detection of a pulse can be difficult (11). Check pulses for sixty seconds, but if no sign of life is detected, then cardiopulmonary resuscitation (CPR) should be initiated (11). Start rewarming, if it can be done without interrupting CPR or delaying transportation to a higher level of care—preferably a center with facilities for interventional core rewarming. Cardiopulmonary resuscitation should be continued, as long as it is safe for the rescuers, until the patient is warm.

# Frostbite

Frostnip is a superficial non-freezing injury of exposed skin that suggests conditions are right for more severe frostbite injury. Ice crystals may form on the surface of the skin and the skin appears red and feels numb to the runner. Importantly, these symptoms resolve quickly with skin covering and no long-term damage occurs (13). Responding to frostnip will help prevent more significant injury. Frostnip is treated by covering the skin and reassessing clothing to protect from further injury.

Frostbite is a direct freezing injury to cold exposed areas of the body. It is best prevented through wear of proper clothing to maintain core body temperature, protection of exposed skin, and response to changing weather conditions. Common sites include the nose, ears, fingers, and toes (2, 13). It is important to recognize weather conditions and skin changes that signal the potential for frostbite injury. The severity of frostbite injury is proportional to the temperature, duration of exposure, and amount and depth of frozen tissue. Runners with superficial frostbite will develop skin numbness and redness followed by a white or yellow slightly raised area of skin (13). Clear or white fluid-filled blisters can

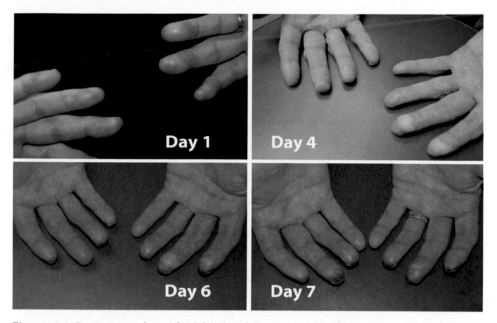

**Figure 13-2** Progression of superficial frostbite following rapid rewarming in a water bath. (Courtesy Jessie Fudge).

occur (Figure 13-2). Deep frostbite extends deeper into the skin layers and results in hemorrhagic blisters, black or darkly hues tissue, and eventual tissue loss (13).

At the first sign of frostbite, remove wet clothing, protect the skin from further cold injury through insulation, and move to a warm and dry location (4, 13). If the injury is to the foot, a runner should attempt to avoid weight bearing on the injured extremity unless the only method of rapid evacuation is walking or running out on it (2, 4, 13). The injured tissue should not be rewarmed until that athlete is in an environment with minimal risk of refreezing. Initial warming can be done using the athlete's own body heat from the axilla, neck, or groin. (2, 4). Care should be taken not to rub the injured skin. Ideally, frostbite should be treated at a medical clinic or local medical facility where rapid rewarming can be done in a hot water bath at 37 to 39 degrees C (2, 13). Spontaneous thawing of skin tissue should be allowed if rapid rewarming cannot be done and there is minimal risk to refreezing (13). Warming of the injured tissue should be continued until the skin is red or purple in color and soft to touch (13). Blisters should initially be left intact and may be covered with dry, loose bandages unless they are at risk of spontaneously breaking open (13). (See Chapter 8 for methods of blister drainage.) Medical evaluation at a hospital should occur as soon as possible to further assess depth of injury and consider higher levels of treatment.

## Non-Freezing Cold Injuries (Trench Foot and Chilblain)

Trench foot and chilblains (pernio) occur when skin is exposed to both cold and wet environments through immersion or damp socks/shoes. Chilblains is a superficial cold injury that results in small red skin lesions that are itchy and painful (1). This can occur after several hours exposed to the cold. As the skin is rewarmed, it can become more painful, itchy, red, hot, and swollen. Blisters and ulcerations can occur (4). The itching and a burning sensation can last for several hours, but there are no usually no long-term effects from chilblains (1).

Trench foot requires more prolonged and repeated exposure to wet-cold conditions (twelve hours to four days) and usually occurs if wet socks are worn continuously for many days without allowing the skin to dry (1, 4). Trench foot results in a painful, swollen red foot. In more severe cases, the foot may appear pale or purple and could progress to gangrene if left untreated (4). Trench foot in running is very rare.

Chilblains and trench foot can be prevented by keeping the feet dry. Ultramarathon runners in a cold, wet environment should change socks two to three times per day. Antiperspirants with aluminum hydroxide can decrease sweating of the foot (1, 3). Treatment requires warming and drying the skin. Wound care may be needed in more severe cases (4).

## Cold Urticaria

Cold urticaria is an allergic reaction to cold temperatures and can result in itchy raised welts on the skin (4). An antihistamine such as Benadryl can be used to control itching and skin symptoms. Runners who develop more severe allergy symptoms in the cold that could present as life-threatening breathing difficulties (anaphylaxis) should carry epinephrine auto-injector and avoid cold exposure (4).

## Cold-Induced Bronchoconstriction

Bronchoconstriction, or reversible narrowing of airways, results in wheezing and is more common when exercising in the cold (4). The exact mechanism of bronchoconstriction in cold weather exercise exposure is not well understood. It is likely that the dry air associated with cold exposure causes irritation of the large breathing tubes in the lungs (bronchioles) and is the cause rather than cold exposure itself (1). Bronchoconstriction results in a cough, chest tightness, shortness of breath, and possibly wheezing (4). This can occur in runners without a diagnosis of asthma. Since running-induced shortness of breath has a broad differential diagnosis, this symptom should be evaluated further by a physician. If exercise-induced bronchoconstriction is diagnosed, then bronchodilator inhalers (i.e., albuterol) fifteen minutes prior to exercises can help prevent symptoms. Other medications are also available if inhalers do not help. Breathing through a thin scarf or bandana will increase the temperature of the inhaled cold air and may decrease symptoms as well (4).

## CHAPTER 14
# High Altitude
## BY TREVOR C. STEINBACH AND ANDREW M. LUKS

## Key Points

1.  The defining environmental feature of high altitude is a non-linear decrease in barometric pressure, which decreases the amount of available oxygen for use in the body.
2.  Normal physiologic responses to low pressure and low oxygen (hypobaric hypoxia) environment, such as increased heart rate and breathing rate, cause individuals to perceive increased exertion while exercising at high altitude.
3.  Athletes traveling to high altitude for leisure or competition face the same risk of acute altitude illness as non-athletes, and should be prepared to recognize the symptoms of high altitude illness and respond to these problems.
4.  Exercise following arrival at high altitude is more difficult than at sea level, but improves with time and appropriate acclimatization.
5.  The benefits of high altitude exposure for improving athletic performance at sea level remain unclear and must be weighed against the logistical challenges of these techniques.

## Introduction

With increasing frequency, athletes are training or taking part in competitions at high altitude, where unique environmental conditions and subsequent physiologic responses may adversely affect exercise performance and place them at risk for developing one of several forms of acute altitude illness. Furthermore, many athletes hope to use the unique features of high altitude to improve sea level performance. This chapter examines each of these situations in depth. After reviewing the key environmental features of high altitude, we discuss the physiologic responses to the low oxygen conditions (hypoxia), and the main challenges faced by runners traveling to high altitude, including the risk of acute altitude illness and the decline in exercise performance. We then review the current understanding of preparations for athletic competition at high altitude and the utility of hypoxic exposure for improving sea level performance.

## The Environment at High Altitude

While many resources define "high altitude" as greater than 2,400 m (approximately 8,000 ft) in elevation, athletes may face challenges with competitions down as low as 1,500 m (approximately 5,000 ft). The defining feature of the environment at these and higher elevations is the exponential decrease in barometric pressure with increasing elevation, resulting in decreased partial pressure of oxygen at all points along the oxygen transport chain from the lungs to exercising muscles. It is this feature of high altitude, referred to as hypobaric hypoxia, which subsequently increases risk for acute altitude illness and may adversely affect exercise performance.

In addition to the decreased availability of oxygen, other environmental factors may also affect well-being and exercise performance. Reduced ambient humidity increases the risk of dehydration, higher UV light exposure increases the risk of sunburn and snow blindness, particularly in snow-covered terrain, and the decrease in ambient temperature increases the risk of hypothermia.

## Normal Adaptations to High Altitude

Exposure to hypoxia causes a number of responses across multiple organ systems that typically help the individual adapt to and tolerate the low oxygen conditions. This process is referred to as acclimatization. Key features of these responses are summarized below and in Table 14-1 (1, 2). While the pattern and time course of responses is generally similar between individuals, there is significant inter-individual variability in the magnitude of the responses with subsequent effects on performance and susceptibility to acute altitude illness.

## The Lungs

Following ascent to high altitude, the low partial pressure of oxygen in the blood (hypoxemia) stimulates respiratory (breathing) centers in the carotid arteries, leading to an increase in the volume of air inhaled and exhaled per minute, referred to as "minute ventilation." With additional time at high altitude, minute ventilation increases further to compensate for the decreased amount of oxygen available in each breath, further aiding acclimatization. Low oxygen levels in the lungs trigger constriction of the local arteries (pulmonary arterioles), causing increased resistance to pulmonary blood flow and increased pulmonary arterial pressure.

**Table 14-1** Selected physiologic responses to high altitude by various organ systems.

| Organ System | Physiologic Responses |
|---|---|
| Lungs | Increased minute ventilation, which rises further with additional time at altitude<br>Increased pulmonary vascular resistance |
| Heart | Increased heart rate<br>Increased cardiac output<br>Reduced stroke volume<br>Variable increases in systemic blood pressure |
| Kidneys | Diuresis and natriuresis (water and salt excretion)<br>Increased erythropoietin (EPO) production<br>Bicarbonate excretion |
| Blood | Increased hemoglobin and hematocrit<br>Initially due to plasma volume loss and hemoconcentration; later due to EPO-mediated increase in red cell mass |
| Muscle | Decreased muscle fiber size<br>Increased myoglobin concentration<br>Increased capillary density<br>Upregulation of mitochondrial genes and glycolytic enzymes |

## The Heart

Exposure to hypoxemia triggers an increase in the volume of blood pumped by the heart each minute, referred to as cardiac output. Driven primarily by an increase in heart rate rather than an increase in the volume of blood pumped with each contraction of the heart, this response helps preserve oxygen delivery to the tissues during hypoxemia. While the contractile strength of the left ventricle is maintained following ascent, the rise in pulmonary artery pressure described above may affect right heart function and contributes to the decrease in exercise performance seen following ascent.

## Fluid Balance

Urine output increases and plasma volume decreases following ascent by mechanisms that remain unclear. Together with increased fluid losses from the respiratory tract due to hyperventilation and reduced ambient humidity, the decrease in plasma volume increases the likelihood of dehydration following ascent.

## The Blood

The concentration of hemoglobin, the main oxygen carrier in the blood, increases following ascent due to the decrease of plasma volume, a phenomenon referred to as "hemoconcentration." Hypoxemia also stimulates the production of erythropoietin (EPO), which, over days to weeks, increases red blood cell production, further increasing hemoglobin concentration, a critical factor in maintaining oxygen delivery to the tissues during hypoxemia.

## How Individuals Experience These Responses

Due to the body's adaptive responses to acute hypoxia, individuals feel different following ascent to high altitude than at sea level. Recognition of these differences is important (Table 14-2), as it will prevent individuals from misinterpreting normal responses as signs of illness. Sojourners will notice a significant increase in the rate and depth of breathing, while exertion causes a sensation of breathlessness, even in well-trained individuals, which improves quickly with rest. Athletes who monitor their heart rate closely will note higher readings both at rest and with any level of physical exertion. Poor sleep quality is common due to alterations in sleep architecture and a form of periodic breathing referred to as central sleep apnea. Many people also report increased frequency of urination and transient lightheadedness upon rising from the sitting position or after bending over.

# Competing or Training at High Altitude

Runners competing or training at high altitude face two distinct challenges, a risk of acute altitude illness in the days following ascent and the effects of hypobaric hypoxia on exercise performance. Each challenge is considered below.

**Table 14-2** Normal symptoms experienced by travelers to high altitude resulting from physiologic responses to the environment.

| |
|---|
| Increased frequency and depth of breathing |
| Increased sense of breathlessness for given level of exertion, typically resolves quickly with rest |
| Increased heart rate at rest and for any given level of submaximal exertion |
| Increased frequency of urination |
| Poor sleep quality, marked by frequent awakenings, vivid dreams, and insomnia |
| Transient lightheadedness when rising to standing position |

Adapted from: Luks AM. Physiology in Medicine: A physiologic approach to prevention and treatment of acute high-altitude illnesses. *J Appl Physiol.* 2015;118(5):509–519.

## Acute Altitude Illness

Regardless of their level of physical fitness, any unacclimatized individual ascending to greater than 2,500 m (approximately 8,200 ft) is at risk for developing one of three forms of acute altitude illness: acute mountain sickness (AMS), a syndrome of non-specific symptoms including headache, fatigue, dizziness, poor sleep, and nausea or vomiting; high altitude cerebral edema (HACE), a potentially fatal illness marked by gait imbalance, altered level of consciousness, and possibly coma; and high altitude pulmonary edema (HAPE), a buildup of fluid in the lungs that results in progressive difficulty breathing with minimal exertion and even at rest, which can also be fatal if not treated promptly. Acute mountain sickness and HAPE can occur at altitudes between 2,000 to 2,500 m (6,600 to 8,200 ft), but are overall uncommon at those elevations (3). High altitude travelers should be able to recognize, prevent, and treat these primary forms of altitude illness, whose features are described in Table 14-3.

Aside from genetic differences that account for individual variation in susceptibility to acute altitude illness, the primary reason people become sick following ascent is they rise too high and too fast, as assessed by the rate of rise in their sleeping elevation. There is an important interaction between the altitude reached and the time spent at that elevation. For example, someone who ascends to 4,000 m (13,200 ft) in a single day may avoid altitude illness if they descend soon after ascent, but would likely become ill if they remain at that elevation for many hours or overnight. Unfortunately, in individuals with no prior high altitude travel, there is no easy way to predict susceptibility. For those who have been to high altitude before, prior performance and vulnerability versus resistance to AMS is a good, but imperfect, predictor of health on future trips. Importantly, while being in good physical condition makes performing physical work at high altitude easier, susceptibility to acute altitude illness is not affected by aerobic capacity; the great athlete is just as susceptible as a sedentary individual (4).

One of the challenges of identifying ill individuals at high altitude is that the symptoms of acute altitude illness are non-specific and can be caused by a variety of other problems (Table 14-4). These other diagnoses should always be considered in ill individuals at high altitude but, in general, illness within a few hours to days of ascent should be attributed to acute altitude illness until proven otherwise.

# Prevention of Altitude Illness

A variety measures can be used to prevent acute altitude illness.

**Table 14-3** Clinical features, prevention, and treatment of high altitude illnesses.

| Condition | Risk Factors | Symptoms and Signs | Prevention | Treatment |
|---|---|---|---|---|
| Acute Mountain Sickness (AMS) | Incidence varies based on altitude reached and rate of ascent<br>Higher risk with more rapid ascent<br>Symptoms onset within 6–10 hours of ascent | Headache plus 1 or more of: nausea, vomiting, lethargy, sustained light-headedness<br>Normal neurological exam and mental status | Slow ascent (limit increases in sleeping elevation to 300–500 m once above 2,500–3,000 m)<br>Avoid overexertion<br>Acetazolamide or dexamethasone if anticipating moderate-high risk ascent profile | Stop ascent<br>Acetaminophen or NSAIDs for headache; antiemetics if needed<br>Mild–moderate illness: acetazolamide<br>Severe illness: dexamethasone<br>Descend if symptoms unresolved after 1–2 days or worse with treatment<br>If symptoms resolve, safe to ascend further |
| High Altitude Cerebral Edema (HACE) | Affects <1% of travelers to > 3,000 m<br>Affected individuals often have preceding AMS symptoms | Occasionally preexisting symptoms of AMS or HAPE (not required)<br>Ataxia, altered mental status, somnolence, coma<br>Focal neurological deficits rare<br>Can be fatal if unrecognized and untreated | Slow ascent<br>Avoid overexertion<br>Acetazolamide or dexamethasone | Descent to altitude at which symptoms resolve<br>If descent is not feasible, supplemental oxygen or portable hyperbaric chamber<br>Dexamethasone<br>Do not ascend further until asymptomatic off all treatment |
| High Altitude Pulmonary Edema (HAPE) | Incidence depends on elevation and ascent rates, but affects 0.2–8% of travelers between 2,500 and 5,500 m.<br>Occurs within 2–5 days of ascent<br>AMS symptoms do not always precede HAPE | Mild: disproportionate dyspnea and hypoxemia when compared to that which is expected, decreased exercise performance, dry cough<br>Severe: Dyspnea at rest or with minimal exertion, cough productive of pink, frothy sputum, cyanosis<br>Potentially fatal if unrecognized and untreated | Slow ascent<br>Avoid overexertion<br>Nifedipine for individuals with history of HAPE (phosphodiesterase inhibitors are an alternative) | Descent to altitude at which symptoms resolve<br>If descent is not feasible, supplemental oxygen or portable hyperbaric chamber<br>Nifedipine or phosphodiesterase inhibitor (do not use in combination) if supplemental oxygen unavailable<br>Do not ascend further until asymptomatic off all treatment |

Adapted from Luks AM. Physiology in medicine: a physiologic approach to prevention and treatment of acute high-altitude illnesses. *J Appl Physiol.* 2015;118(5):509-519 and Luks AM, McIntosh SE, Grissom CK, et al. Wilderness Medical Society practice guidelines for the prevention and treatment of acute altitude illness: 2014 update. *Wilderness and Environ Med.* 2014;25(4 Suppl):S4–S14.

**Table 14-4** Differential diagnosis of acute high altitude illnesses.

| AMS/HACE | HAPE |
|---|---|
| Alcohol hangover | Asthma exacerbation |
| Caffeine withdrawal | Hyperventilation syndrome |
| Carbon monoxide poisoning | Paradoxical vocal cord motion |
| Cerebrovascular accident | Pneumonia |
| Dehydration | Pneumothorax |
| Drug intoxication | Pulmonary embolism |
| Hyponatremia | Severe URI |
| Migraine headache | |
| Physical exhaustion | |
| Transient ischemic attack | |
| Traumatic brain injury | |

URI: upper respiratory tract infection.

## Slow Ascent

Because the primary cause of acute altitude illness is an overly rapid ascent to the target elevation without allowing time for the body to properly acclimatize, the single best means to prevent altitude illness is to undertake a slow ascent. Various published guidelines outline safe ascent rates (4, 5). While the particular details vary between sources, the same general principle applies: slow the increase in sleeping elevation to an appropriate rate and incorporate rest days to allow sufficient time for acclimatization. For example, once above 3,000 m (approximately 10,000 ft), individuals should not increase their sleeping elevation by more than 500 m/day (approximately 1,650 ft); every three to four days, individuals should observe a rest day, sleeping at the same elevation for at least two nights (3, 5). Logistical factors, such as local terrain, sometimes require that individuals ascend more than recommended on a given day. In such cases, it is reasonable to focus on the ascent rate averaged over the entire trip. As individuals make repeated trips to high altitude, they learn their personal tolerance to high altitude and can modify ascent rates accordingly.

## Pre-acclimatization and Staged Ascent

A group of tactics that have garnered recent attention involve exposure to hypoxia on either a continuous or intermittent basis prior to the planned ascent in an effort to aid acclimatization and decrease the risk of maladaptive responses that cause acute altitude illness. "Staged Ascent" involves ascending to and remaining at moderate altitude for several days before the primary planned ascent. For example, a comparison of various physiologic parameters and the incidence of AMS in subjects acutely exposed to 4,300 m (approximately 14,000 ft) in a hypobaric chamber and following ascent on land to an altitude of 4,300 m after six days from an elevation of 2,200 m (approximately 7,200 ft) demonstrated that the latter ascent profile was associated with only minor changes in ventilatory, cardiovascular, and hematologic parameters but a significant decrease in the incidence of AMS (6). Although this study has not been repeated, it suggests this is a useful approach for those with the time to stage their ascent in this manner.

More studies have examined the role of "pre-acclimatization," in which the individual is exposed to hypoxia for a limited period of time on specified number of occasions prior to the planned ascent. For example, in one study, six healthy individuals were exposed to four hours of hypobaric hypoxia equivalent to 4,300 m, five days a week for three weeks, and demonstrated decreased incidence and severity of AMS on a subsequent thirty-hour exposure to 4,300 m, compared to a similar thirty-hour exposure done prior to the three-week protocol (7). Other studies, however, have failed to demonstrate a similar benefit (8, 9). One of the reasons for the conflicting results in the literature is the variability in study protocols for intermittent hypoxic exposure in regards to the duration, frequency, and magnitude of the hypoxic exposure, as well as the method for creating the hypoxic environment. Another challenge with pre-acclimatization strategies for the average individual is the logistical difficulties of implementing these techniques including the extensive time, cost, and resource commitment. Given these issues and the lack of clear guidance on the best recipe for such exposures, preacclimatization cannot be recommended as a standard approach at present.

## Hypoxic Tents

One particular pre-acclimatization strategy that anecdotally is increasingly being used by climbers and others traveling to high altitude are "hypoxic" or "altitude" tents. A sealed tent is erected around a bed in which the person sleeps and the oxygen content of air inside the tent is depleted by pumping nitrogen-enriched air into the tent. Although the benefits of such systems are widely touted in marketing campaigns by product manufacturers, these systems have received only limited scientific study. In the only placebo-controlled study published to date, when compared to those sleeping in sea level conditions, subjects who slept at simulated high altitude for fourteen days encountered a slightly decreased occurrence of AMS upon subsequent ascent to 4,300 m (14,000 ft) (10). Of note, technical difficulties with the system resulted in difficulty achieving and maintaining the intended simulated altitude. The lack of data supporting a benefit will likely not diminish the ongoing use of these systems. They are probably of low risk to individuals using them, aside from the cost of the system and power needed to run them, as well as any potential disruption in spousal relations. Whatever benefit may be derived from their use will not occur with short and/or infrequent exposures and, instead, will likely require sleeping in the tents for at least six to eight hours per night for several weeks prior to the planned altitude exposure.

## Other Non-pharmacologic Measures

Heavy alcohol consumption and opiate pain medications should be avoided, particularly before sleep, as these can decrease minute ventilation and further exacerbate hypoxemia in an already low oxygen environment. Although this recommendation has never been systematically studied, it is an easy behavioral intervention. Given the increased fluid losses at high altitude, it is important to prevent dehydration, whose symptoms can mimic those of AMS. There is no evidence, however, that "forced," or over-hydration, is protective against acute altitude illness. Individuals should simply drink to thirst and avoid excessive intake that can increase the risk of serious problems such as hyponatremia. Chronic users of caffeinated beverages should avoid abrupt cessation of caffeine intake as this could provoke headache, which might be confused with AMS.

## Pharmacologic Measures

While several medications can be used as prophylaxis against acute altitude illness (Table 14-5), they are not necessary in all high altitude travelers. Instead, the use of medications should be based on the estimated risk of the planned ascent (Table 14-6). Pharmacologic prophylaxis should be considered with moderate or high-risk ascent profiles but is not necessary with low risk ascents. Pharmacologic prophylaxis against HAPE is not used in individuals who have not been to high altitude before and, instead, is reserved for those with a prior history of the disease.

Acetazolamide, the primary option for AMS prevention is a diuretic and, as a result, increases urination and potentially increases the risk of dehydration during heavy exertion. Adequate fluid intake should be maintained and will not counteract the protective effects of the medication, which are a function of particular substances eliminated in the urine and their positive impact on increased

**Table 14-5** Dosing and administration of medications used in the prevention and treatment of high altitude illnesses.

| Illness | Medication | Prevention | Treatment |
|---------|-----------|-----------|-----------|
| **AMS** | Acetazolamide | 125 mg orally twice daily | 250 mg orally twice daily |
|  | Dexamethasone | 2 mg orally every 6 hr or 4 mg orally every 12 hr | 4 mg oral/IV/IM every 6 hr |
| **HACE** | Acetazolamide | 125 mg orally twice daily | 250 mg orally twice daily |
|  | Dexamethasone | 2 mg orally every 6 hr or 4 mg orally every 12 hr | 8 mg oral/IV/IM/PO once, then 4 mg every 6 hr |
| **HAPE** | Nifedipine | 30 mg ER every 12 hr | 30 mg ER every 12 hr |
|  | Tadalafil | 10 mg orally twice daily | N/A |
|  | Sildenafil | 50 mg orally every 8 hr | N/A |
|  | Salmeterol* | 125 µg inhaled twice daily | N/A |

IV: Intravenous, IM: Intramuscular, ER: Extended Release formulation.
*Should only be used as an adjunct to other agents and not used as monotherapy.
Adapted from: Luks AM, McIntosh SE, Grissom CK, et al. Wilderness Medical Society practice guidelines for the prevention and treatment of acute altitude illness: 2014 update. *Wilderness and Environ Med.* 2014;25(4 Suppl):S4–S14.

**Table 14-6** Risk assessment for acute high altitude illnesses.

| Risk Level | Characteristics |
|-----------|-----------------|
| Low | Individuals with no prior history of altitude illness and ascent to ≤ 2,800 m<br>Individuals taking ≥ 2 days to arrive at 2,500–3,000 m, with subsequent increases in sleeping elevation < 500 m/day, and allowing an extra day of acclimatization every 1,000 m |
| Moderate | Individuals with a history of AMS and ascending to 2,500–2,800 m in 1 day<br>No history of AMS and ascending to > 2,800 m in 1 day<br>All individuals ascending > 500 m/day (sleeping elevation) at altitudes > 3,000 m, but allowing an extra day for acclimatization every 1,000 m |
| High | Individuals with a history of AMS and ascending to > 2,800 m in 1 day<br>All individuals with a prior history of HACE or HAPE<br>All individuals ascending to > 3,500 m in 1 day<br>All individuals ascending > 500 m per day (sleeping elevation) above 3,000 m without extra days for acclimatization<br>Very rapid ascents (i.e., Mount Kilimanjaro) |

Adapted from Luks AM, McIntosh SE, Grissom CK, et al. Wilderness Medical Society practice guidelines for the prevention and treatment of acute altitude illness: 2014 update. *Wilderness Environ Med* 2014;25:S7 minute ventilation rather than its effect on total body volume status. Several recent studies have raised concern about potential adverse effects of acetazolamide on exercise capacity under normal oxygen conditions (11) and perceived difficulty of exercise at high altitude (12) but this limited evidence has not led to changes in published recommendations on acetazolamide's role in altitude illness prevention (3).

Recent research suggests ibuprofen may have a role in altitude illness prevention. Although it has not been directly compared to acetazolamide or dexamethasone, it was shown to be more effective than placebo in preventing AMS in healthy individuals ascending rapidly by car and then foot to 3,800m (approximately 12,500ft) (13). The dose in this study was 600mg every eight hours starting the morning of ascent (for one day). The safety profile of the medication during heavy exertion or prolonged travel at high altitude—in particular the risk of developing gastrointestinal bleeding or acute kidney injury—remains unclear and is a reason for caution when considering non-steroidal anti-inflammatory agents (NSAID) for altitude illness prophylaxis. Short-term use (approximately one to two days) with cessation prior to heavy exertion is likely safe but given the lack of adequate comparison data, the prescription medications acetazolamide and dexamethasone remain the preferred agents for altitude illness prevention.

## Treatment of Acute Altitude Illness

Descent to lower elevation (approximately 500 to 1,000m; 1,600 to 3,300ft) is the definitive treatment for any acute altitude illness but is not required in all situations. Individuals who develop mild to moderate AMS should stop ascending, rest, and use medications such as aspirin, NSAIDs, or acetaminophen to treat the headache. Acetazolamide or dexamethasone (Table 14-5) can be added for those with moderate to severe symptoms or who fail to improve with conservative measures. If symptoms resolve with appropriate treatment, individuals can resume their planned high altitude activities and ascend to higher elevations.

Descent is indicated if AMS fails to resolve with the measures above or for those with HACE or HAPE. If descent is not feasible, supplemental oxygen or a portable hyperbaric chamber should be used, if available. Patients with HACE should also be started on dexamethasone while those with HAPE should receive a pulmonary vasodilator such as nifedipine or sildenafil (Table 14-5). Diuretics have no role in HAPE treatment, as patients are often dehydrated at the time of their illness and, as a result, at risk for hypotension with diuretic administration. Patients with HAPE who can access health-care facilities in adequately resourced settings, such as a Colorado ski resort, do not need to descend and can often be treated with oxygen alone and observation at the health facility or their lodge.

## Exercise at High Altitude

Unacclimatized runners ascending to high altitude face significant challenges with exercise, particularly during the first few days following ascent. From a subjective standpoint, individuals typically note markedly increased breathlessness, or dyspnea, with exertion. Activities that would not pose difficulty at lower elevation are perceived as considerably more difficult and often require more frequent breaks to catch one's breath.

From an objective standpoint, at any given work rate, minute ventilation, heart rate, and cardiac output are increased relative to sea level values (1, 2, 14). In addition, for reasons that remain unclear despite considerable research, maximum exercise capacity, or $VO_2$ max, decreases following ascent, with roughly 10 percent decline for every 1,000m of altitude gain (1). Because of the decrease in $VO_2$ max, maximum heart rate and minute ventilation are also decreased. With acclimatization over time at high altitude, $VO_2$ max may improve to some extent but does not return to sea level values (15).

A key issue with exercise at high altitude is teasing out normal dyspnea with exertion from the heightened dyspnea and decreased exercise capacity associated with the onset of HAPE. Under normal circumstances, breathlessness resolves within a short time (one to two minutes) of ceasing exertion and individuals have no difficulty keeping up with their travel partners. When individuals develop HAPE, however, they have progressive difficulty keeping up with their group, require frequent rest breaks and much more time for the breathlessness to resolve before they feel as if they are ready to exert themselves again. Severe breathlessness that occurs at rest or with simple activities such as walking slowly on flat ground or going to the bathroom are also concerning signs for disease.

# When to Arrive at High Altitude Prior to the Planned Event

Because exercise performance improves with time at altitude, albeit not to sea level values, athletes often ask when the appropriate arrival time at altitude relative to the planned event is, in order to maximize performance. The bulk of the evidence, which has been reviewed elsewhere (16), suggests two weeks is the optimal duration of stay at the target elevation prior to competition. This allows enough time for the majority of beneficial compensatory responses, such as ventilatory acclimatization, and avoids adverse training effects, such as slower training velocities, that can be seen with longer stays. Shorter durations (e.g., seven days) may also have utility when fourteen days are not feasible but likely do not confer as much benefit (16).

# Sea Level Strategies for Preparing for Exercise at High Altitude

Because spending two weeks at high altitude prior to planned competition is not feasible for many individuals, investigators have examined whether intermittent hypoxic exposure protocols similar to those described above for altitude illness prevention can improve exercise performance at high altitude in lieu of early arrival.

Two types of protocols have been considered, including those with exercise during hypoxic exposure (intermittent hypoxia training) and those in which the individual remains at rest throughout their exposure (intermittent hypoxic exposure). The former has been shown to improve exercise performance in hypoxia, while inconsistent data have been reported regarding the latter. One challenge in the literature on this topic is that, as with preacclimatization protocols for acute altitude illness prevention noted above, the studies employ widely varying protocols as well as different methods for generating hypoxia (a normobaric versus hypobaric). As a result, the optimal approach remains unclear.

## Just-in-Time Arrivals

Given the significant logistical hurdles that arise with either early arrival or intermittent hypoxic training, some have recommended an alternative approach in which the individual arrives as close as possible to the planned event, purportedly for the purpose of minimizing adverse responses to acute hypoxic exposure, such as a decrease in plasma volume or disrupted sleep, that might impair performance. While those reasons seem plausible on the surface and the technique has been used by soccer teams competing in cities located at high altitude (17), there have been no systematic studies of this approach and it cannot be recommended at this time.

## Using High Altitude to Enhance Sea Level Performance

The bulk of this chapter has focused on the challenges with ascending in elevation. Another consideration regarding high altitude is whether it is possible to exploit this environment to improve sea level exercise performance. A variety of approaches have been employed toward this end.

## Live High, Train Low

Interest in extended training at high altitude increased around the time of the Mexico City Olympics in 1968, which were conducted at an elevation of 2,300m (7,600ft). What has been discovered, however, was that while the prolonged exposure to high altitude was associated with benefits such as improved tissue oxygen delivery and utilization, elite athletes were unable to train at the same level of intensity, or training velocities, at which they competed at sea level. As a result, they were at risk for relative deconditioning. Recognition of this problem led to a search for alternative models of high altitude training including those where individuals live at high elevation but descend to low elevation for training.

The potential utility of this live high, train low approach was demonstrated in a seminal study by Levine and Stray-Gundersen in which they randomized a cohort of competitive runners to one of three groups following a four-week sea level training camp: a "high-low" group that lived at 2,500m (8,250ft) and came down to train at 1,250m (4,125 ft), a "high-high" group that lived and trained at 2,500 m, and a "low-low" group that lived and trained at 150m (495ft) (18). Of the three groups, only those in the high-low group demonstrated improved 5,000m time trial performance following return to sea level compared to baseline from the initial training camp. This improvement was sustained over a three-week period. Individuals in the high-low group were also able to reach higher training velocity at $VO_2$ max and a higher maximum steady state following return to sea level, improvements not seen in the other groups. One limitation of this study, which is now referred to as the Live High, Train Low (LHTL) model, was the fact that the runners could not be blinded to their group assignments, thereby raising concern that the results reflected a placebo effect. With this concern in mind, other investigators conducted a randomized, double-blind, placebo-controlled study in which highly trained cyclists were randomized to live for greater than sixteen hours a day for four weeks in either normobaric hypoxia equivalent to 3,000m or ambient air, while participating in training rides in ambient air outside the living facility (19). Contrary to the findings of Levine and Stray-Gundersen, these investigators found no differences in various measures of exercise performance.

Subsequent studies have sought to resolve discrepant results but despite much research, considerable debate persists in the scientific community about the overall utility of the LHTL model and best practices for implementing it (20). Questions persist, for example, as to whether normobaric hypoxia is sufficient, or the exposure should be through terrestrial high altitude (hypobaric hypoxia), as well as the appropriation of time spent in and out of the hypoxic environment. Another important question that has been raised is whether the administered "dose" of hypoxia makes a difference. For example, one study of the LHTL approach showed that improvements were seen in individuals who resided between 2,000 and 2,500m but not in those living at lower or higher elevations (21). Finally, for individuals who do implement the LHTL model, the optimal timing of return to sea level prior to competition remains unclear (22).

## Artificial Means of Hypoxic Exposure

Because the LHTL approach is not widely feasible, elite athletes and their coaches have sought alternative means of creating a hypoxic environment. A variety of models exist for exposing individuals to simulated or artificial hypoxia that vary based on the duration and degree of hypoxia and the means of administration (e.g., hypoxic tent or room versus hypobaric chamber). An example of such an approach would be sleeping in a hypoxic tent at home.

While anecdotal reports suggest such practices are increasingly common, the literature does not provide extensive evidence of benefit. A systematic analysis of available studies examining a variety of artificial hypoxia protocols concluded that a subset of these protocols may lead to benefit in sub-elite athletes, but are likely of no benefit in elite athletes (23). Aside from the expense and time commitment of these approaches, there is likely little risk associated with their use in fit individuals. Whether they provide benefit is not clear. For the elite athlete seeking a reliable means to improve sea level performance, the LHTL approach at terrestrial altitude is likely the best approach at present.

## Elevation Training Masks

In recent years, interest has been raised in the use of "elevation training" or "altitude" masks for the purpose of improving exercise performance. When fit with the mask, individuals breathe through a series of valves that can be adjusted to increase resistance to airflow and, therefore, alter the work of breathing. Despite their increasing use, there is little evidence to suggest these devices improve exercise performance. In one of the few recent studies, subjects were randomized to wear a mask or no mask during a six-week high intensity cycle training protocol. While both groups saw improvement in their $VO_2$ max, there were no differences between the two groups in the magnitude of the responses, suggesting the device adds no further benefit beyond that provided by the training protocol alone (24). There were also no significant differences within or between groups in hemoglobin concentrations or measures of pulmonary function. Importantly, although the devices are purported to simulate the hypoxia of high altitude, they do not actually manipulate the ambient or inspired partial pressure of oxygen and only affect airway resistance. One study did reveal that individuals exercising with the masks experienced hypoxemia, but this was due to an inability to sufficiently increase minute ventilation during exercise rather than due to an effect on inspired air and the degree of hypoxemia was less than what would be experienced at high altitude (25). Given the lack of sufficient data at this time, no recommendations can be made regarding use of these devices or the optimal ways to incorporate them into training regimens.

## Ethical Considerations

Elite athletes engaging in formal competitions must ensure that regular medications, medications taken for acclimation or altitude illness treatment, or other measures undertaken to improve performance do not violate the regulations of the World Anti-Doping Agency (WADA). This issue was raised over a decade ago with regard to altitude tents and other means of using hypoxic exposure to improve performance at sea level. Following considerable discussion and input from the scientific community (26), WADA elected not to ban the use of altitude tents or residence at high altitude. As of the writing of this chapter, these approaches are still permitted (27). Since 2009, WADA has administered the Athlete Biological Passport (ABP). Instead of testing for the presence of banned substances, ABP monitors specific parameters in athletes that may reflect doping, including an individual's hemoglobin concentration. This approach does not take into account trips to altitude or use of simulated hypoxia, and it remains unclear whether ABP correctly accounts for these factors (28).

## CHAPTER 15

# Cardiovascular Care for the Endurance Runner

## BY ANKIT B. SHAH AND AARON L. BAGGISH

## Key Points

1. Exercise-induced cardiac remodeling is an adaptive response to endurance training that is characterized by cardiac chamber enlargement and the ability to generate larger stroke volumes.

2. The purpose of pre-participation screening of competitive athletes is to identify cardiovascular disorders or abnormalities that can potentiate sudden cardiac arrest during athletic participation. The addition of twelve-lead electrocardiograms remains controversial.

3. Routine exercise decreases traditional cardiovascular risk factors including hypertension, cholesterol, body mass, and diabetes, as well as cardiovascular death.

4. Sudden cardiac death is a rare occurrence in the athlete and the cause of death varies by age.

5. Runners should not ignore subtle signs and symptoms such as an unexplained decrease in exercise tolerance or performance as they may be manifestations of underlying cardiovascular disease.

6. At present, there is no definitive data that support advising against "excess" exercise in healthy athletes and recreational exercisers engaged in high-level and extreme doses of physical and athletic activity.

## Introduction

Participation in competitive sport and vigorous recreational exercise, including long distance running, continues to gain in popularity in the United States and abroad. The number of American marathon finishers has increased from 353,000 in 2000 to 509,000 in 2015 (1). It is well accepted that routine exercise promotes favorable changes in traditional cardiovascular risk factors including obesity, diabetes, blood pressure, and cholesterol. However, exercise, irrespective of the "dose," is not completely protective against the development of heart disease. Additionally, the physiologic demands of exercise may precipitate symptoms or even sudden cardiac death in those with underlying heart conditions. The purpose of this chapter is to highlight the pertinent cardiovascular physiology of endurance running, the incidence, causes, and prevention of sudden cardiac death, the impact of exercise on cardiovascular risk factors, and the common cardiovascular symptoms encountered in endurance runners.

## Review of Exercise Physiology

Exercise intensity (external work) and the body's demand for oxygen are directly related. For distance runners, increasing speed and/or incline translates into an increasing need for oxygen. This demand is met by increasing pulmonary oxygen uptake ($VO_2$), the process by which relatively oxygen-deplete blood enters the lungs and refreshes its oxygen content. Transportation of oxygen-rich blood from the lungs to contracting skeletal muscle is the primary function of the cardiovascular system during all forms of endurance exercise and is measured as cardiac output (liters of blood moved per minute). Cardiac output is the product of stroke volume, the volume of blood ejected with each heartbeat, and heart rate. The Fick equation (cardiac output = $VO_2$ x arteriovenous oxygen difference) is used to quantify the relationship between cardiac output and $VO_2$. In healthy persons, there is a direct and inviolate relationship between $VO_2$ and cardiac output. Failure of the cardiovascular system to transport oxygen-rich blood to tissues in need is a common cause of exercise intolerance, the subjective sensation that accompanies diminishing performance, among runners with underlying heart disease.

With maximal exercise effort, coordinated rapid and sustained parasympathetic nervous system withdrawal with concomitant sympathetic nervous system activation can increase cardiac output five- to six-fold. Normal resting heart rate in the athlete may be less than forty beats per minute (bpm) climbing to over 200 bpm in a young athlete with peak effort. Cardiac output augmentation with exercise is predominately attributable to increases in heart rate. Maximum achievable heart rate decreases with age (2), is unaffected by exercise training (3), and varies inherently across individuals. A crude but practical estimate for maximum heart rate (in bpm) is 220 minus your age. This and similar proposed equations carry high standard deviations (very spread out) and are less accurate than values derived from maximal effort-limited exercise testing. We routinely recommend the latter for endurance athletes that use heart rate zones during training or competition.

Endurance-trained athletes commonly experience exercise-induced cardiac remodeling. This is an adaptive response to chronic exposure to the complex combination of intra-cardiac volume and pressure stresses that occur during sustained endurance exercise. Exercise-induced cardiac remodeling in the long distance runner is characterized by marked dilation of all four cardiac chambers, with minimal increase in cardiac wall thickness (4). This adaptive increase in the heart chamber's size enables the heart to generate a larger stroke volume. Despite lower resting heart rates at rest, cardiac output among distance runners is maintained by this increase in stroke volume. During exercise, stroke volume augments due both to an increased ventricular end-diastolic volume (volume of blood in the ventricle immediately before it contracts) and decreased end-systolic volume (volume of blood in the ventricular at the immediate conclusion of contraction). Stroke volume augmentation during exercise works in parallel with increasing heart rate to maximize a runner's ability to maximally increase cardiac output.

## Exercise Performance

For endurance exercises, relative exercise intensity is the most useful metric. Relative exercise intensity is defined as a percentage of some peak or maximal physiological parameter, such as heart rate or oxygen consumption, and thus requires the parameter in use to be measured with considerable accuracy. Relative exercise intensity, when used by athletes and coaches that understand its physiologic underpinnings, provides valuable information for the design of workouts with specific goals.

Maximal oxygen uptake (known as $VO_2$ max or peak $VO_2$), a physiological characteristic determined by rearranging the Fick equation, is the product of cardiac output and the maximal arteriovenous difference. $VO_2$ max is an important determinant of endurance performance and represents a true measure of cardiopulmonary capacity for an individual at a given degree of fitness and oxygen availability (5). $VO_2$ max declines with age (6) and is lower in women (7). In endurance athletes, $VO_2$ max is a not a particularly trainable number and has a physiologic maximum which is largely determined by genetics and perhaps early life exercise patterns. In contrast, ventilatory threshold is exquisitely sensitive to training. Ventilatory threshold, a measure of relative work effort described in terms of a percentage of $VO_2$ max, represents the point at which aerobic capacity can no longer meet the increasing physiologic demands of exercising muscles and effort dependent increases in anaerobic metabolism become a necessary source of energy (8). In untrained people, ventilatory threshold is typically 45 to 65 percent of $VO_2$ max but highly trained endurance athletes often push their ventilatory threshold up to 90 to 95 percent of the $VO_2$ max. During running efforts below the ventilatory threshold, oxygen supply meets or exceeds oxygen demand and athletes can sustain this level of work for extended periods assuming adequate hydration and nutrition. The inspiring performances of elite long distance runners, characterized by sustained high workloads over prolonged periods of time, require each major physiologic system described above: 1) appropriate heart rate recruitment; 2) marked increases in stroke volume due to exercise-induced cardiac remodeling; and 3) exceedingly high oxygen use parameters including $VO_2$ max and ventilatory threshold, to be working in perfect fashion.

## Sudden Cardiac Death: Incidence and Causes

Sudden cardiac death in the athlete is a rare but dreadful event that receives significant attention from the media. Such unexpected deaths are often met with a sense of confusion and bewilderment as athletic prowess is often thought to be synonymous with being healthy and devoid of cardiac disease. Acute bouts of physical exercise transiently increase the risk of sudden death among all people, including elite runners (9, 10). Importantly though, routine, vigorous physical activity lowers overall risk of sudden death in a dose dependent fashion, meaning that the fittest people are at the lowest risk. Among athletes, including long distance runners, absolute risk of sudden death is highest among those with underlying genetic or acquired cardiovascular disease (11, 12, 15). To date, the most definitive sudden death incidence data defining the risk of running come from the RACER study, which cataloged cardiac arrests among United States-based runners participating in organized marathon or half marathon races over a decade long period of study. The overall incidence of sudden death in the RACER study was one per 259,000 runners (13), which has been confirmed in smaller studies (14). This compares favorably to data derived from NCAA collegiate cross-country runners (one death per 41,695 participants/year) (15), triathlon participants (one death per 52,630 athletes) (16), and previously healthy middle aged joggers (one death per 7,620 participants) (9). In addition to demonstrating comparatively low rates of sudden death among runners, the RACER study confirmed higher rates among men, increasing risk with longer race distance, and a strong clustering of events in very close proximity to the finish line. Of note, the incidence of cardiac arrest among male marathon runners increased three-fold during the study period, which almost certainly reflects changes in the underlying health status of men turning to marathon running.

Causes of sudden cardiac death among athletes vary as a function of age. Younger athletes, defined as those younger than thirty-five years old, most commonly succumb to sudden death attributable to underlying congenital or genetic cardiovascular diseases. Primary genetic disorders of the heart muscle including hypertrophic cardiomyopathy (abnormally enlarged) and arrhythmogenic right ventricular cardiomyopathy (abnormal rhythm) are common causes of sudden death in younger runners. Mild forms of these and related diseases of the heart muscle may not impair cardiac function enough to limit exercise capacity, but may sufficiently increase the risk of malignant cardiac electric disturbances that lead to death. Congenital anomalies of the coronary arterial circulation, a form of birth defect that results in improper location of the coronary arteries, is another common cause of sudden death in young runners. Contemporary autopsy series derived from athletic victims of sudden death also routinely include cases with no clear anatomic abnormality. Such cases are presumed to be caused by primary disturbances of the cardiac electrical system, commonly referred to as channelopathies based on underlying defects in cardiomyocyte electrolyte channels.

Sudden death among athletes above the age of thirty-five years is less likely to be caused by congenital or genetic disease, but is more commonly due to disease that is acquired during an athlete's lifetime. In practice, the vast majority of collapse and sudden death among older athletes is caused by atherosclerotic coronary disease. The accumulation of coronary artery plaques may lead to sudden death during running via one of two distinct mechanisms. Coronary plaques, usually those of only mild to moderate severity, may rupture during exercise leading to the formation of an occlusive intravascular clot. In the absence of adequate blood supply, heart muscle downstream of this clot begins to die and may become electrically unstable. In our experience, this pathophysiologic process typically leads to symptoms typical of classic myocardial infarction (heart attack), chest pain, nausea, increases in perspiration, etc., rather than unheralded sudden death. In contrast, moderate to severe coronary plaques rupture relatively infrequently but promote sudden death from "demand or ischemia-mediated arrhythmia." Here, fixed blood supply that is limited by the diseased artery segment may sufficiently supply the heart muscle at low to moderate running speeds but become insufficient at higher workloads. When this threshold is exceeded, a common occurrence during the often unavoidable "finish line surge," oxygen-starved muscle may become sufficiently unstable such that it begins to fibrillate and ultimately disrupts the entire normal electrical activity of the heart. Thus, timely diagnosis and effective management of atherosclerotic coronary artery disease is of paramount importance in aging runners.

## Sudden Cardiac Death: Prevention

Sudden death may be a preventable tragedy. As discussed above, underlying diseases of the heart and blood vessels cause most cases of sudden death during running. Athletes with these conditions may experience warning symptoms including exertional chest pain, inappropriate exertional breathlessness, or the inability to keep up with peers. It is thus of paramount importance that runners of all ages be alerted to the need for vigilance of such symptoms and to report their occurrence immediately to medical professionals. Unfortunately, warning symptoms may be absent and the first manifestation of disease may be catastrophic collapse. Recognition of this fact has been the driving force behind efforts to design, develop, and disseminate pre-participation cardiovascular screening (PPCS) programs. The rationale for PPCS is predicated on the concept that some, if not most, forms of high-risk heart disease fail to produce warning symptoms, but are detectable by some form of screening. The purpose of PPCS is thus to identify cardiovascular disorders or abnormalities that can potentiate sudden cardiac arrest during athletic participation, and to take steps to reduce this risk by sport restriction and/or medical intervention. The American Heart Association and American College of Cardiology recommend a mandatory PPCS protocol for young competitive athletes which includes a focused history and physical examination [17]. The impact of this PPCS approach on sudden death incidence is unknown and its ability to detect culprit diseases may be of limited value [18, 19, 20]. This has led some expert consensus panels to recommend the inclusion of a twelve-lead electrocardiogram (ECG) as part of a more comprehensive PPCS protocol [21, 22]. Indeed, data comparing PPCS is confined to medical history and physical examination to one that includes ECG demonstrate that the ECG significantly increases PPCS's ability to detect high-risk conditions. However, it must be emphasized that the inclusion of ECG comes with increased risk of false-positive testing. This is a problem of decreasing magnitude in the era of increasingly accurate athlete ECG interpretation algorithms is one that will remain substantial in the field for the foreseeable future. As such, the addition of the ECG to a medical history and physical examination-based PPCS remains controversial and the interested reader is directed to several excellent discussions of this topic [17, 23, 24, 25]. All practitioners and organizations considering implementation of a PPCS program, with or without ECG, are urged to consult recent documents that address the strengths and limitations of this process [24].

Screening of runners at older age is less comprehensively dictated and receives comparatively little attention. The authors encourage runners above the age of thirty-five to work closely with primary care and sports cardiology experts to identify and treat cardiovascular disease risk factors. For older athletes planning to embark on or to intensify a training program, exercise testing should strongly be considered based on its ability to screen for many high-risk, often occult forms of acquired cardiovascular disease.

No PPCS approach will eliminate the problem of sport-associated sudden cardiac death. Thus, the ability to resuscitate cardiac arrest victims is a critical component of preparedness for those engaged in or sponsoring races and events. Survivors of cardiac arrest uniformly receive early bystander-administered CPR and have rapid access to automated external defibrillators (AED) at the scene of cardiac arrest (13). AEDs are portable devices capable of detecting and terminating malignant cardiac arrhythmias intended for use by the layperson. An effective resuscitation strategy, one key component of an overall emergency action plan, must include ample team members trained in CPR, the availability of AEDs, and rapid access to Emergency Medical Services with advanced cardiac life support capacities. However, immediate access to all these modalities may be challenging in longer distance races that occur in extreme environments. Therefore, development and practice of an emergency plan based on the race environment that attempts to integrate these key elements. Development and practice of an emergency action plan based on the race environment that attempts to integrate these key elements is mandatory for individuals and organizations that host athletic events including road races and track and field competitions.

## Impact of Exercise on Cardiovascular Risk Factors

Participation in regular- and moderate-intensity exercise confers beneficial cardiovascular risk profiles, reduced cardiovascular morbidity and mortality, and prevention of cardiovascular disease (26, 27, 28, 29, 30). However, daily exercise does not confer a free pass for dietary indiscretion and does not negate the risks associated with bad habits such as smoking and excessive alcohol intake. It is also noteworthy that exercise used in isolation as a risk factor reduction technique is often inadequate and many runners therefore benefit from a comprehensive approach that focuses on exercise dose, dietary modification, stress reduction, and conventional medical therapy. The following sections address the current knowledge base defining the impact of exercise on traditional cardiovascular risk factors.

# Cholesterol

Aerobic exercise training has been demonstrated to have a favorable impact on serum cholesterol. The strongest relationship seems to be with increased levels of high-density lipoprotein (HDL) (31), which is commonly referred to as the good cholesterol because it helps to remove the bad cholesterol from the arteries. While data is less consistent, exercise results in decreased low-density lipoprotein (LDL), the bad cholesterol that contributes to plaque formation and atherosclerosis, and triglycerides (32, 33). It should be noted that lowering total cholesterol by even 10 percent through diet or medication has been shown to result in a 27 percent reduction in the incident of cardiovascular disease (34). Beneficial effects of this magnitude on cholesterol can be seen with adherence to recommended guidelines of 150 minutes of moderate-intensity or seventy-five minutes of vigorous intensity exercise weekly (35). Additionally, incremental benefit may be achieved with exercise routines that exceed the minimum recommended levels (30). It must be emphasized that many runners with a genetic predisposition to high cholesterol will be unable to obtain optimal cholesterol profiles through diet and exercise alone. Thus, many runners will benefit from the addition of medication, most commonly the use of an HMG-Co-A Reductase inhibitor (i.e., a "statin"), which is a safe and effective class of medication that is well tolerated by most athletes.

# Blood Pressure

Hypertension (Systolic Blood Pressure > 140 mm hg or Diastolic Blood Pressure > 90 mm hg) is common among otherwise healthy athletes and is associated with the development of numerous forms of heart disease. While the beneficial impact of exercise training on blood pressure is well established, its impact is typically small with reductions in both systolic and diastolic blood pressure in the 2 to 4 percent range (36, 37, 38, 39, 40). Reductions in blood pressure are more pronounced in those with pre-existing hypertension (36, 37, 41). Long distance runners routinely exceed the minimum-recommended weekly exercise which should confer this beneficial effect on blood pressure. As such, runners with documented hypertension rarely reverse this problem with increasing training mileage and therefore should be treated with antihypertensive medications that have minimal effect on exercise physiology such as ACE-inhibitors or calcium channel blockers.

## Body Mass

The degree of change in body mass related to exercise is dependent on the net energy balance in the individual athlete, and thus requires increased energy expenditure while concomitantly relying on reduced caloric intake. Effective weight loss or stability is best achieved through a weekly exercise dose that is at least double the baseline recommended weekly activity (42, 43, 44, 45). There is a direct dose-response relationship between exercise and body mass with higher exercise workloads resulting in a greater decrease in body mass. Distance running is therefore one very effective component of an overall weight management strategy. It must be emphasized that runners seeking to reduce body mass must couple with deliberate control of caloric intake and should expect sustainable weight loss to occur slowly over months not weeks.

## Metabolic Syndrome and Diabetes Mellitus

Exercise training improves metabolic health, including increased insulin sensitivity and non-insulin-mediated skeletal muscle glucose metabolism (46, 47). The dose of exercise is directly associated with improvements in insulin sensitivity in a graded fashion with greatest improvements seen in those with high intensity and high duration of exercise (48, 49). Studies evaluating the impact of exercise on prevention and treatment of metabolic syndrome (risk factors that include abdominal obesity, high triglycerides, low HDL, hypertension, and elevated fasting blood sugar, all of which increase the risk for cardiovascular disease) and diabetes mellitus have shown that weight loss is the most important determinant to reduce the incidence of diabetes mellitus (50, 51). Athletes with the greatest exercise exposure have the lowest risk of developing diabetes mellitus even after controlling for weight loss and diet (50). Taken together, comprehensive lifestyle choices including exercise, diet, and weight loss have been shown to prevent metabolic syndrome and diabetes mellitus.

## Physical Fitness

There is an inverse relationship between cardiorespiratory fitness and both all-cause and cardiovascular mortality (52, 53, 54). Put simply, fitter people tend to live longer than less fit people. Fitness can be improved by increasing exercise frequency, intensity, or duration among people of all ages and both sexes (55, 56). Physical fitness is determined by many factors in addition to exercise including age, sex, body mass, and genetics (57). Physical fitness is far more responsive to exercise training than any of the traditional cardiovascular risk factors mentioned above. Additionally, routine physical activity attenuates the risk of cardiovascular disease and mortality more than that which can be explained by its impact on individual risk factors.

## Symptoms

Although participation in sport and exercise promotes good health, athletes are not immune to cardiovascular symptoms and disease. Commonly experienced symptoms are discussed below.

### Chest Pain

A differential diagnosis of chest pain in athletes is presented in Table 15-1. Cardiac causes of chest pain are relatively uncommon in athletes under thirty-five years old. While infrequent, cardiac causes include potentially life-threatening diseases such as coronary artery anomalies and hypertrophic cardiomyopathy. In contrast, older athletes with exertional chest discomfort are presumed to have atherosclerotic coronary artery disease until proven otherwise. Cardiac chest pain seen in athletes may be a result of coronary artery disorders, valvular heart disease, diseases of the heart muscle, disorders of the aorta, and electrophysiologic disorders.

Cardiac chest pain in runners generally presents as chest discomfort that reproducibly develops with exertion, resolves with rest, and is located in the substernal and/or left chest area. The discomfort is characterized as an ache, pressure, or tightness that can radiate to the jaw or arm, and can be accompanied with a sense of air hunger. Some athletes may experience chest discomfort during the initial few minutes of exercise that abates with continued exertion. This is commonly referred to as "warm-up angina," a process that reflects focal early exercise coronary artery blood flow insufficiency that is relieved by the subsequent recruitment of collateral arteries. It should not be ignored and should prompt comprehensive assessment for underlying atherosclerotic coronary artery disease. More subtle symptoms such as an unexplained decrease in exercise tolerance or inability to maintain prior race paces should be considered abnormal and medical evaluation should be sought.

In general, symptoms related to a blood flow imbalance in the heart, suggestive of congenital or acquired coronary artery disease, will resolve within several minutes of rest or reduced activity. Common alternative patterns of chest symptoms associated with non-coronary forms of cardiac disease and non-cardiac diagnoses deserved mention. Sudden, sharp tearing chest pain that radiates to the back and is precipitated by intense isometric exercise or body

**Table 15-1** Common non-cardiac causes of chest pain.

| System/Condition | Symptoms | Risk Factors |
|---|---|---|
| **Pulmonary** | | |
| *Asthma* | Exertional chest tightness, cough, wheeze, starts minutes after exercise or in recovery | Cold environment sports, endurance athletes, pool-based athletes |
| *Pneumothorax* | Spontaneous, seen in tall, thin athletes or after trauma, sharp pain worse with deep breathing | Weightlifting, running, SCUBA. Risk factors: smoking, substance abuse |
| *Pulmonary Embolus* | Acute chest pain, new wheeze, pleuritic pain (pain exacerbated with deep breathing), shortness of breath, bloody sputum | Those at risk for blood clots (surgery, trauma, history of clotting disorder, birth control pills) |
| *Pneumonia* | Focal, pleuritic, achy pain, cough, fever | Those with underlying pulmonary issues |
| *Pleurisy* | Sharp pain, worse with deep breath | Can occur after respiratory infections, pneumonia, or blunt chest wall trauma |
| **Gastrointestinal** | | |
| *GERD* | Heartburn, chest, or epigastric pain related to timing of food intake of dietary indiscretion. May be associated with belching, nausea, vomiting, sour taste, dry cough, sore throat | Runners, jumpers, weightlifters. Risk factors: hiatal hernia, NSAIDs, protein supplements |
| **Musculoskeletal** | | |
| *Traumatic Rib Fracture* | Pain, worse with deep inspiration or coughing | Those at risk for body collision/ blunt trauma (cyclists, team sports) |
| *Rib Stress Fracture* | Atraumatic chest wall pain with repetitive activity, ache in region of the rib | Rowers, tennis, basketball |
| *Costochondritis* | Peristernal sharp or pressure-like pain, worse with deep inspiration and upper limb movements. Pain with palpation | Rowers, weightlifters |
| *Intercostal Muscle Injury* | Pain between ribs exacerbated by movement, coughing and deep inspiration. Can generally identify triggering event preceding symptoms | Rowers, throwing motion, forceful twist of upper body |

collision may be manifestations of an aortic dissection, a potential life threatening condition that requires immediate medical attention. Chest pain following a systemic viral illness that is positional in nature, intensifies while lying supine and is not usually intensified by exercise, suggests pericarditis, an inflammation of the lining of the heart. The diagnosis of pericarditis often comes in conjunction with myocarditis, inflammation of the heart muscle with attendant risk of arrhythmia, and accordingly should be not be missed. Chest discomfort, often associated with mild to moderate air hunger, that is provoked by exercise in conjunction with climate extremes or seasonal allergens is often indicative of reactive airway disease (bronchospasm) and not primarily cardiac in nature. Chest discomfort that occurs immediately after a large meal may suggest a gastrointestinal cause. Non-cardiac causes of chest pain including symptoms of reactive airway disease or gastroesophageal reflux disease can last for minutes to hours.

## Syncope

Syncope, defined as a transient loss of consciousness accompanied by loss of postural tone, is common in trained athletes. The vast majority of syncope is unrelated to exercise or occurs after exertion (58). In the minority of athletes who have true exertional syncope, an underlying cardiac cause with associated risk of subsequent sudden death is generally identified. Syncope that truly occurs during intense exercise is a medical emergency and requires further evaluation by a cardiovascular specialist with expertise in caring for athletes. The typical evaluation for exertional history includes at a minimum, a detailed history and physical, electrocardiogram, echocardiogram, and exercise stress testing. Additional testing including the use of ambulatory rhythm monitoring is often indicated.

The majority of syncope in athletes is attributable to neurally mediated mechanisms, a disorder of autonomic regulation of postural tone. An aura with a feeling of warmth, diaphoresis (perspiration), or lightheadedness commonly precedes a loss of consciousness ranging from seconds to a minute. Typically, neurally mediated syncope manifests in the immediate post-exercise setting owing to a sudden reduction in venous return or at times unrelated to exercise when sudden nervous system fluctuations occurs (fright, anxiety, pain, etc.). The reduced venous return that triggers post-exertional syncope is caused by simultaneous cessation of skeletal muscle contraction and altered sympathetic/parasympathetic balance, which results in transient cerebral hypoperfusion (decreased blood flow to the brain). Neurally mediated syncope does not portend a poor prognosis but will recur if steps to avoid the underlying physiology are not taken.

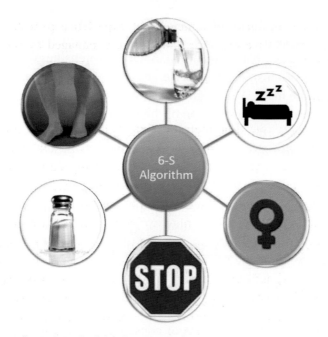

**Figure 15-1** "6-S Algorithm" for the prevention of recurrent neurally-mediated syncope among endurance runners.

Management of the athlete with syncope is dictated by the underlying cause. Those with significant structural or valvular heart disease should be restricted from sport participation until further work-up and management has been instituted. Neurally mediated syncope can be generally treated with conservative life-style measures. In the authors' practice, we use the "6-S Algorithm: Stop, Sips, Salt, Socks, Sleep, and Sex" as a basis for athlete education and therapeutic intervention (Figure 15-1). Initial emphasis should be placed on the principal avoidance tactic, which is to replace sudden termination of running with an active cool down period (Stop). In conjunction, we emphasize the importance of adequate hydration, with use of electrolyte containing fluids (Sips), and liberalized use of table salt or salty snacks, prior to training and races (Salt). In our experience, the use of commercially available athletic compression stockings both during and for a few hours after training and racing often additionally reduces the risk of recurrent syncope (Socks). Adequate sleep and recovery are required, especially during times of higher intensity training (Sleep), an issue that is particularly relevant among student athletes who are routinely forced to balance athletics with academic workload. Lastly, women with syncopal tendencies are often more likely to experience events in conjunction initiation or discontinuation of oral contraceptives (Sex). Recognition of this pattern often provides effective therapeutic options. The small minority of athletes that experience persistent symptoms despite these conservative measures may be best managed by the addition of pharmacologic therapy.

## Palpitations

A slow resting heart rate (less than 60 bpm) is common and normal among trained endurance athletes. Profound bradycardia (less than 40 bpm), a result of heightened parasympathetic activity, can be seen during sleep or rest and is not associated with a poor prognosis. Bradycardia is not concerning in the asymptomatic well-trained athlete. Documentation of an appropriate increase in heart rate with exercise is typically sufficient to exclude a pathologic process.

Premature beats (both atrial and ventricular) may be observed in trained athletes. Palpitations caused by premature beats are a common reason for runners to seek medical assistance. Because endurance runners are typically lean and in sync with their bodies, they may be particularly aware of such alterations in rhythm. Symptomatic premature beats are often described as a slight pause followed by a heavy, single, central thump. Evaluation with an echocardiogram is often required to exclude structural and valvular heart disease. Treadmill exercise stress testing can be utilized to assess the frequency of premature beats during exercise. Absence of structural heart disease in conjunction with suppression of premature beats during exercise is reassuring, and in this scenario premature atrial and ventricular beats are considered benign and without long-term consequences (59, 60).

Tachyarrhythmias (abnormal heart rhythms greater than 100 bpm), specifically atrial fibrillation, may be problematic in the trained athlete. Studies suggest that atrial fibrillation is more common in endurance athletes, especially in the older athlete, compared to their sedentary counterparts (61, 62, 63). The mechanisms responsible for development of atrial fibrillation in endurance athletes are speculative and are an area of active research. Atrial fibrillation in endurance athletes presents in two distinct forms. The first is parasympathetically mediated and is characterized by the onset of atrial fibrillation during times of slow resting heart rate which can potentiate atrial escape (64). Athletes with this form of atrial fibrillation generally experience bouts of arrhythmia during sleep, quiet rest, or after meals. This is commonly referred to as "vagally-mediated" atrial fibrillation and accounts for about 70 percent of atrial fibrillation in athletes (65). Vagally-induced atrial fibrillation almost never occurs with exercise, is four times more common in men (66), and can be precipitated by alcohol (67). The second form of atrial fibrillation is sympathetically mediated and is commonly triggered by exercise or significant psychological stress. The importance of differentiating these two forms of atrial fibrillation lies in their diametrically opposed treatment algorithms, a topic that is beyond the scope of this discussion.

Initial evaluation includes a thorough history and physical followed by blood tests with evaluation of electrolytes and thyroid function. Additional testing to evaluate for cardiac structure and function with an echocardiogram may be necessary. It is imperative to disclose to the use of supplements, caffeine, alcohol, and drugs as use of any of these may increase the likelihood of developing atrial fibrillation. Evaluation and treatment of underlying hypertension at rest and/or during exercise is required. Treatment is based on risk factors and symptoms with treatment options include detraining, which can decrease the number of atrial fibrillation episodes (68), medications, and a catheter-based ablation.

Healthy athletes undergoing exercise testing may demonstrate short bursts of non-sustained ventricular tachycardia. This finding should prompt testing to exclude structural heart disease which, if absent, portends a benign prognosis and does not require medical therapy or sport restriction. Symptomatic or sustained ventricular arrhythmias carry a high risk of adverse events and represent a medical emergency or at least a reason to prohibit run training and competition until a competent sports cardiologist conducts a comprehensive assessment.

## Can You Exercise Too Much?

While the majority of cardiovascular adaptations related to exercise are beneficial and associated with optimal cardiovascular performance, emerging preliminary data suggest that chronic exposure to high levels of exercise training may lead to adverse cardiovascular outcomes in certain subjects. Long-term training and competition have been associated with early-onset atrial fibrillation (69) and increased coronary artery calcifications (70). To what degree the favorable outcomes attributable to exercise apply to individuals who routinely exceed moderate exercise doses remains relatively uncertain. Recent studies suggest that subjects performing the highest amounts of exercise may lose some of the mortality benefits from exercise and excessive exercise may also be associated with adverse outcomes (Figure 15-2) (71, 72, 73). While there is data to support possible adverse outcomes associated with the highest levels of exercise, there are significant limitations in each of these studies. Additionally, it is important to acknowledge that epidemiologic studies of endurance athletes demonstrate reduced mortality and enhanced life span (74, 75, 76).

A thorough understanding of the individual athlete's risk must be considered. The benefits of increased exercise doses may be offset by underlying risk factor profiles in athletes such as family history of early coronary artery disease, risk

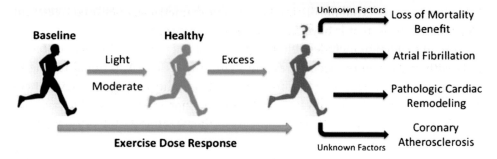

**Figure 15-2** Representation of the exercise dose-response from light/moderate to excess and possible pathologic outcomes associated with excessive levels of exercise. (Reproduced with permission from Kim J, Baggish AL. Physical Activity, Endurance Exercise, and Excess—Can One Overdose; Curr Treat Options Cardio Med (2016) 18:68).

factors such as hypertension and elevated cholesterol levels, and lifestyle choices including smoking, poor diet, and excessive alcohol intake. For the healthy endurance athlete, it may be that greater than moderate amounts of exercise may not have an incrementally better or worse impact on health. Currently available data suggest that high-dose exercise is associated with lower risks of cardiovascular disease and mortality than a sedentary lifestyle. Ideally, the athlete will engage in an open dialogue with his/her physician to make a collaborative decision regarding exercise prescription. This open dialogue will take into account all factors including the athlete's underlying cardiovascular risk, athletic aspirations, and unquantifiable benefits such as stress relief, personal satisfaction, and avoidance of unhealthy habits.

# Conclusions

Regular exercise has many cardioprotective effects including decreasing traditional cardiovascular risk factors and reducing cardiovascular death. The hallmark of an endurance athlete is exercise-induced cardiac remodeling, which is characterized by dilation of all four heart chambers and facilitates increases in stroke volume during exercise. At present, there is no definitive data that support advising against "excess" exercise in healthy athletes and recreational exercisers engaged in high level and extreme doses of physical and athletic activity. However, athletes are not immune to cardiovascular disease and the majority of sudden cardiac death in athletes is in the presence of underlying and previously undetected cardiovascular disease. Medical attention should be sought at the onset of unexplained changes in training patterns or cardiovascular limitations. Runners of all ages are encouraged to seek out cardiovascular care providers with both medical expertise and experience in caring for athletes. Ideally relationships with such providers will be forged during times of health and further relied on during times of concern and illness.

## CHAPTER 16

# Gastrointestinal Symptoms

## BY RICARDO JOSÉ SOARES DA COSTA

## Key Points

1. Gastrointestinal (GI) symptoms are a common feature in endurance running, found in 85 percent of multi-stage endurance races.
2. Running-associated GI symptoms (RAGS) are thought to be due to decreased blood flow to the gut blood vessels and alterations to the GI nervous system that disturbs normal gut structure, motility, and absorption.
3. Interrupted gut integrity and function may lead to both acute and chronic health implications.
4. RAGS may be minimized by maintenance of proper hydration, consuming tolerable amounts of carbohydrate while running, and training the gut to cope with intake during running.
5. The consumption of dietary supplements targeting gut health are not favorable in reducing RAGS.
6. Gluten-free diets in non-celiac runners do not reduce RAGS; however, there is emerging evidence for the positive effects of a diet low in short chain carbohydrates that are poorly absorbed by the small intestine (FODMAP).

## Introduction

In recent years there has been some debate among sport and exercise practitioners and researchers as to whether the gut is equipped to tolerate exercise. This question has arisen as the gut has been identified as a factorial barrier to achieving the "sub-two hour marathon," in regards to the development of gastrointestinal (GI) symptoms and the challenges of nutritional delivery (1, 2, 3). With the exponential growth in endurance running events and participation, ranging from local fun runs to multi-stage ultramarathons, an increasing number of running-associated gastrointestinal symptoms (RAGS) reported to medical teams have been observed in recreational to elite level runners. During an endurance runner's career, most would have suffered from RAGS during competition and training. For some endurance runners, this would be a sporadic occurrence, but for the majority this is more frequently experienced and originates from the body's normal physiological response to exercise. Such frequent occurrence of GI symptoms likely contributes to suboptimal training, poor race performance, or withdrawing from events entirely, and in the elite runner could be the difference in professional income. Indeed, RAGS are one of the key features for reduced running speed during competition, and are one of the leading reasons why runners have to stop during competition or withdraw from the competitive event (4, 5, 6).

More recently, concerns have been raised regarding the causal mechanisms of RAGS, whereby acute and chronic health implications have been identified stemming from exercise-induced gastrointestinal syndrome. This appears to be exacerbated by various intrinsic and extrinsic factors. Links between running intensity, duration, environmental conditions, and GI dysfunction (integrity, function, and symptoms) have now been established (7, 8, 9, 10). Also, training status and sex have been implicated in the occurrence and severity of RAGS (11). Recent investigations into the underlying causal mechanism for exercise-induced gut disturbance and dysfunction have found redistribution of blood flow to working muscles and away from the gut, as well as changes to GI nervous system activity leading to reduced gut function as key factors (12, 13, 14, 15). However, research into prevention and management strategies is scarce. Sporadic field-based studies have attempted to identify relationships between patterns of exercise, dietary behaviors (e.g., nutritional quantity and quality), and external stimuli (i.e., environmental conditions) with symptoms in various running populations. And in controlled laboratory trials some limited research has tried to establish the role of selective nutritional interventions in preventing or attenuating the various gut disturbances seen.

The aims of this chapter are to: 1) identify the prevalence of RAGS during endurance running; 2) provide understanding of the impact of endurance running on markers of gut integrity and function; 3) explore the concept of exercise-induced GI syndrome, the exacerbating factors, and links to GI symptoms; and 4) explore prevention and management strategies for markers of exercise-induced gastrointestinal syndrome and RAGS, as well as provide evidence-based practical recommendations.

## Prevalence during Running

It is well established in the literature that GI symptoms are a common feature of endurance running or endurance events that contain a running element (i.e., triathlon), more so than other endurance sports such as cycling (13, 16, 17). Table 16-1 provides a breakdown of field research assessing the impact of various durations of running exercise of the incidence and severity of GI symptoms. One key feature observed is evidence that the duration of running appears to increase the incidence of RAGS. Another observation is, despite the common belief that running promotes more lower-GI symptoms (flatulence including lower-abdominal bloating, urge to defecate, abdominal pain, abnormal defecation including loose water stools, diarrhea, and blood in stools) compared with upper-GI symptoms (projectile vomiting, regurgitation, urge to regurgitate, gastric bloating, belching, stomach pain, and heartburn), the literature supports the predominant occurrence of upper-GI symptoms and nausea during endurance running. However, there does exist substantial individual variation in symptom incidence and severity, and lower-GI issues during running do occur and induce a considerable burden on runners. Female endurance runners appear to be more prone to RAGS (11), and there has been greater GI issues in female endurance athletes observed during a laboratory controlled gut-challenge protocol, compared with male endurance athletes (20).

From a practical and performance perspective, it is clear that RAGS can impact running performance. Reducing GI symptoms by approximately 60 percent resulted in a 5 percent performance improvement in a one-hour running distance test (20, 21). Besides concerns of running performance, ceasing or withdrawing from competition in response to RAGS is another issues (4, 5, 6). Such gut disturbance can also impact carbohydrate intake during running—if you don't feel well, you are not going to want to eat or drink. For example, carbohydrate intake during running throughout an ultramarathon ranged from 24 g/h to 37 g/h, despite runners carrying and attempting to consume foods and fluids equating to greater than 60 g/h (22, 23). RAGS has also been shown to reduce overall daily energy and macronutrient intake, interfere with optimizing recovery nutrition (19), and led to a longer time (slower race speed) to complete a 230K multi-stage ultramarathon. So, what is causing RAGS? There is now good evidence that suggests a multi-factorial cause consistent with exercise-induced GI syndrome.

# Exercise-Induced Gastrointestinal Syndrome

## Primary Mechanisms

Exercise-induced GI syndrome is a complex array of normal physiological responses that occur at the onset of exercise that agitates and compromises gut

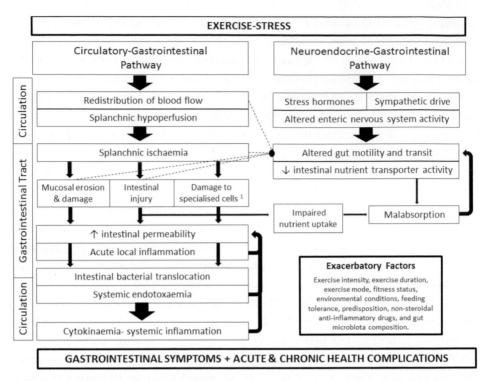

**Figure 16-1** Exercise-induced gastrointestinal syndrome. Specialised antimicrobial protein secreting cells, such as Paneth cells, aid in preventing intestinal originating pathogenic microorganisms gaining entry into the systemic circulation. Splanchnic hypoperfusion, and subsequent intestinal ischemia and injury (including mucosal erosion), results in altered gut motility.

integrity and function. Such responses include a redistribution of blood flow to the working muscle and peripheral circulation that reduces the total blood flow to the gut. Simultaneously, an increase in sympathetic ("fight or flight response") nerve activity and stress hormone production also reduces overall gut functional capacity. The combination of reduced gut blood flow and alterations to nervous system activity lead to a cascade of events that may result in GI symptoms and health issues, as shown in Figure 16-1.

The redistribution of blood away from the gut creates a state of decreased blood flow (hypoperfusion) and results in a lack of oxygen (ischemia) to the intestines (14, 25). At the onset of steady state exercise, blood flow to the gut area has been reported to decrease by 20 percent within ten minutes, with 80 percent reduction reported after one hour of running at 70 percent $VO_2$ max (26). Such a pronounced ischemic situation results in damage and erosion to the intestinal mucosal layer, injury to the intestinal lining cells (epithelium), and damage to specialized antimicrobial protein secreting cells responsible for protecting the internal body against intestinal located pathogenic agents (bacterial communities) (14, 27). The localized damage will initiate a local inflammatory cascade at the epithelium, further contributing to epithelial damage. Additionally, hypoperfusion induced intestinal ischemia also promote heightened intestinal permeability by either damaging the tight-junction protein barrier or promoting dysfunction to these regulatory proteins, subsequently increasing the tight-junction space (28). It has been shown that one hour of steady state running at 70 percent $VO_2$ max is sufficient to substantially increase intestinal permeability (29). Compromise to this integrated partnership of intestinal lining, specialized cells, and regulatory complexes poses a likely threat of invasion by bacterial agents that naturally reside within the gut (the gut microbiome), which can leak into the blood steam. Exercise-induced endotoxemia, or so-called blood poisoning, has been repeatedly observed after endurance running (7, 8).

Despite endotoxemia being a common outcome of exercise, the body has a protective mechanism in the form of antibodies that can tag bacteria with these toxins for destruction and clearance. However, anti-endotoxin antibodies have a limited capacity and tend to show reduced concentrations pre- to post-exercise (30, 31, 32). Therefore, a competent immune system and management strategies to avoid exercise-induced immunosuppression are warranted (33, 34). If the endotoxin load overrides the body's protective capability, a systemic immune response is classically observed, which presents as abnormal acute changes (increases or decreases) in heart rate and body temperature with or without a drop in arterial blood pressure (hypotension), swelling of limbs, and dizziness, delirium, and confusion with or without collapse (7, 8, 35). To counteract such a profound systemic endotoxin and pro-inflammatory response, in healthy individuals, anti-endotoxin antibodies and compensatory anti-inflammatory response are essential. Such responses have been shown to be more competent in endurance-trained individuals compared with sedentary or lower training status athletes (36).

Exercise-induced GI syndrome is also associated with changes that lead to an alteration in gut motility, with potential to reduce both the stomach (gastric) emptying and intestinal transit time (12). Upper-GI symptoms, such as bloating, nausea, and vomiting, are common symptoms reported by running during endurance running and likely reflect poor tolerance to the food and fluid consumed during running in adjunct with altered gut motility (11, 19). There is also evidence to show exercise impairs intestinal nutrient absorption transport mechanisms leading to malabsorption that may contribute to the symptoms (24,

**Table 16-1** Field-based exploratory research assessing the impact of endurance running on the incidence and severity of gastrointestinal symptoms.

| Competition | Occurrence of Gastrointestinal Symptoms [2] | Predominant Symptoms Reported | Upper- vs. Lower-Gastrointestinal Symptoms | References |
|---|---|---|---|---|
| Recreational (10km, 21km, 42km) | 45% | Belching, nausea, abdominal pain, regurgitation, and flatulence. | Upper > lower | (11) |
| Marathon | 4% | Heartburn, belching, bloating, stomach pain, nausea, and regurgitation. | Upper > lower | (16) |
| Half Ironman triathlon | 14% | Heartburn, belching, bloating, stomach pain, nausea, and regurgitation. | Upper > lower | (16) |
| Ironman triathlon | 31%–32% | Heartburn, belching, bloating, stomach pain, nausea, and regurgitation. | Upper > lower | (16) |
| Mountain Ironman triathlon | 93% | Stomach problems, flatulence, belching, bloating, urge to regurgitate, regurgitate, and nausea. | Upper > lower | (5) |
| 161km ultramarathon | 60% | Nausea, abdominal pain, diarrhea, and regurgitation. | Upper > lower | (18) |
| 24 hr ultramarathon [1] (122–208km) | 73% | Regurgitation, urge to regurgitate, belching, bloating, and nausea. | Upper > lower | (19) |
| Multi-stage ultramarathon [1] (5-days, 230km) | 85% | Regurgitation, urge to regurgitate, belching, bloating, and nausea. | Upper > lower | (19) |

[1] Severe gastrointestinal symptoms. [2] Percentage occurrence of gastrointestinal symptoms within the participant cohort.
Upper > lower: greater reports of upper-gastrointestinal symptoms compared with lower-gastrointestinal symptoms.
Upper-gastrointestinal symptoms (gastro-oesophageal and gastro-duodenal originated): projectile vomiting, regurgitation, urge to regurgitate, gastric bloating, belching, stomach pain, and heartburn/gastric acidosis.
Lower-gastrointestinal symptoms (intestinal originated): flatulence including lower-abdominal bloating, urge to defecate, abdominal pain, abnormal defecation including loose water stools, diarrhea, and blood in stools.

38). However, it is unclear if the impaired nutrient absorption mechanisms are due to the hypoperfusion and ischemic injury, or reduced gut activity associated with increased sympathetic drive. This is concerning as carbohydrate intake during endurance running is a common and advised practice, especially when running for more than two hours. Considering exercise has the potential to interfere with intestinal carbohydrate transportation, it has recently been suggested that mal-absorbed nutrients reaching the end of the small intestine (ileum) may promote lower-GI symptoms through increased content being delivered to the large intestine and increasing intestinal pressure (39, 40). This may also suppress gastric emptying and motility via the ileal brake feedback mechanisms (41, 42), thus potentially exacerbating upper-GI symptoms. A strong correlation has been shown between carbohydrate malabsorption and upper-GI symptoms, which supports the novel idea that lower-GI issues (i.e., nutrient malabsorption as a result of intestinal transporter dysfunction) may have implications in the stomach and upper-intestine (20, 21).

Exercise-induced GI syndrome is a complex multi-factorial interaction among the gastrointestinal, circulatory, immune, and nervous systems. It is clear that in assessing whether prevention and management strategies are effective, a global approach should be adapted to assess the impact on the array of GI disturbances arising from exercise stress.

## Health Implications

There is clear evidence that shows exercise-induced changes to gut physiology lead to GI symptoms. However, since exercise gastroenterology is a relatively new area of research, it is less clear how such gut disturbances results in acute and chronic term health complications. For example, acute colitis (injury to the large intestine that results in lower-GI symptoms including lower abdominal pain, abnormal defecation, and blood in stools), is a common feature of endurance running, and is seen to be reversible with recovery time (43, 44, 45). The long-term consequences of repetitive exercise-induced intestinal injury or systemic inflammation are still to be determined; however, its potential link to autoimmune disease, GI disease, and chronic fatigue in high-risk individuals are areas of current research (46, 47, 48). Any potential health implication arising from exercise-induced GI syndrome is likely to come from either: 1) the repetitive injury to the intestinal epithelial and insufficient recovery time between insults; 2) paralysis of the intestinal muscles associated with intestinal hypoperfusion, ischemia, and altered GI nervous system activity during exercise; or 3) local and systemic inflammatory responses associated with intestinal injury and permeability. Table 16-2

**Table 16-2** Potential acute and chronic health complications arising from the physiological alterations of exercise-induced gastrointestinal syndrome.

| Circulatory-Gastrointestinal Pathway | Neuroendocrine-Gastrointestinal Pathway | Performance Implications |
|---|---|---|
| **Acute** | **Acute** | |
| Nausea | Nausea | Longer time to complete |
| Involuntary projective vomiting | Involuntary | running event[1] |
| Involuntary explosive diarrhea | projective vomiting | Reduced total daily intake |
| Gastric lesion and necrosis | Involuntary | Reduced intake during running |
| Intestinal lesion and necrosis | explosive diarrhea | Poorer recovery nutrition |
| Hemorrhagic gastritis | Malabsorption | Reduced running performance |
| Transient intestinal ischemia | Paralytic ileus | (distant test)[1] |
| Reversible ischemic colitis | | |
| Malabsorption | | |
| Systemic endotoxaemia | **Chronic** | |
| Systemic inflammatory response | Ischemic bowel disease | |
| **Chronic** | | |
| Ischemic bowel disease | | |
| Chronic malabsorption (i.e., irritable bowel syndrome) | | |
| Chronic inflammatory conditions (i.e., inflammatory bowel disease) | | |
| Chronic fatigue | | |
| Underperformance (overtraining) syndrome | | |

[1]Symptoms and nutritional status induced.

highlights some key acute and chronic health implications suggested in the current literature, and also potential performance implications.

## Exacerbatory Factors

Besides the primary causal mechanism involved in the development of exercise-induced gastrointestinal syndrome, there are certain extrinsic and intrinsic factors (Figure 16-1 and Table 16-3) that may exacerbate impairment in gastric emptying or intestinal transit, impairment of intestinal nutrient transporters and subsequent malabsorption, intestinal injury and inflammation, intestinal permeability, or systemic endotoxemia.

## Prevention and Management Strategies

There are a substantial amount of anecdotal reports suggesting a wide array of diets, nutritional supplements, and pre-exercise behaviors to prevent RAGS.

Despite a substantial amount of research being conducted to understand the potential causal mechanisms for RAGS, very limited research has been done to determine effective prevention and management strategies. To date, controlled laboratory research have explored the impact of dehydration, nutritional interventions prior to exercise, feeding during running, gut-training, and dietary modification on markers of gut integrity, function, or symptoms.

## Maintenance of Euhydration

Exercise-induced dehydration is a common and accepted feature of endurance running. There is substantial evidence that shows the progression of dehydration during exercise lead to decrements in exercise performance. This is especially apparent when running in hot, ambient conditions (23, 64). Exercise-induced body mass losses greater than or equal to 2 percent (as a proxy for dehydration) have been linked to metabolic dysregulation, heat intolerance, cardiovascular strain, and subsequent inability to maintain exercise workload (65, 66, 67). There is now emerging evidence that dehydration may also have a negative impact on the gut leading to great incidence and severity of RAGS. For example, starting exercise while dehydrated resulted in impaired gastric emptying and greater GI symptoms, including nausea, compared with starting exercise in a euhydrated state (68) (but did not appear to influence intestinal transit time, intestinal permeability, or glucose intestinal absorption in response to exercise). Alternatively, starting exercise euhydrated and developing dehydration during two hours of running at 70 percent $VO_2$ max resulted in higher intestinal injury, malabsorption, and greater gut discomfort and RAGS (predominantly upper-GI symptoms and nausea), compared with maintaining euhydration throughout a run (69). Additionally, mild body water losses during one hour of running at 70 percent $VO_2$ max increased intestinal permeability above resting levels (70). This supports some indirect evidence from exploratory field studies in ultra-endurance runners suggesting that maintaining euhydration during ultramarathon competition may be an important factor in attenuating exercise-induced endotoxemia (7, 8). Furthermore, in hot conditions participants who presented with dehydration showed higher circulatory endotoxin concentrations compared with those who maintained euhydration with ad libitum water intake during two hours of running at 60 percent $VO_2$ max (71).

Starting a run in a euhydrated state and striving to maintain euhydration during running using tolerable feeding regimes can attenuate exercise-induced alterations to gut integrity and function, as well as reduce the incidence and severity of RAGS. Keeping in mind that over-hydration is not recommended because of concerns for exercise-associated hyponatremia, which is also associated with RAGS (9).

**Table 16-3** Extrinsic and intrinsic factors that may exacerbate disturbances to gut integrity and function, and promote greater incidence and severity of gastrointestinal symptoms.

| Exacerbatory Factor | Outcomes and Examples | References |
|---|---|---|
| **Exercise intensity**[1] | – Exercise of moderate intensity appears to promote modest disturbance to markers of gut integrity, function, and gastrointestinal symptoms.<br>– Exercise intensities of equivalent to ≥60% $VO_2$ max are reported to significantly disturbed markers of gut integrity, function, and promote gastrointestinal symptoms, with exercise intensities of >70% $VO_2$ max and intermittent high intensity exercise reported to impair gastric emptying.<br>– High exercise intensities (e.g., ~80% $VO_2$ max equivalent) requires shorter exercise durations to promote gut disturbance. | (12,13,49,50) |
| **Exercise duration**[1] | – Field-based exploratory work has clearly shown that the longer the exercise duration the greater disturbance to markers of gut integrity, function, and gastrointestinal symptoms.<br>– Greater exercise-induced increases in plasma I-FABP (i.e., marker of intestinal injury) after 3 hours of running (pre- to post-exercise peak value 4020 pg/ml) in thermoneutral conditions (~20°C) compared with 2 hours of running (pre- to post-exercise peak value 583 pg/ml) in the same conditions.<br>– Pronounced epithelial permeability, systemic endotoxaemia, systemic cytokinaemia, and symptoms in ultramarathon competition with distances >100km. | (6-8,12,20,51-53) |
| **Exercise mode**[1] | – Running exercise promotes greater gastrointestinal disturbance than other exercise modes (e.g, cycling, swimming, rowing, and gym fitness).<br>– The larger biomechanical vibration in the abdominal region in running compared with cycling, possibly contributing to the greater incidence and severity of gastrointestinal symptoms reported in running.<br>– Longer orocaecal transit time and greater intestinal permeability has been observed in 90 minutes of steady state running compared with steady state cycling, resulting in greater gastrointestinal symptoms.<br>– Mode of exercise does not appear to impact of gastric emptying in response to feeding during exercise. | (17,51,53) |

| Exacerbatory Factor | Outcomes and Examples | References |
|---|---|---|
| Fitness status[1] | – It has been previously reported that fatal health outcomes associated with exertional-heat stress induced gut perturbations (i.e., increased intestinal permeability and subsequent endotoxaemia leading to sepsis and systemic inflammatory response syndrome) are linked to the fitness level of individuals (i.e., individual not fit for task and exertional-heat stress was too great). <br> – Lower anti-endotoxin responses have been observed in sedentary and lower fitness individuals, compared with trained athletes. | (36,54,55) |
| Environmental conditions[1] | – Running in cold to thermoneutral conditions (i.e., $\leq 20°C$) appears to have minimal impact on gastrointestinal status; however, at the onset of heat exposure there is an abrupt increase in the perturbations to gut integrity and subsequent systemic responses (endotoxemia and cytokinemia). For example, greater intestinal injury is observed after 2 hours of steady state running in 30°C and 35°C compared with 20°C. | (7,8,52) |
| Feeding tolerance[1] | – Concerns have recently been raised by sports nutrition practitioners and endurance athletes (especially triathlon, running, ultra-endurance, and adventure athletes) that carbohydrate intake during exercise, when the gut is in a compromised state, is not tolerable, leading to debilitating gastrointestinal symptoms. This intolerance is also dependant on consumption volume (i.e., the higher the intake the more likelihood for gastrointestinal symptoms). <br> – Consuming 90 g/h of multi-transportable carbohydrates (2:1 glucose to fructose ratio) during 2 hours of running at 60% $VO_2$ max in thermoneutral conditions contributes considerably to gastrointestinal symptoms compared with consuming water alone or 45 g/h of a glucose solution during 2 hours of running at 60% $VO_2$ max in 35°C ambient conditions. Such high dosage resulted in symptoms appear 30 minutes into running, peaking post-exercise, with 100% of participants reported at least one gastrointestinal symptom during the gut-challenge trial, with 67% reporting at least one severe gastrointestinal symptom and 28% regurgitation into the oral cavity during the gut-challenge protocol. <br> – Consuming 90 g/h of multi-transportable carbohydrates (2:1 glucose to fructose ratio) during 2 hours of running at 60% $VO_2$ max in thermoneutral conditions resulted in carbohydrate malabsorption in 68% of endurance athletes, which was associated with reported gut discomfort and upper-gastrointestinal symptoms. | (12,16,21-23) |

| Exacerbatory Factor | Outcomes and Examples | References |
|---|---|---|
| | - Total energy density and subsequent osmolality of the consumed bolus (i.e., foods and/or fluids) during running influences the rate of gastric emptying, whereby the higher the energy density and osmolality the slower the emptying rate. | |
| Nonsteroidal anti-inflammatory drugs[1] | - Nonsteroidal anti-inflammatory drugs (NSAIDs) (e.g., aspirin and ibuprofen) are known as gastrointestinal irritants, impacting stomach gastric secretions, bicarbonate release in the duodenum, and erosion of the mucosal lining along the gastrointestinal tract. NSAIDs use has been linked to gastrointestinal injury and dysfunction, including nausea, regurgitation, dyspepsia, gastrointestinal ulceration, gastrointestinal bleeding, and abnormal defecation (e.g., diarrhea). <br><br> - Increases in intestinal injury, and increased gastric and intestinal permeability, can be markedly increased after exercise with the use of NSAIDs before exercise. For example, gastroduodenal permeability was substantially increased, compared with placebo, after 1.3 g of aspirin administration the night before and immediately before 60 minutes of running at 68% $VO_2$ max. Meanwhile, I-FABP was substantially elevated after endurance cycling, in which 400 mg of ibuprofen was administered before exercise (peak I-FABP value 875 pg/ml), compared with no ibuprofen administration (474 pg/ml). | (9,56-58) |
| Predisposition[2] | - Longer orocaecal transit time and increased intestinal permeability has been observed in symptomatic athletes after 90 minutes of steady state running compared with asymptomatic athletes, suggesting there may be some predisposition to exercise-induced gastrointestinal syndrome. <br><br> - There exists two groups of runners, those who experience gastrointestinal symptoms occasionally and those who experience gastrointestinal symptoms repeatedly, suggesting a potential gene variant(s) for predisposition, which warrants further investigation. <br><br> - It is speculated that individuals with predisposition to gastrointestinal diseases or disorders associated with intestinal damage, inflammation, autoimmune responses, and/or sensitivity (e.g., celiac disease, inflammatory bowel disease, irritable bowel syndrome, diverticular disease, gastro-oesophageal reflux disease) may be more prone to exercise-induced gastrointestinal perturbations and associated symptoms. | (17,46,59) |

| Exacerbatory Factor | Outcomes and Examples | References |
|---|---|---|
| **Gut microbiota**[2] | – There is currently evidence to suggest that exercise and diet has the ability to alter the gut microbiota composition, to either enhance gut protective bacterial communities or promote dysbiosis.<br>– Athletes (rugby players) training on a regular basis show higher gut bacterial diversity and higher *Firmicutes* to *Bacteroides* ratio compared to healthy controls. Moreover, regular exercise is associated with higher levels of *Bifidobacterium, Lactobacillus,* and *Clostridium leptum,* which are key short chain fatty acid (e.g., butyrate) producing bacteria, linked to augmented epithelial barrier function.<br>– To date no research has investigated whether the gut microbiota composition influences the degree of exercise-induced perturbations to gut integrity and function, and gastrointestinal symptoms in response to an acute bout of exercise. Considering dysbiosis has the ability to alter the structure and function of the epithelial lining (e.g., mucosal barrier erosion, intestinal injury and permeability, and injury to specialized anti-microbial protein secreting cells), it is speculated that the proportion of *Firmicutes, Bacteroides, proteobacteria,* and *actinobacteria,* and numbers of short chain fatty acid producing bacterial communities may influence gut status in response to exercise. | (60-63) |

[1]Extrinsic factor.[2] Intrinsic factor.

**Table 16-4** Summary of research investigating the impact of nutritional interventions on markers of gut integrity.

| Nutritional Intervention | Exercise Stress and Population | Gut Integrity Outcomes | References |
|---|---|---|---|
| **Antioxidants[1]** | | | |
| Vitamin E 1000 IU/day for 2 weeks vs. placebo (soya lecithin). | – Marathon competition.<br>– 26 male and female marathon runners. | – Vitamin E supplementation did not improve exercise-induced intestinal permeability. | (74) |
| L-ascorbic acid 1000 mg pre-exercise vs. control exercise test. | – Incremental exercise test to exhaustion.<br>– 10 healthy male physical education students. | – L-ascorbic acid supplementation had minimal impact on exercise-induced endotoxemia. | (75) |
| **Amino acids** | | | |
| L-arginine[2] 30 g/day for 14 days vs. placebo (glycine). | – Marathon competition.<br>– 23 male and female marathon runners. | – L-arginine supplementation did not improve exercise-induced intestinal injury or permeability. | (76) |
| Glutamine[3] 0.9 g/kg of fat-free mass per day for 7 days vs. matched placebo. | – 1 hour running at 70% $VO_2$ max in 30°C ambient conditions.<br>– 8 endurance-trained male and female participants. | – Glutamine supplementation attenuated exercise-induced increases in intestinal permeability. | (77) |
| Glutamine[3] 0.9 g/kg of fat-free mass pre-exercise vs. matched placebo. | – 1 hour running at 70% $VO_2$ max in 30°C ambient conditions.<br>– 7 endurance-trained male and female participants. | – Glutamine supplementation attenuated exercise-induced increases in intestinal permeability.<br>– Glutamine supplementation had minimal impact on exercise-induced endotoxemia and cytokinemia. | (72) |
| L-Citrulline[2] 10 g pre-exercise vs. placebo (L-alanine) | – 1 hour running at 70% $VO_2$ max.<br>– 10 healthy male participants. | – L-citrulline supplementation attenuated exercise-induced hypoperfusion and intestinal injury during exercise only, but not recovery. | (78) |

| Nutritional Intervention | Exercise Stress and Population | Gut Integrity Outcomes | References |
|---|---|---|---|
| | | – L-citrulline supplementation had no impact on exercise-induced increases in intestinal permeability. | |
| **Bovine colostrum[3]** | | | |
| 60 g during running training vs. whey protein vs. control. | – 8 weeks running training (x3 sessions per week). Running at lactate threshold for 45 minutes.<br>– 30 healthy male participants. | – Colostrum supplementation increased intestinal permeability in response to exercise, compared with whey and control. | (79) |
| 20 g/day for 14 days vs. placebo (milk protein concentrate). | – 20 minutes running at 80% VO$_2$ max.<br>– 12 healthy male participants. | – Colostrum supplementation attenuated exercise-induced increases in intestinal permeability. | (49) |
| 12.5 g/day for 10 days vs. skimmed milk powder. | – 1½ hours cycling at 50% W max.<br>– 9 male endurance athletes. | – Colostrum supplementation had no impact on exercise-induced cytokinemia or alterations in immunoglobulins compared with skim milk powder. | (80) |
| 1.7 g/kg for 7 days. | – 1½ hours of exercise (cycling and running) of altered intensities in 30°C ambient conditions.<br>– 7 endurance-trained male and 8 untrained male participants. | – Colostrum supplementation had no impact on exercise-induced intestinal injury, intestinal permeability, and cytokinemia. | (81) |
| 10 g/day for 14 days vs. 10 g/day with 37.5 mg zinc carnosine vs. 37.5 mg zinc carnosine only vs. placebo. | – 20 minutes running at 80% VO$_2$ max.<br>– 8 healthy male participants. | – Colostrum supplementation attenuated exercise-induced increases in intestinal permeability. | (82) |

[1]Exercise-induced endotoxaemia may be mediated by free radicals, therefore antioxidant supplementation may ameliorate endotoxaemia. [2]L-citrulline and L-arginine are precursors for nitric oxide production, which is a potent vasodilator, potentially enhancing blood flow into the intestinal microvasculature reducing exercise-induced hypoperfusion and ischaemic. [3]Glutamine and bovine colostrum may enhance the expression of heat shock proteins (i.e., proteins that protect cellular membrane under period of stress), which may protect the intestinal enterocytes, reduce intestinal permeability, and attenuate the development of local inflammatory pathways.

## Nutritional Interventions

Research on nutritional interventions that affect gut integrity in response to exercise has focused on antioxidants, certain amino acids, and bovine colostrum (milk secreted from post-calving cows) (Table 16-4). Considering the overall outcomes, there appear to be some ambiguity with no clear pattern for the improvement in gut status, and no indication of impact on RAGS. Due to the experimental protocols offering moderate exercise stress (72), the observed changes likely do not reflect the substantially greater responses observed in field research (7, 73), thus limiting conclusion and transferability into the practical setting. Since most of the research focus has been on permeability markers of gut integrity, recommendations from these studies are difficult to ascertain and there is risk for misinterpretation. For example, concluding that, "permeability is reduced, therefore this is a good thing," may be inaccurate as there is no evidence of improved gut motility, malabsorption, intestinal injury, systemic responses, and symptoms. And with the limited gut integrity markers used in most studies and absence of symptom data, the ambiguous outcomes, and the modest degree of responses observed, there is no clear evidence that nutritional supplement intervention prevents or reduces exercise-induce changes to gut integrity or RAGS. The exception is for L-citrulline supplementation pre-exercise, which showed a modest decrease in intestinal ischemia and injury during steady state cycling, but failed to maintain the improvements during the gut reperfusion period after exercise, resulting in similar intestinal ischemia and injury as placebo (78).

## Feeding during Exercise

It appears the frequent and consistent consumption of carbohydrate during exercise is a protective strategy against exercise-induced GI alterations. It has been found that consuming 15 g of carbohydrate pre-exercise and every twenty minutes during two hours of running at 60 percent $VO_2$ max in ambient conditions, compared with water alone, abolished intestinal injury, reduced intestinal permeability, and reduced systemic endotoxemia (86). Such quantities of carbohydrate (45 g/h) appear to be well tolerated during exercise. Higher rates (up to 90 g/h) of carbohydrates during running have been recommended (87), but appear to be less tolerable (20, 21).

Outcomes of research on the role of feeding during exercise on gut hypoperfusion and integrity demonstrate that some form of tolerable nutrition within the gut during running appears to maintain intestinal perfusion, reduce ischemia related injury, and changes to the intestinal lining without exacerbating symptoms. Therefore, all runners would benefit from frequently consuming nutrition during exercise, especially carbohydrates. Some runners will find it difficult to consume foods and fluids during running. In this case, training the gut to improve nutritional tolerance would be a valuable option.

# Gut Training

Due to the high adaptability of the gut, there have been opinions that there is an intrinsic ability for the gut to be trained to tolerate carbohydrate intake during exercise and attenuating occurrence of GI symptoms. A recent study investigated a two-week period of daily repetitive gut-challenge, whereby participants consumed 90 g/h carbohydrate (2:1 glucose to fructose ratio) or a carbohydrate-rich food during one hour of running at 60 percent $VO_2$ max, which resulted in a 44 percent and 49 percent reduction in gut discomfort, 60 percent and 63 percent reduction in total Gl symptoms, 64 percent and 62 percent in upper-GI symptoms, respectively, in response to a gut-challenge protocol (20, 21). Despite female runners reporting greater occurrence and severity of RAGS, male runners responded better to the gut training, showing greater improvements in overall gut discomfort, total, and upper-GI symptoms. A history of RAGS and accustomed to training with race nutrition did not appear to influence gut-training outcomes. Gut-training eliminated malabsorption and increased blood glucose availability, thus providing some evidence for mechanistic improvement. The observations also support the protective effect of carbohydrate presence in the gut during exercise on intestinal injury. Considering that RAGS improvements were observed in a wide range of runners (e.g., performance level, sex, and symptom history), research outcomes suggests all runners could benefit from a structured gut-training protocol for two weeks leading into competition. It would also be advised to incorporate gut-training within normal training regimes.

## Probiotics

There is generally advocacy for probiotic supplementation in athletes with the aim of optimizing gut health and preventing gut related issues. It is a common habit for runners to consume probiotics leading into competition, during periods of intensified training, and episodes of ill health. Considering that probiotic bacteria have demonstrated some favorable effects in people with compromised intestinal integrity (i.e., inflammatory diseases of the gut) (88), it is suggested that probiotic supplementation may also show favorable effects in response to exercise-induced gut changes. An observation from a 230K multi-stage ultramarathon conducted in hot ambient conditions reported that runners who consumed high volumes of commercially available probiotic beverages in the competition lead-up week had no RAGS (7). This is suggestive that probiotics may play a role in preventing RAGS, considering that 85 percent of the participant cohort reported severe symptoms during the competition (7).

Previous research has established that as dosage of probiotic supplementation increases, the proportion of specific bacteria numbers also increases (89). This provides a higher probiotic dosage over a short duration of time, or a lower probiotic dosage over a more prolonged time period will create an abundance of specific dosage strains of bacteria and a subsequent protective effect. To date, only three controlled laboratory trials have investigated the impact of probiotic supplementation on markers of gut integrity in response to exercise stress. Four weeks of capsule form lactobacillus, bifidobacterium, and streptococcus supplementation did not affect exercise-induced changes to gut integrity or systemic endotoxemia compared with placebo (50). Similarly, fourteen weeks of multi-species probiotics had no effect on gut integrity (90). A more recent study observed that oral ingestion of a commercially available probiotic beverage containing *Lactobacillus casei* for seven consecutive days before two hours of running at 60 percent $VO_2$ max in hot ambient conditions resulted in a substantially greater endotoxemia during the recovery period, compared with placebo (71). Additionally, no difference in RAGS was evident between the probiotic and placebo groups.

In summary, contrary to common belief, it appears that probiotic supplementation (capsule or beverage) does not result in more favorable outcomes on gut integrity or RAGS. Therefore, it is advised to withhold intake before running, especially if running the hot conditions.

## Dietary Modification

There has recently been an exponential growth in the number of non-celiac athletes following a gluten-free diet. There are also a substantial amount of testimonials and anecdotal evidence, especially from professional athletes, that indicate improvements in GI symptoms and sports performance from following a gluten-free diet. This is supported by an observation that 41 percent of a surveyed athletic population adhered to a gluten-free diet, with the majority being non-celiac. They believed the diet improved their overall gut integrity and enhanced their exercise performance (94). An elegant study analyzed the dietary effect on healthy competitively-trained male and female cyclists. After a ten-day washout period, the study participants followed a gluten-containing or gluten-free diet for seven consecutive days, and then rode at 75 percent maximum exercise intensity for forty-five minutes, followed by a fifteen-minute time trial. There was no observed difference in performance, GI symptoms, or intestinal injury between the two groups (95).

Considering there is not strong scientific rationale or support for the adherence of a gluten-free diet in a non-celiac athlete, it is unlikely that a gluten-free diet will reduce RAGS. However, the application of a low FODMAP diet (short chain carbohydrates that are poorly absorbed by the small intestine) appears to be more convincing. There is now substantial evidence to support the role of a low FODMAP diet in the management of GI symptoms, similar to those experienced by runners, in individuals suffering from irritable bowel syndrome (96, 97). Furthermore, a case study showed that a short-term low FODMAP diet (i.e., reducing the FODMAP content from 81 g/day to 7 g/day) resulted in an elimination of RAGS during running and rest periods in a multi-sport athlete (98). Research into the impact of FODMAP dietary manipulation on markers of gut integrity, function, and symptoms are still in the infancy stage; further studies are needed to determine the impact of a low FODMAP diet in the prevention and management of RAGS.

Exercise-induced endotoxemia may be mediated by free radicals, therefore antioxidant supplementation may ameliorate endotoxemia (2). L-citrulline and L-arginine are precursors for nitric oxide production, which is a potent vasodilator, potentially enhancing blood flow into the intestinal microvasculature reducing exercise-induced hypoperfusion and ischaemic (3) glutamine and bovine colostrum may enhance the expression of heat shock proteins (i.e., proteins that protect cellular membrane under period of stress), which may protect the intestinal enterocytes, reduce intestinal permeability, and attenuate the development of local inflammatory pathways.

# Practical Recommendations

- Consider exacerbatory factors and attempt to minimize their influence on RAGS.
- Reduce heat stress exacerbation by acclimating to heat prior to traveling to competitions in hot conditions.
- Ensure hydration is maintained leading up to competition.
- Avoid using non-steroidal anti-inflammatory drugs (e.g., aspirin and ibuprofen) leading up to and during competition.
- Undertake a full gut assessment in response to exercise stress (gut-challenge protocol) to determine which primary causal factor and exacerbating factors may be contributing to the GI symptoms.

- Test for malabsorption of nutrients commonly used in sports nutrition formulations (e.g., fructose and sorbitol in race nutrition products and lactose in recovery nutrition products).
- Start running in a euhydrated state and maintain euhydration throughout running.
- Prevent both dehydration and over-hydration.
- Avoid overfeeding and overdrinking during running to the point of overwhelming the stomach.
- Identify individual carbohydrate intake tolerance levels during running.
- Consume carbohydrates evenly and more frequently throughout running.
- Avoid long periods without carbohydrate consumption.
- Hypertonic solutions reduce gastric emptying rates, so it is advised to use lower carbohydrate concentration beverages with low osmolality.
- Consider adequate water intake in adjunct with any solids being consumed, including semi-solid forms (i.e., gels).
- Small amounts of protein consumed frequently throughout running appear to have a beneficial effect on gut integrity, but may be less well tolerated than carbohydrates.
- Train your gut to cope with carbohydrate intake during running (both solid and liquid form), using a structured gut-training protocol at least two weeks before a competition that required intake (i.e., greater than two hours).
- Despite the need for more research, a low-FODMAP diet (including the reduction in dietary fiber) in the days leading up to competition or periods of intensified training may decrease RAGS.
- There is no strong evidence to support the consumption of antioxidants, amino acids, or bovine colostrum to reduce RAGS.
- There is no strong evidence to support the acute- and longer-term consumption of probiotics to reduce RAGS.
- There is no evidence to support the adherence of a gluten-free diet in non-celiac runners to reduce RAGS, unless specified by a medical or health practitioner in response to confirmed medical diagnosis.

## CHAPTER **17**

# Environmental Hazards

### BY SARAH TEREZ MALKA AND N. STUART HARRIS

## Key Points

1. Prevention is key! Be aware of weather conditions and local environmental hazards before leaving for a run.
2. Carry a cellular phone in a weatherproof case when running in isolated areas or regions at risk for severe weather.
3. There is no safe outdoor position or location during a lightning storm. If a thunderstorm is approaching, immediately abort your run and retreat to a car or a fully-enclosed building.
4. If caught in a flash flood, keep the body as horizontal as possible, with feet near the water's surface, to avoid foot entrapment in underwater rocks or debris.
5. If submerged in cold water and unable to climb out, float with legs held tightly together and arms crossed across the chest, moving as little as possible, to preserve body heat.
6. In a wildfire, runners should stay low to the ground and cover the face with a moist cloth to avoid inhaling smoke. If on a slope, running downhill is usually a safer option.

## Introduction

The risks of exposure to weather hazards, including severe weather events, are intrinsic to long distance running. Long runs, especially in remote areas, expose a runner to inclement weather and environmental conditions, which can rapidly change from a nuisance to a danger. The National Weather Service reports an average of 300 to 600 deaths per year due to weather in the US (1). The ability to predict, avoid, and safely react to weather hazards, including lightning, flash floods, cold water immersion, and wildfires are essential skills for the long distance runner.

# Lightning

Lightning is a leading cause of weather-related injury and death in the United States, with an average of about fifty fatalities and 150 injuries per year (2). About 100 lightning bolts strike the earth's surface every second, and each bolt can contain up to one billion volts of electricity (3). The rate of death due to lightning strikes is believed to be about 5 to 10 percent, though the true rate is not known, as the strikes that do result in injury are likely under-reported (4, 5, 6). In the US, the incidence of lightning strikes and injuries tends to be greatest in warm and humid areas (e.g., Florida, Gulf Coast, lower Mississippi Valley), where large amounts of warm, moist air rising into the atmosphere create conditions that foster the formation of thunderstorms as the warm, wet air meets the cold, dry air higher in the atmosphere, setting up opposing electrical charges (7). Lightning is also frequent in mountainous regions, where warm, moist air is directed up the mountain face to the higher, freezing air, setting up perfect conditions for thunderstorms to develop just above the mountain peaks (7).

Lightning can cause injury via direct electrical force, by "side splash" (lightning first contacts an object and then arcs to an individual), and by ground current (current can enter a part of the body in contact with the ground and travel through the body to exit another part of the body in contact with the ground). Acute trauma can be caused by the pressure wave created by the blast, or from falls or falling objects. Lightning strike can cause injury to any area in the body from blown ear drums to shoulder dislocations, and the effects of a strike are varied and unpredictable (8). Acute cardiopulmonary arrest is the leading cause of death from lightning injury. Spontaneous resumption of a heartbeat may occur, but respiratory arrest (cessation of breathing) can persist. Even in cases where spontaneous cardiac activity occurs, if respiratory support isn't provided in a timely fashion (i.e., rescue breaths), fatal cardiac arrest is inevitable in a few minutes.

Given the potential severity and lethality of lightning strikes, the best treatment is prevention. Environmental awareness is key. One study found that up to half of lightning strike victims had sufficient time to reach safety prior to their strike (9). Weather reports should be checked prior to embarking on a long run and avoid running outside when severe storms are anticipated. Even with diligent pre-departure awareness, a willingness to continually reassess risk is needed as weather conditions change during a run. It is not at all uncommon for a runner on a summer's afternoon to ascend a mountain trail under blue skies only to suddenly become aware of a threatening thunderhead as they crest a ridge. If a storm approaches, one should consider aborting the run and immediately head toward a safe location (10, 11, 12, 13, 14).

In the US, the vast majority of lightning injuries occur during the summer months and most commonly between noon and 6 p.m.—extra caution should be used during these times or if running in a region known for routine thunderstorms. In mountainous areas of Colorado, for example, long runs would ideally be scheduled very early in the morning as lightning is common by mid-morning and through the afternoon. Subscribe to severe weather alerts on a phone, but be aware that many lightning strikes occur during weaker storms that would not trigger a severe thunderstorm or tornado alert.

If one is caught outside during an approaching storm, definitive shelter should be sought as quickly as possible. Up to one in ten lightning strikes occur when rain is not present, so the absence of rain should not be reassuring. The distance of a storm from an observer may be estimated by measuring the time between the almost instantaneous transmission of the visible lightning strike and the delayed arrival of the sound of the resulting thunder. Sound waves travel roughly one mile each five seconds (i.e., a ten-second period between visualizing a lightning bolt and hearing thunder means the lightning is approximately two miles away). Runners should be aware of the "30–30 rule" (9, 10). The first 30 refers to the time in seconds between seeing a lightning flash and hearing the sound of thunder. If this time is thirty seconds or less, the storm is six or fewer miles away and one is at risk and should move to safety. However, lightning can strike up to ten to fifteen miles from a storm, so this rule does not afford absolute safety. A safer absolute rule is "when thunder roars, go indoors" (11, 12, 13, 14).

Lightning may strike as a storm approaches, is overhead, or as it departs. The second part of the "30–30 rule" reminds individuals to wait 30 minutes after the final lightning is seen or thunder is heard before resuming activities. While this is the safest approach, especially for larger groups where evacuation would take more time, in reality, lightning threat is minimal about fifteen minutes after a storm has passed (11, 12, 13, 14).

There is no definitively safe position or location outdoors in a thunderstorm. If one is caught outside during a storm, the National Weather Service recommends avoiding open fields, the tops of hills or mountains, or a ridge line, staying away from tall, isolated trees or other tall objects, and to avoid water and metal objects. Obviously, it would be difficult to find a location of safety when running through a forest, valley, or mountain trail, and none of these positions provides absolute protection from strike. The only definitive safe location is inside an enclosed, grounded structure such as a house, or inside a car. Partial shelters such as bus stops or tents do not provide protection (6, 8, 11, 12, 13, 14).

There are several myths about "safe" positions that mitigate the risk of injury from a lightning strike, such as standing or crouching on one foot or sitting on a pad or mat. While intuitively sensible, these maneuvers have not demonstrated to provide any significant protection. However, lying flat on the ground should be avoided as this will increase contact between your body and electrified ground (6, 11, 12).

If a runner in a group is struck by lightning, the intervention should be to move all group members to a safe location to minimize the number of potential victims. Then, standard first aid and cardiopulmonary resuscitation (CPR) should be performed. A person struck by lightning does not maintain any electric charge and is safe to touch. Remember that there may be significant internal injuries even without external signs of trauma or burns. If a strike victim is unconscious and requires evacuation, they should be handled with care to keep their head and neck secure (Figure 17-1), as bone, nerves, muscle, and internal organs may be injured without any external signs. Improvised immobilization may be necessary if the patient is unconscious or altered and the rescuer cannot be sure there is no neck injury (Figure 17-2). CPR should be continued as long as practically possible, as a stopped heart caused by lightning strike can potentially be restarted by rescue breaths or defibrillation. If multiple members of a party are struck at one time, institute "reverse triage," that is, give the highest priority to patients in cardiac or respiratory arrest when making decisions about who to treat first. Individuals who have maintained a pulse and spontaneous respirations are likely to survive and can wait for additional providers to arrive. Be aware that unreactive, dilated pupil(s) may occur as a result of transient nervous system instability and should not be mistaken for a sign of brain death or a reason to prematurely cease resuscitative efforts. Even if there are no obvious injuries, all strike victims should seek medical attention.

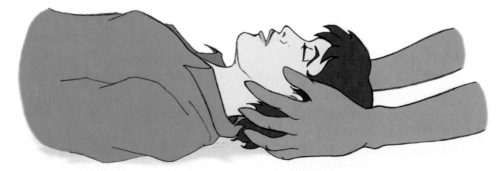

**Figure 17-1** Stabilization of the upper spine. Courtesy of Grant S. Lipman, MD, *The Wilderness First Aid Handbook.*

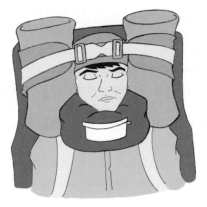

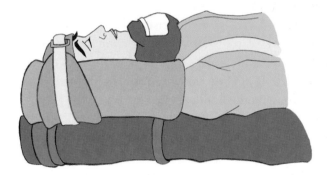

**Figure 17-2** Improvised immobilization of the head and cervical spine. Courtesy of Grant S. Lipman, MD, *The Wilderness First Aid Handbook.*

## Flash Floods

Flooding has historically been the leading cause of death from weather-related hazard. From 1986 to 2015, there have been an average of eighty-two flood-related fatalities in the US per year, which doubled to 176 in 2015 (1). While large-scale floods are easily avoidable with careful attention to weather predictions, backcountry runners may find themselves at risk from flash floods that can strike with minimal warning.

Flash floods can develop within minutes of the triggering event—and not necessarily be accompanied by rain at the downstream site of flooding (15). Common causes of flash floods include heavy rains, ice, or debris jams leading to a dam effect, and levy or dam failures. The most common cause of flash flooding is a storm causing heavy rain or multiple rainstorms within a short time period. As noted, in rocky or mountainous regions, flash flooding may not occur in the area that received the recent rain, but rather downhill or downriver. This is especially true in low-lying areas of the Western US and in any steep area where water can travel quickly downhill and fill up stream and river beds quickly. Areas consisting of rock or clay do not absorb water as well and are more prone to flash flooding. As little as six inches of fast-moving water can sweep an adult off their feet and flash floods may overtake a runner within seconds with little warning (15, 16).

As with all weather-related events, avoidance is the key to injury prevention. Signing up for weather and flash flood alerts is a simple step. If there have been severe or frequent rainstorms in the region within the day or days prior to a run, it may be wise to avoid areas near water, such as riversides, streambeds, canyons, and lower valley areas. In areas of the country that receive daily afternoon storms, morning runs may be a safer option.

If one is in a canyon or by a riverbed during a severe storm, next to a stream or riverbed that is rapidly rising, or suspect that conditions may lead to flash flooding, a search should be made for the quickest path to high ground—and work to quickly climb as high as possible from the bottom of the valley or the riverbed (16, 17). Avoid continuing down in the direction of river flow and attempting to outrun the flood.

If swept up in a flash flood, one should assume the "river safety position": floating on your back, facing upwards with feet facing downstream. If there is a clear point of safety or the shore is close, roll over onto the stomach, and swim aggressively toward shore or safety. Whether floating in the safety position or swimming, the feet should be raised so they are near the surface of the water, and one should keep the body as horizontal as possible at all times. Keeping one's feet pointing downriver and on the surface of the water allows feet to deflect any objects and also prevents feet from getting entrapped in debris or rocks under the water's surface. It is the nature of flash floods that trees and debris are swept along by the rapidly rising waters and their mass and speed pose an additional hazard to drowning. Swimming through or floating into trees in the water should be avoided, as their underwater limbs can act like a strainer and trap a swimmer between branches and the approaching current. Standing in moving water that is deeper than the knees should not be attempted, as a foot can get trapped in a rock or other item on the riverbed and the force of moving water could easily push one over—submerging and trapping the head underwater. It is safe to stand only when calm or very shallow water is reached (18).

## Cold Water Immersion

In the winter, a pond or river may be covered with snow and, thus, may be difficult to navigate while moving quickly down a trail. A simple misstep or fall can lead to cold water immersion. Immersion in cold water poses a significant risk of hypothermia, especially at temperatures below 77 degrees F (25 degrees C). Many rivers fed from by a dam are significantly cooler than this (19). The vast majority of cold water immersion injuries are avoidable with prudent foresight. It is essential to remember that snow cover may hide thin ice and slippery conditions should dictate caution when running near any body of water. While no technology can replace good judgment, access to a cellphone in a waterproof case in high risk areas where cold exposure may occur may allow help to be summoned. There are four stages of the body's response to immersion in cold water, and awareness of these may assist in preventing injury and optimize the opportunity for survival (19, 20).

## Phase 1: Cold Shock

This first phase lasts under two minutes. The shock of the cold water leads to gasping, panic, and the inability to control breathing. Panic makes this reaction much worse. A second response occurs during this phase as the blood vessels in the skin suddenly constrict, trying to minimize heat loss from the cold skin surface and shunt warmth toward the internal organs. This sudden increase in blood flow to the heart and sympathetic nervous system stimulation (the fight-or-flight response) can lead to heart rhythm disturbances, which in turn may lead to heart attack and sudden death. In this initial phase, a focus on calming the breathing rate, trying to relax, and maintaining the head above the water can prevent a victim dying.

## Phase 2: Cold Incapacitation

This second phase lasts from ten to fifteen minutes. As cold numbs the nerves and muscles, the fingers become stiff and muscles lose the ability for meaningful movement. It thus becomes hard to swim effectively or to pull oneself out of the water. In this phase, all effort should focus on self-rescue before strength is lost and coordination becomes poor. If unable to self-extricate and if there is ice or snow, attempting to throw arms and upper body onto the bank may result in them freezing there—essentially keeping the head above water. If unable to do so, remaining as still as possible with arms crossed over the chest and legs pressed together may maintain a small thermal gradient and slightly slow the rate of heat loss and onset of hypothermia.

## Phase 3: Onset of Hypothermia

The internal body temperature slowly cools as heat is lost to the surrounding cold water. (For symptoms and signs of hypothermia refer to Chapter 13.) Depending on water temperature, onset of hypothermia may take thirty minutes or more. Even in very cold water, most adults can survive up to an hour before loss of consciousness and subsequent drowning. Neurologically intact survivals following cardiac arrest from prolonged cold water immersion have been documented—especially in children. Rescuers should continue resuscitative efforts until a victim has been fully rewarmed.

## Phase 4: Circum-Rescue Collapse

For reasons unknown, some survivors of cold-water immersion will suffer unexpected death shortly after rescue or during rewarming. This may be due to body core temperature continuing to fall as the blood vessels open up during the warming process, bringing cold blood from the extremities toward the heart, and causing a fatal cardiac rhythm. But the definitive cause is unknown. For this reason, all victims of cold water immersion should consider receiving medical attention after rescue. If possible, transport to the hospital should be performed by ambulance rather than private vehicle so that optimal warming techniques can be initiated and the victim can be monitored.

# Wildfires

Wildfires have historically been common in the dry (summer) months in the Western US and Canada, and are becoming increasingly common in the spring and fall, as well (21). Wildfires may be difficult to avoid for the distance runner, as fires can be unpredictable and may rapidly spread or change directions. A surface forest fire can spread at fifty to eighty-three feet per minute (fifteen to twenty-five meters per minute) and grass fires can spread up to 1,263 feet per minute (385 meters per minute), many times faster than most runners can sprint (22).

Fires pose a risk to runners via multiple mechanisms. Flames or radiant heat can cause thermal injury from direct burns, lung injury due to smoke inhalation, or hyperthermia. Indirect effects may be seen due to decreased oxygen or increased levels of toxic gases such as carbon monoxide and carbon dioxide. There is the risk of trauma from falling trees or unstable ground. Additionally, smoke can irritate the eyes and respiratory system, even when not in close proximity to the actual blaze. The presence of a "smoke wave," defined as two or more consecutive days with fine airborne particles specific to wildfires, can lead to severe respiratory pollution exposures, even when the fires are hundreds of miles away (22).

If running in a region prone to fires, pay attention to fire risk levels before setting out. Be aware of conditions that increase risk of fire spreading: high winds, dry ground and vegetation, and the condition of the brush. In an area near active fires or in a high-risk region, one should opt for natural fabrics, such as wool or cotton. Synthetic fabrics melt in heat and can cause additional burns (22).

If in an active fire or in close proximity, it is important to stay calm and seek an area to shelter from the heat, such as in a trench, crevice, behind a large rock, or near a stream or water source. Covering the head and exposed skin as much as possible may provide some protection from the flames. Crouching low to the ground and keeping the head and mouth close to the ground will reduce smoke and gas inhalation. If possible, wet a piece of cloth or shirt, and hold it over the mouth to serve as a filter. In extreme circumstances, urine could be used as a moisture source (22).

When choosing an escape path, remember that hot air rises. Move downhill and away from the fire at a 45-degree angle when possible, as this will tend to help to move away from the direction of fire spread and out of the flame's path. Move slowly to avoid heat exhaustion, and constantly monitor the direction of fire spread. Maintain awareness of the surroundings and be on the lookout for any safe shelter areas. If you are able to see through the flames and they are less than three feet deep, consider quickly passing through the flames into the already burnt area. If unable to flee and one is at risk to be overtaken by the fire, attempt to completely cover the entire body as well as possible and lie face down on the ground (22). Any victim of a wildfire should be quickly evacuated to medical care, as thermal injury and burns often progress and even small injuries may have long lasting repercussions.

## CHAPTER 18

# Skin Problems

## BY NATALIE BADOWSKI WU AND KENDALL WU

## Key Points

1.  Trauma-related conditions can be avoided with the appropriate use of properly fitting equipment, non-irritating fabrics, lubricants, and protective barriers.
2.  Skin infections in runners often have a characteristic appearance and nearly always require treatment with prescription medications.
3.  Contact dermatitis, whether allergic or irritant, is common in runners and requires preventative measures and early treatment.
4.  Runners need to be aware of chemicals, medications, and environmental conditions that can predispose them to sun sensitivity and should be meticulous with sunscreen use to help avoid sunburn and skin cancer.

The skin is the largest organ of the body and as such is the most common source of injuries for athletes (1). It consists of three main layers: the epidermis, the dermis, and subcutaneous tissue. Skin lesions and rashes vary and are characterized by their size and general appearance. There are four main classes of skin conditions that runners can encounter: trauma related, infectious, immunological and inflammatory, and environmental reactions (1).

## Traumatic Conditions

### Chafing and Pack Rash

Chafing occurs as a result of rubbing between two surfaces of the skin (i.e., between the thighs) or between the skin surface and some other material (2). "Pack rash" describes the specific chafing that occurs when a pack rubs against the skin (Figure 18-1). Runners can prevent chafing by wearing dry clothing that fits properly (Table 18-1) (2). Drying agents such as talcum powder can be used to

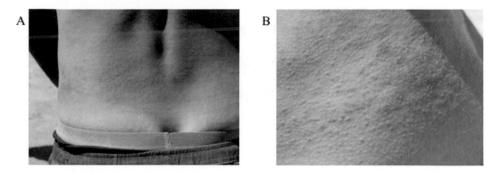

**Figure 18-1** Examples of pack rash injury. A represents a runner with pack rash injury on the lower back; B represents a close-up of the pack rash injury. Photos courtesy of Grant S. Lipman, MD.

help to reduce moisture while lubricants (petroleum jelly, zinc oxide, BodyGlide, etc.) can be used to reduce friction and improve the ease that surfaces slide next to each other (2, 3).

Should chafing occur, one can treat the affected area by cleaning it with luke-warm tap water and a mild soap (2, 4). If there is any debris, the area should be flushed with water. Both scrubbing and using hydrogen peroxide should be avoided, as they can injure the underlying healthy tissue and worsen the wound (2). Once the wound has been cleaned and dried thoroughly, the athlete can apply a topical anti-biotic or petroleum jelly and then cover the area with sterile gauze or a pad (2, 4). If there is any inflammation (red raised and swollen area), a topical steroid can also be applied (4). If the injured area experiences a great deal of movement, a stretch Band-Aid or gauze roll can be wrapped around the area to keep the pad from moving (2).

There are also newer technologies that cover abrasions and chafing injuries such as semi-permeable and hydrocolloid dressings (e.g., Tegaderm, Spenco 2nd Skin, Compeed/Blister Block), which can increase the rate of wound healing and potentially decrease scarring (2). These types of product can typically be left on the skin for prolonged periods (2). It is normal for excess fluid from the wound to accumulate under these types of dressings; in these cases, the dressing should be removed and replaced daily to keep it dry and assist with healing (2). For cases where there is severe pain, the runner should seek the care of their medical provider. Runners should also ensure their tetanus shots are up-to-date to avoid subsequent tetanus infection (2).

## Nipple Bleeding (Jogger's Nipple)

Nipple bleeding (also known as Jogger's Nipple) is a result of repetitive fric-tion between the nipples and the shirt material in contact with the skin (1,

**Table 18-1** Prevention and treatment of trauma-related skin conditions.

| Condition | Prevention | Treatment |
|---|---|---|
| Chafing and Pack Rash | Properly fitting equipment<br>Drying agents (i.e., talcum powder)<br>Lubricants (e.g., petroleum jelly, zinc oxide, BodyGlide) | Water and mild soap<br>Topical antibiotic (i.e., bacitracin)<br>Topical lubricant (i.e., petroleum jelly)<br>Topical steroid (if inflammation)<br>Sterile gauze and pad<br>Semipermeable and hydrocolloid dressings |
| Nipple Bleeding a.k.a. Jogger's Nipple | Properly fitting equipment<br>Synthetic materials<br>Anti-moisture products (i.e., antiperspirant)<br>Drying agents (i.e., talcum powder)<br>Lubricants (e.g., petroleum jelly, zinc oxide, BodyGlide)<br>Tape (e.g., patches or Band-Aids) | Water and mild soap<br>Topical antibiotic (i.e., bacitracin)<br>Topical lubricant (i.e., petroleum jelly) |
| Talon Noir | Lubricants (e.g., petroleum jelly, zinc oxide, BodyGlide)<br>Heel pads<br>Changing socks and/or shoes | Resolves with rest |
| Calluses and Corns | Properly fitting equipment<br>Synthetic materials<br>Lubricants (e.g., petroleum jelly, zinc oxide, BodyGlide)<br>Pads, shoe inserts | Soak in warm water and grind down area with pumice stone or callus remover<br>Urea cream (20% or 40%) |
| Abrasions | Avoid injury | Water and mild soap<br>Topical antibiotic (i.e., bacitracin)<br>Band-Aid, sterile gauze, or pad |
| Lacerations | Avoid injury | Water and mild soap<br>Closure via Steri-Strips, butterfly closures, stitches, or staples |

2, 5, 6). This type of chafing tends to occur at a higher frequency in runners who wear clothing made of coarse fibers, such as cotton, due in part to these materials retaining moisture and further exacerbating the frictional injury (2, 5, 6). The repeated rubbing between the material and the affected region of the body results in painful chafing which may lead to bleeding with continued irritation (2, 5). Other factors including temperature, moisture, material type, activity level, and individual skin characteristics can all affect susceptibility as well (6).

Prevention of nipple bleeding starts with wearing dry, synthetic, well-fitting, and moisture-wicking clothes (5). Synthetic materials, unlike cotton, wick away moisture and tend to reduce the likelihood of occurrence (1, 2, 5). Nipple bleeding can also be prevented with the use of anti-moisture products (i.e., antiperspirant), moisture absorbing products (i.e., talcum powder), lubricators (i.e., petroleum jelly), and taping prophylactically using commercially available patches or Band-Aids. In some cases, a combination can also be used (1, 2, 5, 6).

In the event that nipple bleeding occurs, treatment includes cleaning the affected areas gently with water, drying the areas thoroughly, and applying a lubricant such as petroleum jelly or a topical antibiotic ointment (1, 2, 5).

---

## Talon Noir

---

Some runners develop a blue-black or brown discolored area of the skin—most commonly seen over the heel area—called talon noir (also known as calcaneal petechiae or sometimes "black heel") (Figure 18-2) (3, 5). The color change results from the damaged dermal capillaries due to repeated trauma from the stop-start motion during running, changes in direction, or repeated hard pounding (2, 3, 5, 6). This coloration is typically asymptomatic and will gradually resolve on its own within two to three weeks once the activity is stopped (3, 5, 6). Skin lubricants, pads, changing socks or shoes, or taking a rest from running can reduce the incidence (2, 5, 6). In some cases, the talon noir may appear like a melanoma (skin cancer) (5). If there is any question that it may be a melanoma, the runner should consult their health-care provider for a more definitive diagnosis.

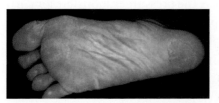

**Figure 18-2** Example of talon noir as well as a blister on the heel.

## Calluses and Corns

Calluses occur when the skin thickens as a protective response to chronic and repeated friction and are especially common over bony areas of the foot (Figure 18-3) (1, 2, 4). These may be prevented by wearing synthetic socks and using properly fitting shoes. If calluses develop due to anatomical abnormalities, pads or other orthotic devices can be used to reduce and prevent friction (2).

Calluses should be removed to avoid either developing blisters deep underneath which are painful and difficult to drain, or run the risk of ripping the callus off leaving a painful ulcer. To remove calluses, runners can soak their feet in warm water for several minutes and grind down the area with a pumice stone or callus remover (1, 2, 4). Afterward, the runner can apply urea cream (20 percent or 40 percent) and cover the area with duct tape, paper tape, or a smooth layer to alleviate friction and minimize formation of a callus (2). Other abrasives, topical salicylic acid, or urea preparations can also be used to remove the thickened skin (4).

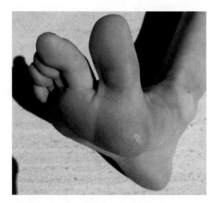

**Figure 18-3** Example of a callus on the ball of the foot.

Corns are areas of skin thickening that are the result of repeated unequal forces on the foot during a running stride (2). Corns are differentiated from calluses by a differentiated type of skin in the center (central core), whereas calluses represent thickened skin with no alteration in the appearance of the skin. There are two different types of corns, distinguished by their texture: they may be hard or soft. Hard corns are typically located on the sole of the foot and can be painful, thereby limiting athletic activity. They have a similar appearance to calluses but are typically smaller and more localized. Soft corns tend to be located between toes and appear as white macerated plaques (2).

As ill-fitting shoes cause corns, switching to properly fitting shoes with room in the toe box can help decrease their occurrence (2). Shoe inserts and pads can also be used to help distribute weight and relieve the pressure responsible for corn development (2, 3). Over-the-counter toe separators or moleskin can be used to relieve soft corns (2). Treatment of corns involves paring down the corn carefully (2). Additional treatment options include using callus-removing medications or surgery, and runners should consult a podiatrist for definitive care.

# Abrasions

An abrasion is an area of the body with skin scraped or sloughed off (Figure 18-4). Occasionally, the abrasion may also have embedded dirt, gravel, and debris. The injured area should be treated as soon as possible—preferably within twelve hours. The skin should be scrubbed to remove any dirt and debris, and sometimes tweezers are necessary to pick out any embedded rocks (7). Water under pressure may also help irrigate the wound and flush out any potential disease-causing bacteria that can lead to infections. Antiseptic ointment or antibiotic gel can be applied to create a protective layer. Ideally, the wound should be covered with a non-adherent dressing (i.e., Spenco 2nd Skin) and then secured with a bandage (7). The area should be kept clean and dry and observed for signs of infection, which include surrounding redness and tenderness, pus drainage, swelling, fevers, and chills.

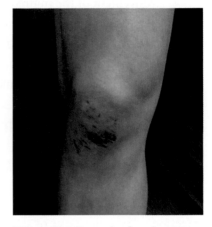

**Figure 18-4** Example of an abrasion on the knee.

# Lacerations

A laceration is a cut or puncture into the skin that breaks all the layers of the skin's surface and results in bleeding. Lacerations over a joint, a broken bone, deep puncture wounds, deep wounds on the hands or feet, wounds with large areas of crushed tissue, and any animal or human bites to the hand, wrist, or foot are all considered "high risk" for infection and require a runner to stop immediately and seek prompt medical attention (7). Lacerations are time sensitive as they are at higher risk for infection due to inoculation of bacteria the longer they are left open. Extremity lacerations should be closed within eight hours, those on the torso within twelve hours, and those on the face or scalp within twenty-four hours (7). All wounds require considerable irrigation to remove any dirt, gravel, and pathogens. Many result in X-rays to evaluate for any foreign objects deep in the tissue or to evaluate for underlying fracture. Most wounds will result in closure in a medical setting, either with stitches or staples. If the laceration is small and only through the top surface of the skin, Steri-Strips, or butterfly closures may be sufficient for closing and have a good cosmetic outcome. Occasionally, a medical provider may choose to leave wounds open to minimize infection. The assessment of a laceration has several steps:

- Bleeding is usually controlled with direct pressure.
- The extremity distant to the area of injury needs to be evaluated to ensure there is adequate blood flow, which can be checked by squeezing then letting go of the finger tips or toe tips. These should blanch then regain color in a few seconds.
- Sensation should be checked to ensure it is intact.
- Movement of the injured area needs to be evaluated for both nerve and tendon function. The areas around and distant to the injury should move appropriately with full strength.
- If there is any concern about blood flow, sensation, tendon integrity, or excessive blood loss, prompt medical attention is required.

# Infections

## Bacterial Skin Infections

The runner's skin is the perfect environment for the development of bacterial infections. The outer layer of skin becomes repeatedly moist and warm allowing for an optimal medium for the growth and passage of organisms. Runners are also frequently exposed to skin trauma from blisters to abrasions further allowing routes for bacteria to enter the body.

The most common bacterial infections are caused by *Staphylococcus* and *Streptococcus* species that exist as part of the natural skin flora, but may create a local infection with disruption of the skin barrier. Both strains present in a variety of clinical conditions including: impetigo, folliculitis, furuncles, and cellulitis, among others. All of these bacterial infections may be prevented by using clothing that wicks away moisture, showering soon after exercise, following good hand hygiene, and avoiding the sharing of equipment, clothing, towels, and tape (2). If infection occurs, there are a number of options for treatment (Table 18-2). Cautious observation is warranted for any bacterial infection to ensure that it does not progress to sepsis—which is a full body infection that presents with fevers, chills, and fatigue with the potential for very serious complications including death. Any spreading, streaking infection, association with systemic symptoms (fevers, chills, malaise), and/or poor response to antibiotics warrants prompt medical attention and possible IV antibiotics.

## Cellulitis

Cellulitis is a spreading reddened, tender, and warm patch of skin that is caused by a bacterial infection (Figure 18-5) (8). It is usually the result of bacteria passing through a break in the skin, often from wounds or minor trauma such as blister or abrasions (8). Occasionally, the infection may spread to large areas of skin and may be associated with systemic symptoms such as fevers and chills (8). Treatment involves taking a prescription antibiotic (8). Large areas of skin infection, circumferential infections, or infections with systemic symptoms warrant prompt medical attention and may require intravenous antibiotic treatment.

One particularly dangerous type of cellulitis is caused by an antibiotic-resistant strain of bacteria called methicillin-resistant *Staphylococcus aureus* (MRSA). This is considered "an emerging epidemic" in the infectious disease world (9), with athletes (including runners) at increased risk for acquiring this infection due to sport-associated skin damage, sharing of equipment, and the presence of a warm, moist skin environment (10).

The infection itself presents as a red tender area, often with an associated abscess, but presentation can also include red papules, nodules, pustules, and plaques. Many runners may interpret their initial infection as a "spider bite" (10). An abscess can be drained and treated without antibiotics if less than five centimeters, but many physicians obtain cultures of the wound and choose antibiotic

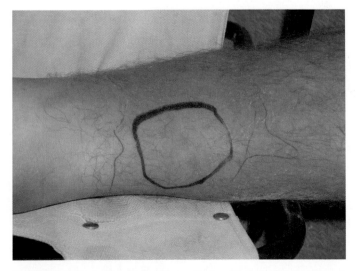

**Figure 18-5** Example of cellulitis on the leg. Photo courtesy of Grant S. Lipman, MD.

**Table 18-2** Treatment options for infections.

| Category | Condition | Over-the-Counter Options | Prescription Only |
|---|---|---|---|
| Bacterial | Impetigo | Antibiotic ointment (i.e., bacitracin) | Topical or oral antibiotics |
| | Folliculitis (Inflammation of Hair Follicles) | Antibiotic ointment (i.e., bacitracin) | Topical or oral antibiotics |
| | Furunculosis (Boils) | Antibiotic ointment (i.e., bacitracin) | Topical or oral antibiotics |
| | Cellulitis | See your provider | Oral antibiotics |
| | Methicillin-Resistant Staphylococcus Aureus (MRSA) | See your provider | Oral antibiotics |
| | Erythrasma (General) | Antibacterial soap | Oral antibiotics |
| | Erythrasma (Interdigital Form) | Whitfield's Ointment | Topical and/or oral antibiotics |
| | Pitted Keratolysis | Aluminum subacetate (Burow's Solution or Domeboro) | Oral antibiotics |
| | Acne Mechanica | Topical benzoyl peroxide 10%<br>Salicylic acid 2% | Retinoid<br>Topical or oral antibiotics |
| Viral | Plantar Warts | Pare down<br>Salicylic acid 17% | Surgical excision, cryotherapy |
| Fungal | Tinea Pedis (Athlete's Foot) | Clomitrazole 1%<br>Miconazole 2%<br>Terbinafine 1%<br>Butenafine 1%<br>Tolnaftate 1% | Topical and oral antifungals |
| | Tinea Cruris (Jock Itch) and Tinea Corporis (Ringworm) | Clomitrazole 1%<br>Miconazole 2%<br>Terbinafine 1%<br>Butenafine 1%<br>Tolnaftate 1% | Topical and oral antifungals |

treatment either before or after cultures are positive. Most MRSA infections respond well to specific oral antibiotics (10).

## Erythrasma

Erythrasma is a red, scaling plaque often found in the armpit, groin, or in between the toes caused by the bacterium *Corynebacterium minutissimum* (2). The rash is often asymptomatic and well defined initially, but may later appear brown and raised with some the middle of the rash clearing (11). The interdigital type may present as scales, fissures, and constant skin breaks between the toes, and up to 30 percent of people with this bacterial infection have a concurrent fungal infection (11). Risk factors for all types include body moisture, warm climate, increased sweating, and diabetes (11). It is usually diagnosed clinically but clinicians may use a Wood's lamp (which will reveal a fluorescent red color) or a culture of the skin scrapings to confirm diagnosis (2, 11). Traditionally, this infection has been treated with antibacterial soaps or oral antibiotics (2). However, in a recent double-blind, placebo-controlled study, a complete response was must successful with fusidic acid 2 percent cream. For the interdigital form, oral antibiotics are supplemented with topical treatments such as Whitfield's ointment, 2 percent clindamycin, or fusidic acid 2 percent (also known as 2 percent sodium fusidate) (2).

## Pitted Keratolysis (Stinky Foot or Sweaty Sock Syndrome)

Pitted keratolysis is common in runners. It is caused by the *Corynebacterium* species strain of bacteria that feeds on thick keratin (especially calluses) and prefers feet kept in the warm, moist environment of the shoe (12). The foot develops characteristic yellow-brown, one to seven millimeter crater-like pits on the weight bearing sole of the foot that is distinct from the more central locations of tinea pedis or plantar warts (2). These pits emit a foul odor and can become secondarily infected due to the open skin (2). The lesions are usually diagnosed clinically but may also be cultured for definitive diagnosis (12).

The runner can treat the infection with aluminum subacetate (Burow's Solution or Domeboro) soaks up to three times a day as well as topical benzoyl peroxide and topical antibiotics (2). Combination of topical fusidic acid with prescription oral antibiotics has also been successful (13) as has mupirocin 2 percent ointment (14). More serious or secondarily infected feet can benefit from more broad oral antibiotics (14). Runners can prevent infection by washing socks and shoes at high temperatures (greater than 60 degrees C), wearing shoes with good ventilation, and avoiding callus formation (13). Pitted keratolysis can be prevented with the use of aluminum chloride to dry out the feet before exercising (2). Some individuals have also benefitted from treatment with low-dose botulinum toxin injection to the plantar foot to create anhidrosis (the stopping of sweating) (13).

## Acne Mechanica

Acne mechanica is a well-defined popular and pustular lesion that is caused by friction, pressure, squeezing, stretching, and occlusion related to the runner's clothing or equipment (i.e., running packs) (Figure 18-6) (2). A few cases have also been seen due to the use of topical skin care products and with vigorous massages (15). It is thought that the mechanical disturbance of the skin causes skin cell thickening and disrupts the normal skin flora prompting bacterial infection and the development of this acne (15). Recently, one review has proposed two subtypes of the lesions: one, folliculitis mechanica, independent from the typical acne, caused by local inflammation; and the other, acne mechanica, a "flare up" of the acne in individuals prone to the disease (15).

Diagnosis is often made clinically with the careful evaluation of the location of the acne and the runner's clothing and equipment (2). Acne mechanica can clear spontaneously when the triggering factor is removed (occlusive clothing, packs, etc.). The lesions tend to be more resistant to medication than traditional acne. Treatment includes using retinoids (i.e., retinoic), topical antibiotics (i.e., clindamycin) and other topical compounds such as benzoyl peroxide and salicylate (2). One review suggests no medication for folliculitis mechanica outside of mild cleansers and moisturizers, but supports traditional acne treatments for acne mechanica (15). More resistant

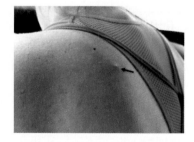

**Figure 18-6** Acne mechanica on the back (arrow).

cases may require oral antibiotic therapy though the runners are then at risk of sun rashes while on these medications (3). Prevention is important and includes showering immediately after activity, using mildly abrasive soaps, application of salicylic acid lotions after showering, moisture wicking materials during exercise, and avoiding the triggering factors (2).

# Viral Infections

## Plantar Warts

Plantar warts (verruca vulgaris, mimesis, and verruca plantaris) are hard, grainy growths on the sole or toes of the foot caused by the *human papillomavirus* (HPV). They also sometimes grow under calluses (2), but can be differentiated by paring away the area. Warts typically have "black seeds" that represent clotted capillaries (2). Plantar warts range in size from a few millimeters to several centimeters (2).

In general, plantar warts are not a serious health concern. However, they can be a source of discomfort or pain due to increased pressure placed on the region (3). Runners can choose to have the warts pared down, or apply over the counter topical salicylic acid for treatment (3). Other methods such as burning them off with cryotherapy or surgery can be used but may require taking time off from running (1, 3).

# Fungal Infections

The most common fungal infections in runners are called dermatophytes. These infections are categorized by the part of the body that they affect: tinea pedis (foot), tinea cruris (groin), and tinea corporis (body). These fungi live off of keratin, one of the main proteins that make up the structure of skin, hair, and nails (16). Several antifungal treatment options are available for fungal infections (Table 18-2).

## Tinea Pedis (Athlete's Foot)

Tinea pedis is one of the most common problems in athletes including runners (Figure 18-7). Active individuals are more likely to develop superficial fungal infections (16). Tinea pedis is more common in those running ≥ 65 km weekly (50 percent of runners) with a trend showing increased running distance resulting in increased occurrence (17).

The warm, moist, and occlusive environment of sweaty athletic shoes and socks, coupled with the increased carbon dioxide levels and impact-related

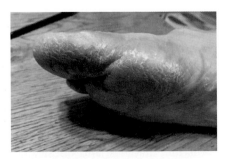

**Figure 18-7** Tinea pedis (Athlete's Foot).

epidermal damage is optimal for the growth and development of the fungus (18). Fomites (nonliving objects capable of transferring disease) help spread the disease and infect athletes through shared showers, locker rooms, and pool floors.

The infection has three main presentations. The first and most common is the interdigital tinea pedis, which consists of itchy, swollen erosions or even scales in the web spaces between the toes, especially in between the third and fourth toe (19). The runner may have macerated skin or associated fissures that cause pain. The second is hyperkeratotic (or moccasin) tinea pedis, which presents as a sheet of diffuse scales on the sole and the sides of the foot, sometimes with some underlying redness (19). This presentation is often chronic (19). The last type is vesiculobullous (inflammatory) tinea pedis, presenting with itchy and painful vesicles and redness, usually on the inside of the foot (19). More severe symptoms present in cases where there is overgrowth of bacteria on top of the fungal infection. Tinea pedis can be diagnosed clinically or with prepared skin scrapings (19).

This fungal infection is treated with topical antifungals. An athlete can initiate treatment with over-the-counter antifungals (e.g., clomitrazole 1 percent, miconazole 2 percent, terbinafine 1 percent, butenafine 1 percent, or tolnaftate 1 percent) that are available in cream, lotion, or even powder forms (20). These are applied two times daily for four weeks, and optimally for a week after the disappearance of the lesions (20). If the infection is very severe and resistant to topical antifungals, the athlete can be prescribed stronger topical antifungals or oral antifungal medication (20). One recent review suggested that topical terbinafine for four weeks as the treatment of choice for limited tinea pedis and oral regimens for the more resistant strains (21). In addition, runners with the interdigital type of tinea pedis can use 20 percent aluminum chloride to dry the toe webbing and kill bacteria and fungi (18).

Runners can prevent athlete's foot with frequent sock changes, the use of moisture wicking synthetic socks, wearing ventilating shoes, using drying foot powder after showers and before running, and always wearing sandals in public locker rooms and showers (5).

## Tinea Cruris (Jock Itch) and Tinea Corporis (Ringworm)

Tinea cruris, also known as "jock itch," is a fungal infection involving the upper inner thigh and around the genitals that is more common in men than in women (19). It is often associated with tinea pedis and risk factors include sweating, moisture, diabetes, and obesity (19). The rash appears as an elevated, red rash with clear borders and vesicles. The rash starts medially and spreads outward, sometimes affecting the perineum, the buttocks, and the anal area but sparing the scrotum (19).

Tinea corporis—also known as ringworm—is the fungal skin infection that occurs on the body (other than feet, groin, face, or hands). It may occur through contact with affected people, animals, fomites, or from contact with other sites of fungal infection (such as tinea pedis). The rash appears as an itchy, red scaling patch or elevated circular lesion that spreads out. The center may clear up, but the raised border remains. The patches and lesions may coalesce to form larger patches, and skin vesicles may also appear.

Both infections can be formally diagnosed like tinea pedis with prepared skin scrapings. Both tinea cruris and corporis can be initially treated with the same topical antifungals as in tinea pedis. In an analysis of sixty-five trials for topical antifungals, no difference was noticed between the different options in terms of a cure at the end of the treatment course, but prescription antifungals of butenafine, terbinafine, and naftifine were most effective in a sustained cure (22). Occasionally, patients will need treatment with oral antifungal medications especially in cases involving large areas of the body, more than one body area at the same time, or with ineffective topical treatment (21).

# Immune and Inflammatory Conditions

## Irritant Contact Dermatitis

Irritant contact dermatitis results from direct contact with an irritant resulting in pruritic erythema (itchy redness) and often with blistering or a vesicular (fluid-filled) rash (Figure 18-8). There are many irritants that can cause a reaction in runners from plants to lotions and clothing or equipment components. It is a response to direct damage of the skin and the inability of the skin to repair itself fast enough (23). It manifests itself

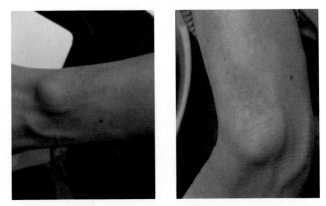

**Figure 18-8** Examples of irritant contact dermatitis on the wrist.

**Table 18-3** Treatment options for immunological and inflammatory conditions.

| Condition | Over-the-Counter Options | Prescription Only |
|---|---|---|
| Irritant Contact Dermatitis | Emollient/moisturizer (e.g., Cethaphil, Theraplex)<br><br>Soap substitutes (i.e., shea butter)<br><br>Topical corticosteroid (i.e., Cortisone-10)<br><br>Antihistamines (e.g., diphenhydramine, ranitidine, cimetidine, loratidine) | Topical and oral corticosteroids |
| Allergic Contact Dermatitis | Barrier products (e.g., Stokogard, Hollister Moisture Barrier, Hydropel, Ivy Shield, Shield Skin, Dermofilm, Uniderm)<br><br>Removal products (e.g., Tecnu, Zanfel, Dr. West's Ivy Detox Cleanser)<br><br>Emollient/moisturizer (e.g., Cethaphil, Theraplex)<br><br>Topical corticosteroid (i.e., Cortisone-10)<br><br>Aluminum subacetate (Burow's Solution or Domeboro) | Topical and oral corticosteroids |
| Cholindergic Urticarias (Hives) | Antihistamines (e.g., diphenhydramine, ranitidine, cimetidine, loratidine) | Antihistamines |
| Solar Urticarias (Hives) | Broad spectrum/high SPF sunscreens<br><br>Antihistamines (e.g., diphenhydramine, ranitidine, cimetidine, loratidine) | Anthistamines |
| Cold Urticarias (Hives) | Antihistamines (e.g., diphenhydramine, ranitidine, cimetidine, loratidine) | Anthistamines Antibiotics |

from minutes to hours from initial exposure (23). The rash usually has the shape and sharp margins of the item that caused the reaction, but may also have unusual geometric or linear shapes (3). It is localized to area of contact but diffuse rashes can also occur (23).

Irritant contact dermatitis is often diagnosed through history and physical exam, though patch tests from an immunologist can be helpful when the cause is not clinically obvious or if an allergic contact dermatitis is suspected (23). However, patch tests are often negative in irritant contact dermatitis. The key to treatment is to identify the irritant and prevent exposure. This may include wearing non-allergenic clothing under uniforms or equipment or using nail polish on metal surfaces (24). Some authors have suggested using absorbent cotton socks and frequent sock changes to prevent shoe-associated contact dermatitis or buying non-allergenic shoes with polyurethane insoles (5). One can also substitute hypoallergenic paper tape for athletic tape.

Once a runner has developed irritant contact dermatitis, he or she can apply an emollient or moisturizer to enhance the skin barrier and improve healing (Table 18-3) (23). Soap substitutes (i.e., shea butter) may also prevent further irritation (23). More severe rashes can be treated with a gel, lotion, or spray preparation of corticosteroids (5). For even more severe cases, a dermatologist should adjust the strength and duration of topical corticosteroid treatment (23). A systemic burst of prescription oral steroids may be used for large affected areas, involving the genitals or face, or particularly symptomatic or severe cases. Antihistamines may also provide symptomatic relief (24).

## Allergic Contact Dermatitis

Allergic contact dermatitis is an immune reaction in which contact with an allergen results in a delayed rash with blistering and/or vesicles. It occurs when those that have been sensitized to the allergen with are exposed to it again (23). The reaction can occur anytime from eight to ninety-six hours after exposure though typically is seen within forty-eight hours (23).

One common allergic contact dermatitis is from the species of plants which include poison ivy, poison oak, poison sumac, and stinging nettle (Figure 18-10). The rash of allergic contact dermatitis appears initially as an area of redness and itchiness that evolves into vesicles and bullae. Specifically, the lesions appear in a linear array (from the brushing of the plant on skin during activity) (25), but can also manifest as a "handprint pattern" from transfer of the plant's oils from the palm (26). Some individuals present with rare asymptomatic black spots on the skin that cannot be washed off and later produce the same vesicles and blisters. The fluid in the vesicles does not contain antigen and does not spread the rash. However, repeated contact with exposed clothing, tools, or even pets, can result in a subsequent or worse reaction (25).

Allergic contact dermatitis is often diagnosed through history and physical exam. Unlike in irritant contact dermatitis, patch testing will show a positive test if the allergen has been identified. Treatment is similar as in irritant contact dermatitis. Prevention of the offending allergen is key. The same strategies of using emollients, topical corticosteroids, and for severe cases, systemic steroids can also be used for treating allergic contact dermatitis (Table 18-3).

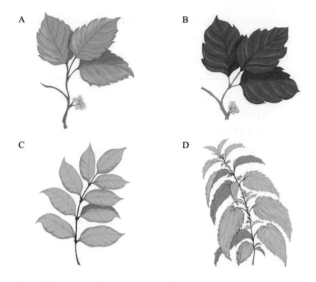

**Figure 18-9** Some plants that cause allergic contact dermatitis.

All components of these plants have a chemical called urushiol that is highly allergenic and to which sensitization may be genetically determined (25). Some individuals may also notice cross reactivity with other plants including the following tree species: Japanese Lacquer, Mango, Cashew Nut, Brazilian Pepper, Florida Holly, and Ginkgo.

A. Poison ivy
B. Poison oak
C. Poison sumac
D. Stinging nettle
Courtesy Grant S. Lipman, MD, Skyhorse Publishing, New York 2013.

Studies have found that urushiol degrades easily in water if applied immediately—up to a 50 percent improvement if applied within ten minutes (25). In addition, proprietary products (e.g., Tecnu, Zanfel, and Dr. West's Ivy Detox Cleanser) have been helpful to reduce rash development though these products have limited studies supporting their efficacy (25).

After the rash has appeared, a runner can treat the itch with aluminum subacetate (Burow's Solution or Domeboro), soaks with baking soda, cool compresses, calamine lotion, and/or topical corticosteroids (25). The moderate strength steroid creams are most useful in early, local reactions before vesicles appear, but due to skin thinning and adrenal suppression with long-term topical use, the mainstay of treatment is prescription oral corticosteroids for an extended ten- to twelve-day course (25).

Few studies have evaluated prevention tactics to prevent urushiol exposure. Dry, loose fabrics are protective (25). In addition, commercial barrier methods have been found to decrease dermatitis by as much as 59 percent with Stokogard (27). Despite local anecdotes, there have been no studies showing efficacy of sunscreens or other lotions in preventing Toxicodendron dermatitis.

## Physical Urticarias (Hives)

A physical urticaria is a skin outbreak of hives that is caused by some environmental stimuli—whether exercise, heat, cold, vibration, or sunlight (Figure 18-11) (28). Cholinergic urticaria which can occur with exertion, exercise, a hot bath, high ambient temperature, or even strong emotion appears as two to four millimeter wheals (red, swollen marks) with surrounding general edema that develop two to thirty minutes after heating of the body (5). The runner may notice generalized tingling and itching before the rash and then note that the rash typically begins on the trunk and neck and spreads distally to involve other parts of the body (28). In rare cases, systemic symptoms such as abdominal cramps, nausea, and vomiting, can also be associated with this reaction (5).

Solar urticaria is the itching and the presence of wheals after exposure to sunlight, especially to UV-A (320 to 400nm) and visible light (400 to 600nm). It is more common in normally unexposed areas (such as the trunk) and less common in frequently exposed areas (face, arms) (18). Cold urticaria presents with itching and wheal-like lesions that are smaller than those in the other physical urticarias, minutes after exposure to cold air, water or objects (29). The lesions will often be found on the inner arms and legs and the lateral flank (24).

The cause of all of these physical urticarias is not well understood, but thought to result from the histamine release by inflammatory mast cells. For cholinergic urticaria, one study suggests that this histamine response is a possible reaction to one's own sweat (28), although sweat pore occlusion or sweat gland destruction have also been proposed as mechanisms (30). In solar urticaria, the histamine

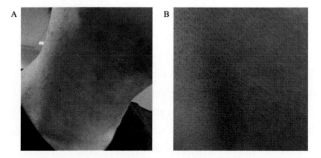

**Figure 18-10** Examples of physical urticarias (hives) on the neck (A) and back (B).

response is thought to be the result of a photo allergen being produced on the skin when the right wavelength of light is absorbed (31).

Diagnosis is often through both medical history and physical exam as well as testing by exposing the patient to the potential triggers (28), including photo testing (32) for solar urticaria and the ice cube test in cold urticaria (18). Treatment is based on avoidance of known triggers. Those with solar urticaria need to seek out sunscreens with a broad spectrum and a high sun protection factor (SPF) and perhaps those that filter out even visible light with products containing iron oxide, titanium dioxide, and zinc oxide. Medical management is typically done with oral antihistamines, either after the rash appears or prophylactically before situations that may cause the rash (24, 32). In addition, for cold urticaria new evidence suggests that antibiotics could be helpful even if no underlying infection is diagnosed (32).

## Exposures

### *Photodermatoses*

Photodermatoses are skin reactions to UV light (Figure 18-12) (24). They are classified into immunological responses, photo-aggravated disorders, chemical or drug reactions, or genetic disorders (33). Immunologically-mediated photodermatoses include entities such as solar urticaria (previously described). Photo-aggravated dermatoses are skin conditions that are present but are exacerbated by UV light and these include acne vulgaris, lupus erythematosus, atopic dermatitis, rosacea, psoriasis, among others and are treated with sun exposure prevention and treatment of the underlying condition (33). Chemical and drug photosensitivity is the primary focus of this section.

Chemical and drug photodermatitis has a variable presentation, ranging from hives and nodules (sun poisoning) to patches (large raised lesions) to solar urticaria with generalized edema (24). Certain medications or products can make the skin more sensitive to the sun. Runners should check all their prescription and over-the-counter medications for possible photosensitivity side effects. Once present, the condition is difficult to treat. Antihistamines can provide symptomatic relief and topical corticosteroids can be tried initially (33). However,

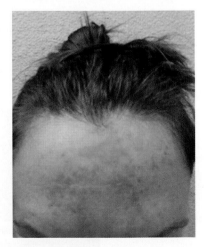

**Figure 18-11** Photodermatosis on the forehead.

severe cases may require systemic steroids (24). Prevention is key. Runners should use sunblock without PABA and avoid sun-sensitizing medications (24).

## Runner's Purpura

Purpura is the discoloration of areas of skin that appear as a purple rash or patch that can been seen in runners' lower extremities and face during vigorous exercise in hot weather conditions (5, 34). Studies suggest it is due to the overloading of the body's thermoregulation (5, 34). Local excessive dilation of blood vessels in the skin and stagnant blood flow (5, 34) which, when combined with the repetitive pressure of every running step, results in further skin swelling, inflammation, and subsequent injury (2, 5, 34). Pre-existing sun damage to the skin can also increase the possibility of occurrence of purpura due to a decrease of collagen in that area of the skin (2). The condition and discoloration typically resolves spontaneously within three to ten days with rest (5, 34). Compression (such as the use of compression stockings), prescription medications, or steroids creams or lotions taken before running may help to prevent purpura from forming (5, 34). Additionally, those who suffer from purpura should wear sunscreen to prevent sun damage to the skin and worsening of the underlying injuries.

## Sunburn

Sunburn is when the outer layer of the skin becomes damaged from the exposure of the skin to UV light. It often appears as painful redness, tightness, and swelling (first-degree burn) but can progress to blisters (second-degree burn) and more systemic symptoms (headache, generalized weakness). Sunburns often progress to skin peeling and itching. Risk factors include light colored skin, outdoor sports, and sun-sensitizing medications.

Treatment is geared toward alleviating symptoms. Athletes can use cool compresses, aloe, antibiotic ointments (for blistered skin), oral analgesic medications (acetaminophen or non-steroidal anti-inflammatory drugs), and increased fluid intake (24).

Prevention is key and runners should use sweatproof and waterproof sunscreen as well as protective clothing (24). Runners can also choose to avoid the harshest sunlight times from 10 a.m. to 4 p.m. (24).

---

## Actinic Damage and Skin Cancer

---

Repeated sunburns can put a runner at risk for developing actinic damage (precancerous lesions) or skin cancer. Other risk factors include fair complexion, unprotected sun exposure, geographic location (for example, Australia has the highest skin cancer rate), and high altitude. As runners spend many hours outdoors and may have suboptimal use of sunscreen, they are at greater risk for developing these types of lesions. In addition to UV radiation, high physical strain and high training intensity has been purported to create an environment of immunosuppression predisposing to more nevi (moles), and thus may be more likely to develop malignant melanoma (35, 36).

Prevention of sunburn and dangerous sun exposure is key for runners. They should utilize a broad-spectrum sunscreen that blocks both UVA and UVB as well as high-SPF lip balm (24). A sun protective factor (SPF) of at least 30 is optimal and the sunscreen should be generously applied at least thirty minutes before running so that the product may set and dry and will not be immediately washed away in sweat (3). Ideally, the product should be water or sweat resistant and should be reapplied every two to four hours with activity and immediately after sweating, water exposure, or towel drying (37). There are also spray and gel formulations of sunscreens available as well as non-comedogenic sunscreens for those prone to acne outbreaks. Appropriate clothing, such as clothing with a UV protection factor (UPF) of at least 25, hats, and eyeglasses with adequate UV protection can also be helpful. In the future, runners can possibly also elect to monitor their UV exposure in real time, utilizing wearable technology applications (38).

Regular physician skin checks are also highly encouraged, especially in those with fair complexions, questionable nevi, or lesions. Runners should also monitor their own skin lesions for suspicious changes. The mnemonic ABCDE is useful, denoting concerning characteristics of pigmented lesions as seen in Table 18-4 (37). A doctor should evaluate any new or changing lesion immediately, which may require surgical excision (37). Many runners may ask about maintaining vitamin D levels through sun exposure. The American Academy of Dermatologists, however, recommends maintaining adequate levels with dietary supplementation rather than with sun exposure or tanning booths (39).

**Table 18-4**  ABCDE of skin lesions.

| A | Asymmetry |
|---|---|
| B | Border, irregular or uneven |
| C | Color, irregular or uneven coloring |
| D | Diameter > 6 mm |
| E | Evolving lesion |

## CHAPTER 19

# Ocular Problems

BY MORTEZA KHODAEE AND KARIN VANBAAK

## Key Points

1. Eye injuries and problems are uncommon among distance runners.
2. Red eye is a relatively common condition that can be caused by many traumatic and non-traumatic eye disorders. Red eye with any visual problems should be taken seriously and be evaluated by a physician.
3. Ultraviolet protection with sunglasses particularly in high-altitude and snowy conditions is strongly recommended.

## Ultra Runners

Visual disturbance is an uncommon occurrence among distance runners (1). While running is in general considered a low risk or "eye safe" activity, it is important for runners to understand common and dangerous injuries that could occur especially in remote environments (2, 3, 4, 5). Ultra runners in particular may be subject to injury due to the environmental factors they encounter more than the nature of the activity itself (6). One study showed that about 3 percent of runners developed vision problems severe enough to impact race performance during 161 ultramarathons (7). According to another study, most of these athletes report painless blurry vision and cloudiness (8). The underlying etiology in most cases is still unknown, but it may be due to corneal edema, a swelling of the clear layer covering the pupil of the eye (Figure 19-1) (9). Red eye is another common condition that can be present in many traumatic and non-traumatic eye disorders (Figure 19-2). Although, conjunctivitis (inflammation of the thin layer covering the white part of the eye and inside the eyelids) is the most common cause, other uncommon conditions can cause red eye (Table 19-1).

In this chapter the authors discuss eye conditions that runners and medical team members providing coverage for running events should be aware

**Human eye anatomy**

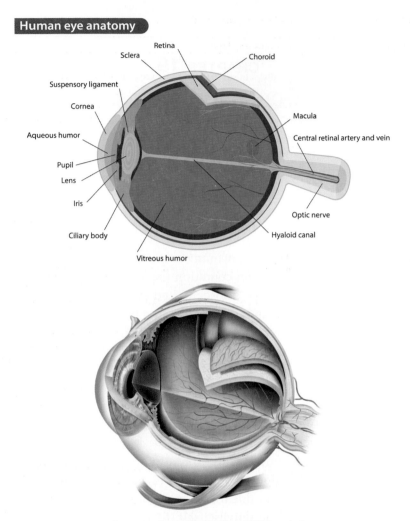

Figure 19-1  Eye Anatomy. Photo Credit: Getty Images (US) istockphoto.com

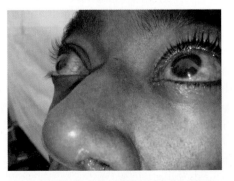

Figure 19-2  An example of red eye. Photo Credit: Mortezza Khodaee

**Table 19-1** Differential diagnoses/various causes of red eye.

| Condition | Symptoms and Signs |
| --- | --- |
| Conjunctivitis<br>Viral | Typically painless (herpes is an exception which causes severe pain); diffuse conjunctival redness; mild itching; watery discharge; unilateral or bilateral; normal vision and pupillary reactions |
| Bacterial | Mild pain with stinging sensation; conjunctival injection with foreign body sensation; may have mild purulent discharge; unilateral or bilateral; normal vision and pupillary reactions with occasional eyelid edema |
| Chemical | Mild–moderate pain; diffuse conjunctival injection; watery discharge; sensitivity to light; unilateral or bilateral; normal vision and pupillary reactions |
| Allergic | Painless diffuse conjunctival injection with significant tearing; intense itching; bilateral; normal vision and pupillary reactions |
| Subconjunctival hemorrhage | Painless; bright red area in the white part of the eyeball; usually one eye only; no discharge; normal vision and pupillary reactions |
| Trauma (corneal abrasion, foreign object, hyphema) | Usually painful (depends on the type); redness intensity and diffusion varies by cause; may or may not have visual disturbance or pupillary reaction abnormality |
| Scleritis | Severe pain radiating to area around the eye, worse with eye movements; diffuse redness; watery discharge; light sensitivity; intense pain at night and pain upon awakening; diminished vision, tenderness, scleral edema, corneal ulceration |
| Blepharitis | Painless or mildly painful red and irritated eye; itchy; crusted eyelids; usually bilateral; dandruff-like scaling on eyelashes; normal vision and pupillary reactions |
| Episcleritis | Mild to no pain; limited patches of redness; mild clear discharge; normal vision and pupillary reactions; dilated episcleral (a thin membrane covering the sclera) blood vessels, edema of episclera, tenderness over the area of injection, confined red isolated patch |
| Keratitis (corneal inflammation) | Painful red eye; diminished vision; light sensitivity; mucopurulent (slimy, pus-like) discharge; foreign body sensation; diminished vision, corneal opacities/white spot; fluorescein staining shows corneal ulcers; eyelid edema |
| Iritis | Constant radiating eye pain developing over hours; watering red eye; blurred vision; light sensitivity; diminished vision; poorly reacting, constricted pupils |
| Uveitis | Severe pain particularly with eye movement; light sensitivity; unilateral or bilateral with tearing ; decreased vision |
| Keratoconjunctivitis Sicca (dry eye) | Mild pain; itchy eyes with foreign body sensation; occasional tearing; bilateral; mild conjunctival injection (appears bloodshot) with no corneal involvement; normal vision and pupillary reactions |
| Glaucoma (acute closed-angle) | Acute onset of severe pain; watering diffuse red eye; halos appear when patient is around lights; unilateral or bilateral; significant reduction in visual acuity; dilated pupils react poorly to light; tender eyeball |

1. Beal C, Giordano B. Clinical Evaluation of Red Eyes in Pediatric Patients. J Pediatr Health Care. 2016;30(5):506–514.
2. Cronau H, Kankanala RR, Mauger T. Diagnosis and management of red eye in primary care. Am Fam Physician. 2010;81(2):137–144.

of for appropriate management. Also discussed is general considerations for injury prevention.

# Non-traumatic Eye Problems

## Ultraviolet (UV) Injury/Keratoconjunctivitis

This is commonly referred to as "snow blindness," and is an inflammation/irritation of the surface layer of the eye (cornea and conjunctiva) due to prolonged exposure to high levels of UV radiation. It is important to remember that the quantity of UV exposure increases with higher altitude, lower latitude, and in reflective environments (6). We see this injury most commonly in water, snow, and high altitude sports (2, 5). Symptoms of snow blindness typically start four to ten hours after the UV exposure and include pain, eye redness, and sensitivity to light (2, 5). Treatment includes closing the eyes and resting in a dark place. Symptoms typically resolve in twelve to fourteen hours after onset (6). Some doctors will also consider treating it with lubricating drops, topical anti-inflammatories, and/or topical antibiotics (1, 6).

## Wind/Cold injury

This has also been referred to as "frozen cornea," and actually looks like a corneal abrasion over the whole eye. It is usually seen in athletes exposed to high winds and low temperatures, notably mountaineers and parachutists (10). Symptoms include pain, sensitivity to light, and eyelid spasm (10). For treatment, athletes should be removed from the extreme environment and allowed time to heal. They should also be thoroughly examined for the presence of foreign bodies in the eye (10, 11).

## High Altitude and the Eye

Exposure to high-altitude racing conditions brings with it inherent challenges of dehydration, excessive sun exposure, low oxygen levels, cold, wind, and low barometric pressure (12, 13, 14). Some immediate effects of high altitude on the eyes include corneal edema high altitude retinopathy (damage to the retina), and UV-induced keratoconjunctivitis (inflammation of the cornea and conjunctiva) (12). It is a well-known phenomenon that central corneal thickness increases in extremely high altitude (greater than 6,000 m) (13, 14, 15, 16). The corneal thickening seems to be a result of hypoxia (low oxygen) and/or a corneal metabolism dysfunction (12, 13, 14). High altitude retinopathy consists of hemorrhage, cotton wool spots (abnormal finding of fluffy white patches on the retina), and papilledema (swelling of the optic disk) (12). Athletes that have had refractive eye surgery (like Lasik) may be adversely affected by high altitude, wind, and excessive exposure to sunlight and UV radiation (8, 12, 16). Long term exposure to high altitude can cause dry eye syndrome which often requires chronic use of artificial tears or lubricants (12).

## Corneal Edema (Opacity)

Painless blurred vision is the most common eye complaint in long distance runners (1, 8, 9). The absence of pain helps distinguish corneal edema from a corneal abrasion. Cases of partial or unilateral (affecting one eye only) corneal edema are not common (9, 17). However, the exact incidence of unilateral or bilateral corneal edema among ultra runners is unknown. There are many possible causes for corneal edema among ultra runners. In general, corneal edema can be as a result of an acute or chronic trauma, chemical exposure, inflammatory process, and hypoxia (low oxygen) (18). The likelihood of trauma to corneal tissue is enhanced by airborne debris along dirt roads where high altitude endurance events are held. Impurities in the air caused by flying dust particles and strong winds can traumatize already sensitive tissues. Using aerosol and pump action sunscreen canisters can be a potential source of eye problems. In addition, sweat may inadvertently drip down into the eyes of racers causing eye problems and corneal irritation (9). While hard contact lenses are more often associated with corneal pathology, soft contact lenses too may confer increased risk of corneal edema and opacity under racing conditions of heat, dirt, sun, and wind exposure (9).

Corneal edema among ultra runners typically resolves within a few hours without intervention. (1, 8, 9). Some athletes have been able to prevent recurrence of the visual dysfunction with protective eye glasses and hydration lubricant eye drops (1). Visual dysfunction can be so severe that athletes are unable to complete the race. The risks versus the benefits of racing with even a modicum of lost peripheral vision or depth perception needs to be seriously considered during high altitude sporting events. Even minor visual dysfunction increases accident risks. Low-level light poses an increased hazard for those with corneal edema and should be taken into consideration when determining whether or not it is advisable for an athlete to continue racing. Based on the reported natural course of endurance exercise-related corneal edema, if symptoms worsen or fail to resolve within twenty-four hours, a full ophthalmologic examination is warranted (1, 9).

## Runners with Chronic Disease or Existing Eye Problems

Due to the growing popularity of distance running, the average age of recreational runners has been increasing in the recent decades. This means, many runners may have existing chronic diseases (e.g., hypertension/high blood pressure) or ophthalmologic conditions which can affect their eyes. Individuals with well-controlled hypertension or diabetes should be able to continue running as long as there are no visual symptoms during or after running.

Regular dynamic exercise is not harmful to eyes in individuals with well-controlled glaucoma and regular running should be encouraged in this population (19). In fact, vigorous physical activity may reduce the risk of glaucoma (20).

There is no evidence that individuals with corrective eye surgery are at risk for eye injuries in general. However, the risk of corneal edema may be slightly higher at high altitude in individuals with corrective eye surgery (particularly radial keratotomy) in comparison to runners with no history of eye surgery (6). Runners should be able to wear their contact lenses during the race. The main issue is to keep the contact lenses clean and lubricated (6).

# Eye Injuries

## Corneal Abrasion

A corneal abrasion is essentially a scratch on the surface of the eye. This is a common injury which is often a result of mild trauma (2, 21). Runners in particular can get a corneal abrasion solely from dry eyes (2). Common symptoms include pain and a "foreign body sensation"—or feeling like something is stuck in one's eye—eye redness, tearing, and sensitivity to light (2, 21). This injury is almost never dangerous, and is typically expected to heal in twenty-four to forty-eight hours (21). In the clinic setting, physicians often do not use any medication treatment, but injuries sustained in wilderness environments may carry a higher risk of infection. Because of this, some physicians recommend treating these corneal abrasions with antibiotic eye drops (2, 5). Wearing contact lenses carries an increased risk of infection, so this should be avoided until the injury is healed (2, 21). This injury should not be treated with an eye patch, as this has been shown to slow healing (2, 4).

**Table 19-2** Eye Problems Among Distance Runners

| Condition | Cause | Symptoms | Signs | Management | Return to Running |
|---|---|---|---|---|---|
| Non-traumatic | | | | | |
| UV injury/ kerato- conjunctivitis | Prolonged high intensity UV exposure | Delayed symptoms onset (4–10 h); pain, sensitivity to light | Diffuse punctate staining with fluorescein | Close eyes and rest in a dark room; consider lubricating drops, patch, oral analgesics and/or antibiotics | Once symptoms resolved (no functional or binocular loss of vision) with full spectrum UV protection |
| Cold/Wind injury | Freezing of the outer cell layer of the cornea, abrasion from high wind | Pain, sensitivity to light, eyelid spasm | Eyelid spasm, small foreign bodies/debris, eye redness | Remove from offending environment, check for foreign body, consider topical eye lubricants and oral analgesics | Once symptoms resolved, with full wind/cold protective eyewear |
| Corneal edema | Acute/chronic trauma, chemical exposure, inflammatory process, high altitude, and hypoxia | Painless blurred vision | Corneal opacity | Remove possible causal factors, check for foreign body, consider topical eye lubricants | Avoid contact lens use while healing; can participate right away if no functional or binocular loss of vision |
| Traumatic | | | | | |
| Corneal abrasion | Scratch, usually from minor trauma | Pain, redness, foreign body sensation, tearing | Red eye, scratch can be seen with fluorescein dye/black light evaluation | Do not patch; antibiotic and/ or cycloplegic eye drop use at the discretion of physician; oral analgesics | Avoid contact lens use while healing; can participate right away if no functional or binocular loss of vision |

| Condition | Cause | Symptoms | Signs | Management | Return to Running |
|---|---|---|---|---|---|
| Eyelid laceration | Blunt or sharp trauma to the eye | Pain, bleeding, tearing | Laceration visible | Repair by general practitioner or ophthalmologist depending on location and severity; refer for repair if laceration at lid margin or involving lacrimal/tear duct system | Once repair is completed, with proper eye protection if no functional or binocular loss of vision |
| Foreign body | Usually small foreign body from environmental conditions | Pain, irritation, tearing, redness | Red eye, foreign body often found under upper eyelid | Removal by irrigation or with moist cotton swab | Follow up treatment as per corneal abrasion |
| Subconjunctival hemorrhage | Spontaneous, minor trauma, or Valsalva | Usually no symptoms | Bright red area in the white part of the eyeball | Watchful waiting, may take 2 weeks to resolve | No restriction |
| Preorbital contusion | Blunt trauma to eye | Pain, swelling, may have visual disturbance from eyelid swelling | Bruising and swelling in the soft tissues around the eye | Cold compress, oral analgesics | Once comfortable, as long as no serious underlying injury |
| Orbital blow-out fracture | Blunt trauma to eye | Pain, swelling, bruising around eye; may have pain with eye movement and/or double vision with upward gaze | Tenderness to palpation around bony orbit; restricted extraocular movement | Diagnosis with CT scan; referral to ophthalmology; may require surgical repair | To be determined by ophthalmologist |
| Globe rupture | Blunt or sharp trauma to the eye | Pain, deformity, visual disturbance | Hyphema, 360° subconjunctival hemorrhage, penetrating foreign body, pupillary deformity | Shield eye, avoid Valsalva; immediate referral to ophthalmology for treatment based on severity of injury | |

| Condition | Cause | Symptoms | Signs | Management | Return to Running |
|-----------|-------|----------|-------|------------|-------------------|
| **Hyphema** | Blunt trauma to the eye | Pain, red eye, blurred vision | Blood in the anterior chamber (colored part of the eye) | Referral to ophthalmology; traditional treatment of bed rest with head of bed elevated for first few days may or may not be necessary; no athletics participation; close monitoring of intraocular pressure and for rebleeding; Sickle Cell status (particularly in African Americans) should be checked | To be determined by ophthalmologist |
| **Retrobulbar hemorrhage** | Blunt trauma to eye | Pain, swelling, bruising, visual disturbance, limited eye movement | Bulging eye, tense soft tissues around the eye | Referral to ophthalmology for potential surgical management | To be determined by ophthalmologist |
| **Retinal hemorrhage and detachment** | Blunt trauma to eye (sometimes minor) | Partial loss of visual field, floaters, and flashes of lights, ± pain | Partial loss of visual field, funduscopic evaluation is needed | Referral to ophthalmology for potential surgical management | To be determined by ophthalmologist |

1.  Aerni GA. Blunt visual trauma. Clin Sports Med. 2013;32(2):289-301.
2.  Cass SP. Ocular injuries in sports. Curr Sports Med Rep. 2012;11(1):11–15.
3.  Olsen DE, Sikka RS, Pulling T, Broton M. Eye Injuries in Sports. Netter's Sports Medicine. Philadelphia, Pennsylvania, USA: Saunders, an imprint of Elsevier Inc.; 2010:332-339.
4.  Rodriguez JO, Lavina AM, Agarwal A. Prevention and treatment of common eye injuries in sports. Am Fam Physician. 2003;67(7):1481–1488.

## Eyelid Lacerations

An eyelid laceration is a cut to the eyelid. A recent study of eye injuries at an eye hospital in Finland found that injuries to the eyelid were the most common injuries seen in orienteering (sports engaging navigational skills while covering unfamiliar terrain at speed) (3). These cuts can occur after blunt or sharp trauma to the eye, and because of this, someone should undergo a thorough evaluation for more complex injuries to the eyelid or the underlying eye itself (5, 21). Depending on the depth and location of the cut, these can be repaired by a general practitioner or may need to be referred to an ophthalmologist (2, 5). It is recommended that these be repaired in twelve to thirty-six hours (2).

## Foreign Body

While this certainly could refer to a sharp object stuck in the eye, it is common for outdoor sports participants to get small foreign bodies such as dirt, grass, or insects in their eyes. Symptoms usually include pain, redness, and sensitivity to light (21). These are commonly missed under the upper lid, so this area should be examined by everting the upper eyelid (2, 4). Small foreign bodies can often be removed with simple irrigation, but a moist cotton swab can be used if this does not work (2). As with corneal abrasions, antibiotics are not typically used in the clinic setting, but may be considered in the wilderness setting (2, 4).

## Subconjunctival Hemorrhage

Subconjunctival hemorrhage is the injury which we see as bright red blood in the white part of the eyeball (sclera). This usually results from minor trauma or Valsalva (cough, heavy lifting), and is almost always a benign injury (21). It is usually painless with no visual deficiency (5). The bleeding may look frightening, but should resolve in about two weeks (5, 21). Those who had a major trauma, or have bleeding which completely surrounds the iris (colored part of the eye) should be evaluated for serious injury (21).

## Preorbital Contusion

This refers to what is commonly known as a "black eye," which is bruising and swelling in the soft tissues around the eye. Vision is usually preserved. If the injury and exam do not suggest any underlying fracture or eyeball injury, preorbital contusion can be treated with a cold compress. If the contusion is severe, consider follow up with an ophthalmologist for evaluation of the back of the eye (21).

## Orbital Fracture

The bones which form the structure of the eye socket are referred to as the bony orbit. One of the purposes of this structure is to absorb energy from a blow to the eye area by breaking. About a third of orbital fractures seen in the United States happen during sports. However these tend to occur in contact and high-velocity ball sports (4, 21). The symptoms of an orbital fracture are nonspecific with pain with eye movement and swelling, but a particular fracture location will result in double vision with looking up (21). This injury needs a CT scan for diagnosis, should be referred to an ophthalmologist, and may require surgical repair (2, 4).

## Globe Rupture

The eyeball is a ball filled with a jelly-like fluid, and globe rupture refers to any injury which results in a tear or hole through the entire surface of the eyeball. This is an uncommon, but very serious, injury. It can be difficult to identify, however. Symptoms which should raise suspicion for this injury include subconjunctival hemorrhage of 360 degrees around the iris, blood in the iris, irregularly shaped pupil, and vision loss after a significant injury (2, 4). If this injury is suspected, the eye should be shielded with something, like a Styrofoam cup, which will not put any pressure on the eyeball. A flat patch should not be used, and an ophthalmologist should be consulted as soon as possible (2, 4).

## Hyphema

Hyphema refers to blood in the anterior chamber, or in front of the iris. This is caused by blunt trauma to the eye and a tear in peripheral iris blood vessels (4, 5, 21). Symptoms include pain, a red eye, and blurred vision. This injury can result in long term visual complications, so if this injury is diagnosed, the athlete should be followed by an ophthalmologist. The eye should be protected with a shield not a patch (4, 5, 21).

## Retrobulbar Hemorrhage

This potentially serious injury refers to bleeding behind the eyeball. Because that is a fully confined space, too much bleeding can result in an increase in pressure which can permanently damage someone's vision (2, 4, 21). This injury comes from blunt trauma to the eye, and symptoms can include pain, swelling, vision changes, and limited eye movement (21). You may notice that an individual's eye tissues seem tense or their eyelid appears to be bulging (21). If a significant injury is suspected, removing the blood should occur as quickly as possible or high compartment pressures can lead to permanent vision loss after only sixty minutes (2, 21).

## Retinal Hemorrhage and Detachment

This injury is primarily caused by a pulling between the vitreous tissue (Figure 19-1) and retina as the result of a blunt trauma (2). However, cases of non-traumatic retinal hemorrhage and detachment have been reported in endurance athletes (2, 22). Symptoms include partial loss of visual field, floaters, and flashes of light. Pain may or may not be present. A funduscopic evaluation is necessary to examine the retina. Immediate referral to an ophthalmologist is needed. Often time, surgical intervention is indicated (2, 4).

## Warning Signs for Serious Injury

Athletes participating in extreme environments should be aware of certain eye symptoms which should prompt them to get a medical evaluation (Table 19-3).

**Table 19-3**  Eye Conditions Requiring Immediate Referral.

| |
|---|
| Sudden decrease or loss of visual acuity |
| Sudden loss of visual field (partial or complete) |
| Pain with eye movement |
| Diplopia (double vision) |
| Flashes of light, floaters, or halos around lights |
| Significant injury to the eye and surrounding structures (e.g., eyelid laceration) |
| Photophobia (sensitivity to light) |
| Decrease or inability of eye movement |
| Inability to remove foreign objects in the eye |
| Traumatic subconjunctival hemorrhage |
| Pupil asymmetry |

1. Olsen DE, Sikka RS, Pulling T, Broton M. Eye Injuries in Sports. Netter's Sports Medicine. Philadelphia, Pennsylvania, USA: Saunders, an imprint of Elsevier Inc.; 2010:332–339.
2. Rodriguez JO, Lavina AM, Agarwal A. Prevention and treatment of common eye injuries in sports. Am Fam Physician. 2003;67(7):1481-1488.

These include a sudden decrease in or loss of vision, loss of one field/region of vision (e.g., left peripheral vision), painful eye movement, double vision, flashes of light or floaters, halos around lights, or significant injury to the eye and surrounding structures (4, 5).

## Injury Prevention

Especially for ultra runners, the most important tool for preventing common and serious injuries is proper eye protection. The American Society for Testing and Materials standards has guidelines for eyewear material, but only for high risk/contact sports (5). In general, 2 mm polycarbonate lenses are recommended for low-risk sports (3 mm for moderate- and high-risk), in an impact resistant frame (5). Full spectrum UV protection is important as well as sunscreen to soft tissues surrounding the eyes (6). Contact lenses do not offer protection against injury (5). Risk factors for eye injury in wilderness activities include UV light exposure, strong wind, small flying particles (ice, sand), high altitude, cold and dry conditions, night activity, activity in woods and bushes, contact lens wearing, and having only one functional eye (6). Glasses with corrective lenses and UV protection in a wraparound style are the preferred eye wear for racing at high altitudes and in dusty and windy conditions.

## CHAPTER 20

# Bites and Envenomations
## BY JEREMIAH W. RAY

## Key Points

1.  Prevention is the best strategy in avoiding animal bites and envenomations. Never intentionally engage a wild animal.
2.  Avoid reaching under boulders or into foliage, as it may cause a defensive strike.
3.  For all animal bites, standard first-aid wound cleansing with soap and water is of paramount importance to minimize infection.
4.  Ensure up to date tetanus immunization and discuss with your health-care provider the utility of pre-exposure immunization to rabies when competing in areas where local animal populations have a notable rabies virus burden.
5.  If safe, attempt to take a photograph of the offending animal. This will aid in expert identification at a medical facility and facilitate the most appropriate treatment strategy. This is particularly helpful in the case of snake envenomations.
6.  When an envenomating snake is suspected to be of the rattlesnake, cottonmouth, and copperhead family, seek medical care immediately as intravenous administration of anti-venom is the only reliable treatment.
7.  For snake bites in North America, do not apply a tourniquet or pressure bandage; do not suction the wound; and do not cut or incise the wound.
8.  To prevent bites from flying insects, wear permethrin embedded clothing in conjunction with a topically applied insect repellent.
9.  When running in remote regions with a known population of large predatory carnivores, run in groups of three or more and carry capsaicin-based spray for defense.

## Mammals

Animal bites and envenomations pose a significant hazard to any outdoor enthusiast, particularly during trail running in venues that involve exposure to natural wildlife habitats. In a review of animal-related fatalities in the United States from 1999 to 2007, there were on average two hundred animal-caused fatalities a year, with an annual incidence of 6.9 fatalities per ten million population (1). Several large carnivores that are native to North America and have resulted in human fatalities include the black, brown (grizzly), and polar bear, coyote, wolf, and mountain lion (puma) (2).

## Prevention

It is strongly recommended that prior to running through any wilderness area, to check with local wildlife officials regarding fauna specific to that region. While not evidence-based, an accepted general rule is to stay at least a hundred yards from all wild animals. When running through remote regions, it is highly recommended to have at least one running partner as this will decrease the chances of a predatory attack by carnivorous mammals such as bears, wolves, and mountain lions (2). Capsaicin-based bear repellent spray wards off all North American bear species (3). In a review of eighty-three North American capsaicin-based bear repellent spray incidents, bear spray was 96 percent effective in warding off unwanted bear advances and there were no fatalities (3). If a large carnivore is encountered and it attempts to engage, attempts should be made to scare off the animal by displaying aggressive human behavior such as shouting, swinging sticks, waving arms, and throwing rocks (4). If a black bear or other large carnivore charges, one should attempt to run away and escape as this is predatory behavior. This is true for all North American carnivores with the exception of the brown bear, also known as the grizzly bear. Brown bears usually have a lighter colored fur than the black bear, have a large shoulder hump, a concave nose, and long, light-colored claws. If a brown bear is encountered, a submissive approach is recommended: keeping silent or speaking in a soft monotone voice, avoidance of eye contact, and slowly backing away, not running. If attacked, the victim should play dead and attempt to protect the head by covering it with hands.

Rabies is a preventable viral disease that is most commonly transmitted when the saliva of an infected host is introduced through broken skin, such as in a bite (5). Rabies affects mammals by causing swelling of the brain, and if not treated is nearly always fatal. The majority of its reservoirs in the United States are within carnivores such as foxes, skunks, and raccoons, but also insect-eating bats. Domesticated animals in the United States have much lower prevalence of rabies infection due to mandatory vaccination laws, but rabid cats and, less commonly, rabid dogs, still exist. Although there is no definitive way to tell if an animal has rabies virus by its appearance, possible clues to an active infection are: staggering

**Table 20-1** Reported cases of rabies in animals by the Centers of Disease Control and Prevention in the United States in 2014.

| Animal | Reported Number of Cases in 2014 | Dominant US Distribution |
|---|---|---|
| Raccoon | 1,822 | Eastern US and Texas |
| Bats | 1,756 | Distributed throughout most of North America |
| Skunks | 1,588 | Central and Eastern US, California, Arizona |
| Foxes | 311 | Eastern US, Texas, Arizona |
| Cat (domesticated) | 272 | Northeastern US, Texas |
| Dog (domesticated) | 59 | Eastern US, Texas, Puerto Rico |

gait, unsteady movements, partial paralysis to hind quarters, profuse salivation, bewildered or confused behavior, and avoidance of water. See Table 20-1 for reported rabies cases in the United States of America listed by animal.

Those who knowingly travel to areas where rabies virus is endemic should consult with their care provider to discuss the utility of rabies pre-exposure prophylaxis according to the Advisory Committee for Immunization Practices, a branch of the Centers for Disease Control (CDC) (with free online resources). Rabies pre-exposure prophylaxis provides an important degree of immunity to rabies virus and allows fewer vaccinations post-exposure (two booster immunizations instead of the four) and provides a longer time period in which to safely seek this care (9). It is important to note that this immunity provides some degree

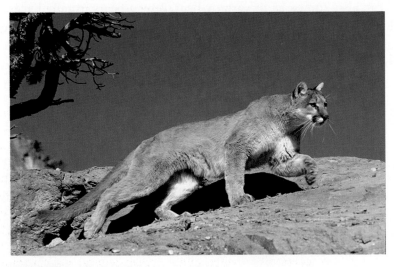

**Figure 20-1** A mountain lion.

of protection but medical care should be sought to measure antibody titers and evaluation for further booster immunization if there is potential exposure (5).

When running in more urban regions, particular attention should be paid to domesticated dogs. Outside of agriculture-related incidents, domesticated dogs produce more deaths than any other mammal in North America, accounting for an average of 17.6 fatalities each year (1). Extra caution must be maintained around pit bulls, as this breed accounts for 29 percent of all dog bites in the United States (1).

## Treatment

When bitten by a mammal, one should ensure safe distance from the animal, so as to avoid subsequent attacks. Once the bite victim is safe from further animal exposure, it is important to promptly clean the wound to prevent infection. Thorough wound cleansing with soap and water and copious irrigation is of paramount importance to minimize the chances for wound infection. All potable water is satisfactory for wound irrigation (6). Special wound cleansing solutions are not required and offer no significant prevention of wound infection rates when compared to water irrigation alone (7). Copious tap water irrigation has been shown to reduce bacterial load with equal efficacy of sterile saline (8). Wound cleansing is also the most important step in prevention of both rabies and tetanus (9).

The role of prophylactic antibiotics after dog or cat bites is controversial (10). After a mammalian bite, prophylactic antibiotics are administered if the wound is high risk for infection such as bites that are deep, large, contaminated with debris or lots of crushed tissue, on the hand or foot, or if the victims health is compromised (11). Consultation with a medical provider is encouraged.

## Insects

It is estimated that there are four to six million species of insects and that they comprise approximately half of all life on Earth (12). Insects (arthropods) are invertebrates with an exoskeleton, segmented bodies, and jointed appendages. A bite is described as a mechanical disruption of the skin due to oral apparatus, where a sting is the introduction of venom, as with scorpions and bees (13). Many arthropods display predatory behavior and cause notable disease to humans (14). A bite at best will cause a simple local inflammatory response and at worst can cause more severe local tissue death or systemic symptoms as a result of envenomation. Spiders and scorpions are often solitary creatures and will commonly flee an encounter with a larger animal such as a runner. Conversely, the blood feeding arthropods (mosquitoes, flies, fleas, mites, midges, chiggers, and ticks) actively seek hosts for blood meals (15).

## Mosquitos, Ticks, and Other Biting Insects

### Prevention

Habitat avoidance is the most efficient modality of bite prevention. When running outdoors, however, this is not always feasible thus lending to the utility of clothing modification and topically applied insect repellents. Special attention should be paid to protecting lower extremities as 77.3 percent of mosquito bites occur below the level of the knee (16). When traveling to regions with heavy burdens of biting arthropods, the CDC recommends utilizing as much clothing barrier protection as able, such as long-sleeved shirts and pants (17). In 1946, the US Armed Forces began to use DEET (diethyl-3-methylbenzamide) as an effective and safe topically-applied mosquito repellent (18). DEET was marketed to the general public ten years later in 1956 and has been a mainstay of topically-applied mosquito repellence throughout the latter half of the twentieth century (19). From 1956 to 2008 there were forty-three cases of DEET toxicity most of which manifested as headache or skin irritation, but also six reported deaths (intentional overdoses or unintentional overuse in children) (20, 21). Most DEET containing products range in concentrations of 30 to 40 percent, which is an effective concentration (31). As human studies have shown a plateau effect of insect repellent ability of DEET at about 50 percent (22), higher concentrations are not recommended as there is increased risk of skin irritation with minimal benefit (33). DEET has species specific repellent profiles and when traveling to areas endemic with malaria carrying mosquitos, more frequent applications are required (23).

A newer repellent, picaridin (icaridin in Europe), has several advantages over DEET. Whereas DEET can damage spandex, rayon, plastic, and vinyl, picaridin is non-corrosive on all surfaces; is less greasy; less irritating; and lacks a chemical odor (18). At 20 percent concentration picaridin is proven to be as effective as DEET, with longer acting repellency against mosquitoes, flies, chiggers, and ticks (23). The third available chemical repellent in the United States is IR3535, produced by Avon. Field studies show IR3535 has superior insect repellency over DEET, particularly against sandflies and biting midges with longer duration of efficacy (24).

Most plant-based repellents exhibit limited efficacy but there are two with moderate efficacy and worth considering for bite prevention. The first is an extract of the leaves of lemon eucalyptus (PMD) that is also available in a synthetic formulation. Formulations containing PMD with concentrations of 10 percent to

40 percent are as effective as DEET against mosquito bites, but superior to DEET at preventing tick bites (25). The second repellent is permethrin, derived from dried chrysanthemum flowers, and has been shown to kill ticks on contact (18). Permethrin embedded clothing is superior to topically applied DEET for bite prevention of bites from ticks, gnats, and chiggers (19).

Various essential oils (e.g., citronella, geranium, clove, mint, nutmeg, soybean, and pennyroyal) are substantially less efficacious than DEET at reducing mosquito bite rates and offer approximately twenty minutes of decreased bite frequency compared to the 301 minutes of protection afforded by DEET (26). Essential oils, particularly mint derivatives, should be avoided in children younger than two years of age due to seizure risks (27). Consumption of garlic has long been touted as a natural method of mosquito bite prevention, but a controlled trial found it ineffective (28).

In summary, the ideal insect prevention strategy would be utilization of permethrin embedded clothing in conjunction with a topical application of picaridin, IR3535, or DEET for mosquito bite prevention; or permethrin embedded clothing with a topical application IR3535, picaridin, or PMD for prevention of bites from ticks, black flies, sandflies, and biting midges (20). The majority of insect bites typically results in mild, local, allergic reactions and require no further medical care outside of routine wound cleaning (13).

---

## Bees, Wasps, and Ants

---

### *Prevention*

Of the non-domesticated animals in North America, the hymenoptera (which includes wasps, bees, and fire ants) are the most lethal to humans (1), accounting for an average of 56.6 deaths per year in the United States (1). The vast majority of these fatalities are due to an emergent swelling of the airways called anaphylaxis, and are only rarely due to swarming attacks from Africanized honey bees—where the average lethal number of stings are 500 to 1,200 per victim (29).

Most hymenoptera do not display aggressive behavior, with the exception of the Africanized honeybees and the yellow jacket, also known as a "meat bee," which is an aggressive scavenger and responsible for the majority of hymenoptera envenomations (30). The Africanized honey bee is exceptionally defensive of its nest and recruits colony members for a swarming stinging defense (31). The generally accepted strategy in fleeing from bees is to run away from the nest, ideally protecting oneself in a sealed environment such as a house, car, or tent. If shelter is not available, running through trees and bushes may impede the insects.

Submersion under water is not an optimal escape strategy, as hymenoptera are attracted to exhaled carbon dioxide in human breath (32).

## Treatment

If an individual has a personal history or a family history of hypersensitivity to stings, including anaphylaxis, they should seek the care of an allergist or immunologist to be tested for hymenoptera hypersensitivity (33). In those cases, venom immunotherapy reduces severity of the reactions and should be considered in individuals with severe reactions (34). Additionally, it is prudent that highly sensitive individuals should always carry an epinephrine auto injector—as deaths from anaphylaxis are a preventable, but tragically common, occurrence (35).

Bees have barbed stingers that imbed in the skin, thus eviscerating the insect as a consequence of the sting (29). Once the stinger is lodged in flesh, it continues to inject venom for up to sixty seconds and must be removed prior to this in order to minimize venom burden (36). Once stung, the stinger should be quickly removed from the flesh by firmly flicking or scraping the stinger with any available object such as credit card, knife blade, sharp rock, or stick. Wasps are divided in to either hornets, yellow jackets, or other subdivisions. They possess a smooth stinging apparatus that is capable of multiple stings per encounter (29). The same is true with fire ants and there will be no stinger to remove after these attacks.

Cold packs and an over-the-counter medication called diphenhydramine (i.e., Benadryl) are often helpful to reduce symptom severity (37). It is common to experience streaking after envenomation but this is generally reactive, not infective, and it is exceedingly rare for hymenoptera stings to require antibiotics (38).

---

## Scorpions

---

Like spiders, scorpions are in the class arachnid and are characterized by grasping pincers and segmented tail with a telson (stinger) (39). The pincers are purely for holding prey and have little ability to harm humans (40). It is the scorpion's telson in their terminal tail segment that contains the stinger and venom glands that must be avoided.

## Prevention

While menacing in appearance, scorpions are leery of larger animals and rarely show aggressive behavior toward humans (41). Most scorpion envenomations are defensive and occur when the creature is accidentally pressed upon while it is sheltering in clothing, shoes, or bedding (42). Thus the best preventative strategy for scorpion envenomation is utilization of protective footwear and to shake out clothing, shoes, and bedding when in endemic regions.

## Treatment

In North America, the only scorpion that is considered dangerous to humans is the Bark Scorpion (43). The Bark Scorpion is found throughout New Mexico, Arizona, southern California, and Mexico (44). Scorpion venom has a number of toxins, most of which are lethal to insects, but some that may cause problems in humans, particularly children (45). Ninety percent of scorpion envenomations cause simple local inflammatory responses similar to that of a severe bee sting, resolve spontaneously on the order of hours to days, and require no further medical care (40). Nearly all of the envenomations that result in systemic illness occur in children due to their relatively high venom to body mass ratio (46). The effects of scorpion envenomation are dictated by the offending species, with the most dangerous scorpions residing in the Near and Middle East, North Africa, Brazil, and India (47). The dominant systemic effect of scorpion envenomation is neuromuscular agitation as manifested as muscle twitching, gait disturbance, uncontrolled limb movements, and eye movements (48). More dangerous nervous system excitation can occur such as: hypersalivation, sweating, tearing, diarrhea, vomiting, and increased airway secretions that can interfere with breathing (40). The pain of a scorpion sting will manifest quickly, and signs of envenomation usually progress to maximum severity within five hours. Anascorp is the only FDA-approved scorpion antivenom available in the United States (49). Its use is controversial given its unclear efficacy coupled with undesirable side effect profile, but may be of benefit when symptoms are severe or when the victim is small (50). Due to the often delayed progression of symptoms after a scorpion envenomation (especially outside of North America), definitive medical care should be quickly obtained and often a period of observation is necessary to ensure no progression of symptoms.

# Snakes

## Prevention

Snakebites are estimated to lead to 9,000 emergency room visits annually in the United States (51). Venomous snakes account for approximately one-third of these visits (52). The United States averages 5.2 to 7.4 snake-related fatalities annually (1). In North America, there are two families of snake that are venomous: the Viperidae family, which includes the rattlesnake, cottonmouth (water moccasin), and the copperhead; and the Elapidae family, containing the coral snake (51). Trail running exposes athletes to the snake's natural habitat and therefore increases risk of injury and envenomation. Wearing thick protective clothing such as denim pants or leather boots may reduce venom volume injection by as much as two-thirds (53), but this is impractical to the runner. Generally, during a defensive strike, less venom is delivered than an offensive strike, and 25 percent of defensive strikes are "dry bites" in which no venom is delivered (54). Pit vipers are deaf to airborne noise but are responsive to vibration, so stomping the ground to alert the snake from a distance and avoidance of cornering them will reduce the chances of a strike (55). The strike distance of a snake is roughly two-thirds of the total length of the snake (55).

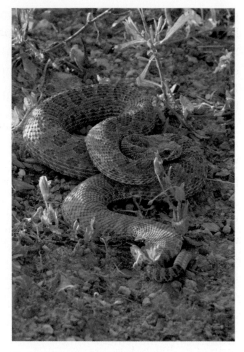

**Figure 20-2** Prairie Rattlesnake.

## Treatment

If bitten by a snake, one should move beyond striking distance. If safe, a photograph should be taken of the offending snake to assist the health-care providers in providing the appropriate medical therapy. If the snake is deemed non-venomous, there is no need to seek medical care, simply wash the wound and ensure up-to-date tetanus status. Symptoms of envenomation include bruising, swelling, redness, and severe pain in addition to systemic symptoms such as nausea, vomiting, diarrhea, passing out, rapid heart rate, and cold, clammy skin (54). There have been documented cases of sudden death from anaphylactic reaction to the envenomation, so any sudden shortness of breath from a snakebite should be treated with epinephrine injection. The swelling and bruising start locally at the bite site then spread centrally as the venom spreads. After a bite, any jewelry should be quickly removed as it may become constricting if there is progressive swelling.

The standard therapy for all North American pit viper bites that manifest any signs of envenomation (local or systemic) is the rapid administration of antivenom (56). As it may take six to twelve hours for signs of envenomation (such as bruising and progressive swelling), all venomous snakebites should be promptly evacuated to definitive medical care for observation for at least eight hours (56). If any early signs of envenomation in the field, the decision should be made as to the quickest route of a hospital: making the journey on one's own, or having the victim stay put and alerting emergency medical services. Envenomations from the coral snake are rare, but the neurotoxin it delivers can be fatal if not treated with snake specific antivenin (57).

There are several snakebite treatment myths that have permeated popular culture and are often applied to the detriment of the victim. Oral suction of the bite area provides no useful extraction of venom (58). Mechanical suction should be avoided as there is questionable increase in venom removal and the suction can increase local tissue damage (59). Intentionally cutting or bleeding of the snakebite site has no benefit (60). Application of an electrical current does not alter snake venom, but it does cause pain to the victim and should be avoided (61). Tourniquets should be avoided in pit viper bites, as they have been shown to lead to higher rates of amputation and have no proven benefits (62). Veno-occlusive tourniquets are of use in some Elapidae (e.g., cobras, black mambas, adders) envenomations as they possess potent neurotoxins and benefit from slowing neurotoxin spread, but anyone who applies this type of tourniquet should be trained in the application.

## CHAPTER 21

# Chronic Medical Conditions

## BY ERIN DRASLER AND TRACY A. CUSHING

## Key Points

1. Runners with heart disease need to advance training slowly and consistently.
2. Regular running decreases risk of death from heart attacks and increases quality of life.
3. Runners with lung diseases such as asthma or COPD should incorporate a slow warm-up into their training, which can boost running performance to levels of those without underlying lung disease.
4. Regular running can benefit those with neurologic disorders such as seizures, multiple sclerosis, and headaches, by reducing both the frequency and severity of disease-related symptoms.
5. Digital technology has revolutionized diabetes management such that diabetic runners can get real-time feedback while running to optimally manage their blood sugars.
6. The myth that distance running causes degenerative arthritis has been debunked; runners have about half the rate of hip and knee replacements as non-runners.

## Introduction

Living with a chronic disease doesn't have to mean letting go of one's running goals. Runners should be empowered to become expert in managing their chronic illness while attaining these goals. As a common theme, sufferers of most chronic conditions benefit significantly from regular exercise like running. This chapter focuses on several chronic medical conditions that challenge runners, and current recommendations for managing these conditions while continuing to run.

# Heart Disease

## Coronary Artery Disease

Coronary artery disease (CAD) is the leading cause of death of both men and women in the United States, and concern for CAD may complicate many runners' lives, particularly as they age (1). CAD occurs when the major blood vessels supplying the heart with oxygen and nutrients become narrowed with cholesterol-containing plaques, decreasing their ability to adequately supply the heart. According to the Centers for Disease Control and Prevention, 11.5 percent of the population carries a diagnosis of CAD. Many more people remain undiagnosed, and they live with partial blockages within the blood vessels of their heart (2). Most studies of people with CAD show that regular aerobic exercise such as running decreases risk of death from heart attacks, and also increases quality of life (3, 4). In this section, we will discuss conditions that make one prone to development of CAD, CAD, medications that could interfere with running, and current recommendations for running with CAD.

Many medical conditions contribute to developing CAD, including high blood pressure, high cholesterol, diabetes, obesity, and a sedentary lifestyle (5). Some data suggests that regular running improves all of the other five risk factors (6), leading to a lower incidence of CAD, a 29 percent lower all-cause mortality, and a 50 percent lower cardiovascular death rate (mortality) in runners compared to non-runners (7). Family history is also an important factor in the development of CAD, and unfortunately cannot be modified.

But there is some contradictory evidence in regard to the development of CAD. While regular aerobic exercise, including distance running, leads to a seven-year increase in life expectancy, there may be an upper limit to the amount of exercise that is beneficial (8, 9). It is hypothesized that chronic training for and participating in extreme endurance events can cause microtrauma to blood vessels and actually increase stiffening and calcification of the coronary arteries (10). More research is needed to clarify the optimal "dose" of exercise, but at this time consensus suggests consistent moderate exercise as extremely beneficial in the prevention and management of CAD.

Managing CAD, as well as underlying hypertension, high cholesterol, diabetes, and obesity, is done in conjunction with a physician and often requires prescription medications. These medications can result in decreased exercise tolerance, so adjustment may be needed when training for distance running. High blood pressure medications such as: ACE inhibitors, calcium channel blockers, and central alpha agonists are generally considered to be the best tolerated medications while exercising (10).

In patients with known CAD, multiple studies have shown exercise for cardiac rehabilitation lowers your risk of cardiac mortality (4). If one has risk factors for cardiovascular disease, the American Heart Association recommends consulting a physician and considering an exercise stress test to examine the heart's ability to respond to the stress of exercise prior to beginning running (11). Training should be advanced more slowly and consistently in this population, to avoid excess stress on the heart. Patients with known CAD should consider avoiding additional stresses such as extremes of heat or high altitudes, which place additional strain on an already challenged heart. Most importantly, listen to the body's cues and slow down or stop if you develop chest pressure, shortness of breath, nausea, or extreme fatigue; as many runners may have undiagnosed CAD, these symptoms may be the "early warning signal" of cardiovascular disease (12).

## Congestive Heart Failure

About 5.7 million people in the United States currently live with congestive heart failure (CHF) (2), which occurs when the heart's ability to function as a pump fails to supply your body with adequate blood and oxygen. While running puts the heart under additional stress and can cause worsening heart failure, regular aerobic exercise can be beneficial in patients with heart failure. Most experts suggest working with a physician to optimize an individual's medication regimen prior to initiation of a regular running schedule.

Most patients with heart failure take medications called diuretics or "water pills" as a first line treatment to remove the excess fluid that can collect in the lungs and other tissues (13). This may put runners at an increased risk of electrolyte imbalances while running, particularly in the heat. Runners with CHF need to be much more diligent about appropriate hydration, as well as avoiding overhydration during running. However, in the setting of heart failure, appropriately taken diuretics may actually increase exercise performance (14).

Runners with CHF should increase their mileage slowly and in consultation with a trainer, so as not to cause additional damage to their heart or worsening cardiac function (14). Running with stable heart failure usually isn't a problem—as long as you keep your effort level at or below the heart's ability to compensate for increased demand.

## Abnormal Heart Rhythms

There are conflicting opinions on endurance running as a risk for abnormal heart rhythms (arrhythmias). Several studies report that endurance training increases the risk of arrhythmias such as atrial fibrillation or atrial flutter by two to ten times (15, 16). This has garnered attention within the running community, as these arrhythmias put patients at higher risk for stroke and decrease exercise tolerance (15). Some researchers believe that the endurance training of long distance runners results in overgrowth of muscle tissue in the left side of the heart, making one prone to developing arrhythmias (16). Another theory is that transient volume overload of the heart may form fibrous tissue that acts as a nidus for arrhythmias. Other studies have not supported this: a 2013 study of runners showed that when adjusted for daily energy expenditure, those who exercised consistently had a lower incidence of arrhythmias than cohorts who completed the same amount of exercise but less consistently (17). In this study, authors noted that the observed runners had been running on average for over ten years, so if the long-term physiologic changes discussed above had occurred, they expected to see increased frequency of arrhythmias. As with CAD and CHF, consistency seems to be the most important aspect of endurance exercise to minimize the risks to the cardiovascular system (18, 19).

# Lungs

## Asthma

Asthma, particularly exercise-induced bronchospasm (EIB), afflicts up to 23 percent of athletes compared to 4 percent of regular people (20). Experts speculate that this may be because of prolonged high rates of breathing during intense exercise. Long distance running exposes athletes to factors that can contribute to worsening asthma symptoms including pollen, hot or cold weather, and poor air quality. Controlling these variables may not always be possible, and prolonged exposure may result in airway spasm. Several studies have shown that many people seem to have mild EIB and be unaware (21, 22).

Fortunately, runners perform quite well despite their asthma. Asthmatic athletes studied during the 2008 Olympics won a disproportionate 29 percent of the individual medals. While several studies show that lung function improves with use of asthma inhalers, this doesn't necessarily translate to faster race times. Researchers believe this discrepancy is because lung function isn't usually the limiting factor to running performance (23).

Runners with asthma should warm up thoroughly, for at least twenty minutes, to help minimize the chance of bronchospasm during a race (24). This warm-up should consist of both easy running as well as high intensity exertion at approximately 90 percent of maximum effort—this may significantly decrease

EIB during a race (20, 21). If pollen, smoke, or cold weather typically trigger an asthma exacerbation, breathing through a balaclava or scarf to filter inhaled particles and increase humidity may also help minimize bronchospasm (24). Experts recommend having a thorough evaluation with a physician prior to participating in distance running or other endurance athletics to make sure asthma is optimally controlled. Some researchers believe that EIB differs from standard asthma slightly and can be treated more effectively with short-acting beta-agonist inhalers without the addition of steroid inhalers (which are often used for asthma maintenance) (25). Most importantly, an inhaler should be carried on long runs in case of an emergency.

## Chronic Obstructive Pulmonary Disease (COPD)

COPD (emphysema) results from progressive destruction of lung tissue, most commonly due to smoking (26). Similarly to asthma, lungs with COPD often respond to the stress of running with bronchospasm. Treatment and considerations are the same as discussed above for asthma. The biggest difference is that patients with COPD often have decreased lung volume and less pulmonary reserve. This means that at high altitude or at maximum exertion, runners with COPD are more likely to have low oxygen levels compromising performance (27).

COPD causes patients to have lower exercise capacity and, similarly to those with CAD, affected patients should participate in slow progression of low-intensity training in order to increase this exercise capacity (28). In 2015, Russell Winwood, an Australian fitness enthusiast, became the first person ever with stage IV (very severe) COPD to complete a marathon (29). An inspiration for many who struggle with COPD, Winwood showed that he could thrive as a runner despite his disease. The American Thoracic Society recommends working with your pulmonologist (lung doctor) to develop a personalized exercise plan to optimize lung function, especially in patients with more severe disease (30).

# Neurological Disorders

## Seizures

Seizure disorders affect about 2 percent of the population; epileptics have historically been advised to avoid participation in athletic ventures for fear of provoking seizures (31). While there are case reports of seizures brought on by exercise, most recent research shows that exercise actually decreases seizure frequency and seizure threshold, particularly when not done to the point of exhaustion (32, 33).

When coupled with the other benefits of long distance running to the runner's psyche and overall physical fitness, the benefits of running with a seizure disorder likely far outweigh risks.

Seizures result from an area of the brain with focal overactive neurons, and some types of seizures result in a sudden loss of consciousness. People with focal seizures without associated loss of consciousness are typically at less risk of adverse events because they are conscious during the episode and can avoid a dangerous fall. The potential for falls while running should be considered, particularly if the terrain is remote or treacherous. However, the International League Against Epilepsy (ILAE) classifies running as no significant additional risk posed to the participant should they have a seizure during participation (31).

Certain factors can precipitate seizures, such as fatigue, overheating, and electrolyte imbalances, which can be exacerbated by running. Runners with epilepsy must be extra vigilant to their food and fluids intake to avoid such situations (34).

Runners with a seizure disorder should consult their physician to make sure their seizures are optimally controlled on medications prior to starting a training regime (31, 35). Runners should consider carrying medication to stop a seizure if it occurs, such as a benzodiazepine. If a bystander witnesses a runner having a seizure, the most important focus should be preventing trauma by removing rocks from the area or pulling the person away from a drop-off (31).

## Multiple Sclerosis

Multiple sclerosis (MS) is an auto-immune disorder that causes the body to attack and destroy the protective coating around nerves. Flares of MS can be predictably triggered by heat (36). Therefore, a diagnosis of MS has historically made most sufferers shy away from nearly all exercise, including running. Runners with MS need to be particularly careful about exertion in extreme heat. Some runners opt to pre-cool themselves with ice packs or have their support teams bring cool packs to aid stations. While the initial effects of exercise on MS can lead to worsening symptoms, over time the effect on MS symptoms can actually be beneficial (36, 37). According to a recent review, endurance training improves many symptoms of MS including function in walking, balance, cognition, fatigue, depression, and quality of life (38).

## Migraine/Headache Disorders

Headaches represent the most common neurologic disorder, with almost 20 percent of the population suffering from headaches according to the CDC (39). Ranging in severity from mild to incapacitating, headaches can prevent people from running due to fear of triggering a headache. Migraine sufferers are often aware of their triggers, some of which can be linked with running such as sun exposure, heat, or dehydration (40). Several recent studies, however, show that regular aerobic exercise including distance running can prevent migraines (41, 42).

The exact mechanism by which exercise prevents migraines remains elusive; researchers hypothesize it may be due to increased release of brain endorphins, improved neurotransmitter function, decreased inflammation, or increased serotonin production (43, 44). Several comparative studies of migraines randomized to treatment with aerobic exercise or preventative medications showed that both were equally effective at reducing frequency and severity of migraines, but with fewer side effects in the exercise group (44). Most major medical organizations including the American Academy of Neurology and the National Institute of Neurologic Disorders and Stroke recommend regular exercise in management of headache disorders (43).

# Endocrine Disorders

## Diabetes

According to the American Diabetes Association, 9.3 percent of the US population lives with diabetes (45). Since it affects the body's normal ability to process and utilize sugar, long distance running with diabetes can be challenging. Divided into two subcategories, type 1 diabetes occurs when the pancreas does not secrete enough insulin to process sugar; type 2 occurs when the body becomes less sensitive to the insulin produced by the pancreas. Both result in elevated glucose (sugar) levels, and both require significant attention to manage while running. However, many marathoners and ultramarathoners with diabetes perform at elite levels despite their illness, as they have adjusted their insulin needs to fit their planned goals (45, 46).

Though digital technology is not strictly necessary for glucose management, devices including insulin pumps and continuous glucose monitors make it more convenient to run with diabetes. With these devices, diabetics can track their blood sugars in real time (47). In general, intense physical exercise such as distance running causes a decrease in blood sugar due primarily to enhanced glucose uptake by multiple organs during exercise (46). Diabetic runners generally need to eat about 15 to 30 g of carbohydrates per hour of running to keep their glucose levels steady (48). Increased carbohydrate needs often continue for several hours after running, called the "lag effect" of exercise (49). This occurs because the body uses glycogen, or sugar stores in liver and muscle, while it is running. After running, your body replaces this glycogen, which can take up to twenty-four hours.

After exercise, it is important to continue checking blood sugars frequently. Many physicians also recommend exercising at least two hours before bedtime, to avoid overnight low sugar (hypoglycemic) episodes (49, 50).

Prior to beginning a regular running schedule, diabetic runners should consult a physician specialized in diabetes management (endocrinologist) to help adjust their insulin schedule; long-acting insulin doses typically need to be lowered by about 80 percent on days with long runs. During exercise, blood glucose should be kept at least 100 mg/dL (50).

## Thyroid Disorders

The thyroid, a large gland in the neck, secretes hormones that regulate your body's metabolism and are essential to the function of every organ in your body. Up to 12 percent of the population will have disordered thyroid function at some time in their lives (51). Those who produce too much thyroid hormone can experience diarrhea, tremors, and heart palpitations, while those who produce too little have constipation, fatigue, and depression. Runners with both low and high thyroid hormone levels may need to adjust their hormone replacement during intense training. Not much data is available regarding the specific effects of training on hormone levels, and there appears to be a lot of individual variability (52, 53). There is some debate over whether prolonged and intense training causes low thyroid function. At this time, experts recommend close monitoring of thyroid hormone levels with an endocrinologist during training. In addition, consistency in training allows the body to keep thyroid hormone levels from fluctuating (53). There appears to be a transient decrease in thyroid function during the adjustment period with increased exercise stress (54). The same trend has also been observed with intense exercise without appropriate increase in calorie intake. There is concern about treating "subclinical hypothyroidism," which means symptoms possibly related to low thyroid without demonstrably low thyroid hormone levels. While thyroid medication has been recommended by some running coaches as a performance-enhancing drug, there have been no studies that reliably show thyroid hormone has any performance benefits (55).

## Gastrointestinal (GI) Disorders

### Inflammatory Bowel Disease (IBD)

Inflammatory bowel diseases such as Crohn's disease or ulcerative colitis cause an auto-immune attack on the lining of the intestinal wall (56). Sufferers have frequent bouts of diarrhea coupled with abdominal pain which can progress to needing surgery in certain cases. These symptoms can make distance running seem daunting; it can be difficult and painful to run with abdominal cramps and distance from a convenient bathroom may dictate the day's running plan. Yet the best available research suggests that regular exercise can decrease both pro-inflammatory modulators of the disease, as well as improving symptoms of colitis (57, 58). Though more research is needed, runners with IBD can safely continue participating in their sport without fear of a worsening of their disease. While there are no specific recommendations for running with IBD, experts suggest postponing particularly difficult or stressful workouts to a less symptomatic day (59).

## Runner's Colitis

Nearly all long distance runners experience at least occasional GI distress while running (60, 61). When running longer distances the body responds by shunting blood away from the intestines to the heart, muscles, and lungs—where it is currently needed. This often causes difficulty in digesting food taken in during the race, leading to diarrhea. More seriously, it can lead to the walls of the intestine being so deprived of blood that they actually begin to slough off (62).

Many distance runners have this to some degree. One study showed that 23 percent of marathon participants had stool positive for blood after the race, most of whom were not symptomatic (62). Fortunately, this condition usually resolves spontaneously with simple hydration, and causes no long-term consequences.

To avoid succumbing to runner's colitis, experts recommend maintaining adequate hydration, careful consideration of food intake choices during the race, and timing of food intake during a race. Being aware to not push yourself past your aerobic threshold for extended periods of time during a long race can also help to avoid this complication (61).

# Musculoskeletal Disorders

## Arthritis

In 2015, a groundbreaking article came out challenging the conventional wisdom that distance runners will inevitably get osteoarthritis from repetitive trauma to the knees and hips. This article showed that, in 75,000 study participants, those who ran had about half the rate of hip replacements than those who did not (63). Runners with higher mileage had an even lower incidence. While this difference can be explained by the lower weights of the more fit runners, it still exposes the causative link between running and arthritis as a myth.

Arthritis seems to be provoked by an initial injury to the joint (63). There is minimal evidence that osteoarthritis worsens with activity, and no research that shows improvement with rest. However, continuing to run through serious pain on an injured joint could contribute to the development of arthritis.

Experts recommend that runners with osteoarthritis, especially after joint replacement, consider running more trails and less roads, providing more variability and less repetitive stress (64, 65). Runners can consider using trekking poles to lessen pressure on the knees on the steeps. Runners should consider participating in cross-training activities with less impact as well as core strengthening activities. However, there is no data to suggest that runners should stop running after a diagnosis of osteoarthritis.

## Rhabdomyolysis

While some breakdown of muscle is inevitable during intense exercise, exertional rhabdomyolysis (ER) represents an extreme form. Defined as a blood creatinine kinase (CK) level of five to fifty times the normal limit, ER often results in urine the color of cola, as the kidneys excrete these proteins (66). Caused by prolonged and/or repetitive exercise, distance runners are prone to developing ER. Particularly in trail running, which involves a lot of eccentric muscle contraction as the muscles lengthen while contracting during steep downhills, many if not most runners will have an elevated CK level if checked immediately after a race (67, 68). However, while non-exertional rhabdomyolysis progresses to kidney failure 20 to 40 percent of the time, ER causes kidney failure in only about 1 percent of cases. This is likely because as long as appropriate urine output is maintained, the kidneys are able to clear the muscle breakdown products without damaging the kidneys themselves. Factors that predispose to kidney failure in ER include: dehydration, excessive heat, NSAID (nonsteroidal anti-inflammatory drug) use, and recent viral illness.

Some runners unfortunately suffer from recurrent cases of ER, and there are many underlying environmental and genetic variables that can be a predisposition (69, 70). Several classes of medications such as diuretics, antipsychotics, antidepressants, and antihistamines have been implicated in the development of ER. Statins have likewise been blamed, though several studies suggest that though they only cause minor muscle pain. Consultation with a doctor is recommended to adjust medications prior to competing to lower the risk. Additionally, avoiding alcohol and recreational drugs prior to a race can decrease chances for developing

ER. Many different genetic mutations in muscle such as autoimmune myopathies, disorders of glycogen metabolism, or sickle cell trait can also provoke ER, though these disorders are quite rare. If suspected, genetic testing or muscle biopsy may be required for additional evaluation. If one has had ER previously, particularly with kidney injury or elevated CK lasting beyond two weeks, experts recommend additional work-up for underlying medical conditions.

Based on expert consensus, one can limit the chances of developing ER by following the above recommendations. Consider postponing a race if a recent viral or bacterial illness or an injury that has limited training. During the race, avoid NSAIDs such as ibuprofen or naproxen, as these can inhibit the kidneys' ability to clear muscle breakdown products (71). Most importantly, maintain appropriate hydration status with water and electrolyte replacement.

# SECTION 4
# After the Run

## CHAPTER 22

# Nutrition for Recovery and Prevention
## BY ALICIA KENDIG

## Key Points

1. Proper nutrition can be used to an athlete's advantage to speed recovery and optimize the adaptation of the body to key training stimuli.

2. During heavy phases of training intensity and volume, proper recovery nutrition practices can prevent injury by decreasing time needed for recovery. Chronic under-recovery can lead to overuse injuries.

3. Carbohydrate stores (glycogen) is a limited resource of energy stored in the liver and muscle. During longer endurance activity, these glycogen stores will become depleted and need to be spared by consuming nutrition during activity, or replaced after the activity is completed. The recovery is most effective within thirty to sixty minutes after activity is completed.

4. Exercise-induced muscle damage (EIMD) naturally occurs during training. Dietary protein consumed in the recovery phase (thirty to sixty minutes post-exercise) can increase muscle protein synthesis (MPS) and decrease muscle breakdown during this time.

5. Natural sources of antioxidants can help to decrease stress markers increased during activity, but dietary supplement forms of these nutrients may actually inhibit the natural training response and be detrimental to performance markers.

6. Rehydration after longer endurance activity not only replaces fluids lost during exercise, but can also actively cool core temperature.

7. Planning and packing recovery snacks for consumption immediately post-exercise can help to efficiently address this ideal recovery time, optimize training adaptations, and jumpstart the recovery process to prepare for the next training session.

In the world of high performance sport, one thing is for sure: athletes learn to take care of their bodies so their bodies can take care of them. Typically, this comes with increased importance the older an athlete gets, but when recovery time is of the essence, various modalities can make a significant difference. Research in the field of enhancing recovery has proposed various ideas, with many having been adopted over the years, although only a few have withstood the test of time. Some examples of this include massage therapy, cold and hot plunges, sauna, compression pants, and cryotherapy compression. Although there is limited research regarding some of these modalities, there is significant literature supporting the use of nutrition to improve recovery time, prevent injury, and enhance adaptations to training. This chapter aims to outline the long distance runner's need for recovery nutrition and explain the role that food and nutrition can have on an athletes training and recovery plan.

## Why the Need for Recovery

Without enough rest and recovery, an athlete may feel sluggish and far from high performance. A harsh reality is that inadequate recovery can also increase risk of injury. A recent Scandinavian study demonstrated that athletes sleeping more than eight hours on weekdays reduced their chance of injury by 61 percent, and those reaching recommended nutrition intakes reduced their odds for injury by 64 percent (16). Without appropriate recovery, a body may ache, muscles may feel more fatigued, and motivation to continue can be derailed. There are physiological explanations for all of these signs and symptoms, and when selecting recovery modalities, these explanations can help you choose and prioritize what you need in order to recover quickly and efficiently.

Although often referred to as "recovery nutrition," post-training meals can also maximize adaptation from the training already completed, and prevent injury in the next training session. Using nutrition to an athlete's advantage can help achieve all of these functions. In previous chapters, the importance of fueling appropriately for training has been outlined in detail, both before training begins and during longer training sessions. Recovery nutrition is arguably equally as important if not more so, especially during high volume and intensity training phases.

For endurance training athletes engaging in higher training volumes, muscle glycogen represents an important fuel source during prolonged moderate-to high-intensity exercise. Muscle glycogen is the stored form of carbohydrate, metabolized in the recovery phase by a process called glycogenesis. These glycogen stores are found in the liver and muscle, and broken down when energy is needed to sustain higher intensity aerobic activity for up to two hours of energy. Carbohydrates and essential fatty acids are the main fuels oxidized by skeletal muscle during exercise, with their contributions to energy production varying based on intensity level and previous meals and snacks consumed. Even the leanest athletes have a large store of fatty acids, without much need to replenish during heavy phases of training; however, carbohydrate stores have limited capacities, with the general timeline to exhaustion being approximately two hours of higher intensity activity.

---

### Practicing the 4 Rs of Recovery

**R**eplenish muscle glycogen (carbohydrate stored in muscle) after practice by eating as much as 1 g of carbohydrate per kilogram body weight.

**R**epair and regenerate muscle with high quality protein by eating 0.25 to 0.30 g of protein per kilogram body weight (approximately 15 to 25 g protein for the average sized athletes—no improvement of recovery seen in protein intakes higher than 40 g of protein, regardless of body size).

**R**einforce muscle cells and immune system with colorful and antioxidant-rich foods (e.g., fruits, veggies, whole grains, fish, nuts, olive oil). Athletes should consider eating at least 2 to 3 cups of fruit and 3 to 4 cups of vegetables daily, which is in line with dietary recommendations for physically active individuals (12).

**R**ehydrate with fluid and electrolytes based on sweat losses in training/competition (150 percent of fluid losses, or three cups fluid per pound of sweat lost). Urine color can be used as a hydration guide in the hours after training, with a goal of maintaining light yellow color (not clear nor dark).

---

# Replenish Energy Stores

## Why Carbohydrates for Recovery and Injury Prevention?

After cessation of exercise, muscle glycogen is typically restored to pre-exercise concentrations within twenty-four hours, provided that sufficient amounts of carbohydrates are ingested. However, athletes training numerous times a day will likely need to replenish energy stores more quickly than that, especially if quality of the workouts is of priority. Carbohydrate intake is the rate-limiting factor for recovery/restoration of glycogen stores. The rate of glycogen resynthesis is dependent on a few factors including provision of exogenous carbohydrate intake (eating/drinking carbohydrate) factors regulating glucose transport into the cell, such as insulin, exercise-stimulated protein transport, and other enzymes (2).

For most runners, incorporation of moderate- and high-intensity training sessions is at the core of their training regimens. For long distance runners, successive days of high-volume training increase the importance of using recovery nutrition to prevent over training and reinforce the immune system. Relative Energy Deficit Syndrome (RED-S) is a term used by medical professionals to describe the imbalance of overall caloric intake in relation to the amount of energy being expended. Recovery nutrition is one way that athletes with heavy training volume can prevent this imbalance from happening.

## Recovery Nutrition Occurs in Two Phases

**Phase 1:** The first thirty minutes is independent of circulating insulin levels, and the second has been observed to be insulin dependent. Insulin is naturally secreted by the pancreas to facilitate blood glucose absorption and storage. Glycogen levels after exercise are a far more important regulator of glycogen resynthesis than insulin levels during the initial phases of recovery. In other words, glycogen synthesis occurs much quicker after longer, exhaustive training sessions.

**Phase 2:** After this, muscle glycogen synthesis increases with the sensitivity of muscle glucose uptake due to circulating insulin levels. Because of this role that insulin plays in regulating muscle glycogen synthesis during this second phase, much emphasis should be put on refueling within the first sixty minutes following glycogen-depleting activity.

## How Much Carbohydrate for Recovery?

The amount of ingested carbohydrate needed to optimize increased glycogen resynthesis after exercise has been tested by numerous researchers. Ultimately, no additional improvement in glycogen synthesis activity was seen in amounts higher than 1.2 g of carbohydrate per kilogram body weight. In addition to the amount, timing and frequency of ingestion have also been tested (17). More frequent intakes of carbohydrates can further stimulate post-exercise skeletal muscle glucose uptake, and optimize muscle glycogen levels, especially during the first couple hours post-exercise recovery (17). Because of this, athletes looking to complete more than one workout per day should look to replace carbohydrates after each workout. This can help an athlete be performance-ready for the latter training session and can help prevent fatigue related injuries (muscle strains, joint injuries, decreased focus, and improvised nervous system function).

> In the field of elite sport, adjusting the before, during, and post-training snacks are a very easy way to adjust caloric intake. Meals should be nutrient-dense, focusing on raw and lightly cooked vegetables (50 percent of your plate), lean proteins (approximately 25 percent of your plate), and whole grain carbohydrates (approximately 25 percent of your plate). As training intensifies, snacks before and after training should increase in caloric size, and with training sessions over ninety minutes, snacks of easily digestible carbohydrates should be added. For recovery days, one can eliminate training snacks, or at least on easy days, eliminate a few of these snacks. This can be a simple way to help adjust caloric intake and assist in meal planning.

## Just Carbohydrate, or Carbohydrate + Protein for Recovery?

More recently, it has been suggested that the addition of protein ingestion may be an effective way to improve muscle glycogen resynthesis. Co-ingestion of protein with carbohydrate can further raise the stimulated insulin levels, almost three times higher than carbohydrates alone. However, this addition of protein has not been shown to increase glycogen synthesis above that of carbohydrate alone, despite this increased insulin response. Any incorporation of protein intake during this initial recovery nutrition phase is not to benefit glycogen resynthesis, but may have other recovery and injury prevention effects (4). Additional factors should be considered when combining protein with carbohydrate to encourage recovery, not just due to its effect on insulin levels.

The relatively recent concept of "Train Low and Compete High" posits that endurance athletes should train with low glycogen/low carbohydrate availability to enhance the training response, but exercise with high carbohydrate availability when performance is important, such as during competitive events, should be

**Table 22-1** Ways to "Train Low and Compete High": How to reduce carbohydrate availability to alter responses to endurance-training-based sessions.

| Nutrition Strategy | Desired Outcomes |
|---|---|
| Morning run after an overnight fast | • Reduced availability of carbohydrate for the specific training session |
| Long low-intensity run without carbohydrate intake during the session | • Reduced stores of carbohydrate/glycogen restoration following previous days training |
| Withhold carbohydrate in the first few hours of recovery | • Acute reduction of carbohydrate available for central nervous systems depending on duration of training session and extent of carbohydrate restriction |

considered at the elite level. Exercising with low muscle glycogen stores amplifies the activation of signaling proteins that promote mitochondrial biogenesis and other training adaptations (13). These preliminary findings have been seen in the research lab and not necessarily out on the trail or track. Because of this, the application of this principle can be tricky and should be explored only after discussion with a coach and/or sport dietitian to identify what training sessions would be best to trial this concept.

Some examples of ways to accomplish this can be found in Table 22-1. Notably, a suggested way to lower this glycogen availability is to reduce the intake of carbohydrates after the first training session, to reduce reliance of the muscle on carbohydrate as a fuel source for the second training session. It is important to factor in this alteration to prevent chances of injury and illness when exercising in this glycogen-depleted state. It is highly advised to consult with a sport dietitian prior to applying this to a training regimen, as these suggestions can be detrimental to training if carbohydrate intake is already low or severely insufficient.

# Repair and Regenerate Muscle Fibers

## Why Is Protein Important for Injury Recovery and Prevention?

Exhaustive or unaccustomed intense exercise can cause muscle damage, resulting in muscle soreness, temporary decrease in muscle force, swelling, inflammation, and an increase of intramuscular proteins in the blood. The degree of the severity of muscle damage is influenced by the type, intensity, and the duration of training. The most undesirable consequences of this exercise-induced muscle damage

(EIMD) is negative impact on muscle function and decreased muscle force. This may lead to injury when athletes continue training through EIMD. Onset of this damage starts immediately after training and can last for several days post-exercise, with most of the symptoms appearing within twenty-four to forty-eight hours (known as delayed onset muscle soreness or DOMS). Nutrition including the consumption of dietary proteins are one of the most common strategies used to prevent and treat this acute muscle damage.

There are two phases proposed in this damage process according to Sousa et al. (4). First is the primary damage that occurs during the exercise, involving mechanical and metabolic alterations. Secondary to that is damage associated with the inflammatory response. Both of these lead to structural damage in the muscle cell (4). Ingestion of protein has been shown to both prevent this damage and repair the muscle cell by stimulating muscle synthesis (3). Amino acids and/or protein administration has been shown to increase muscle protein synthesis rates after endurance type exercise. It appears that milk proteins and their isolated forms, whey and casein, offer an anabolic advantage over soy protein in promoting muscle hypertrophy. Whey protein especially has a fast intestinal absorption rates, while casein is much slower which delays the release of amino acids.

## How Much Protein Is Needed for Recovery?

Current data suggest that dietary protein intake necessary to support metabolic adaptation, repair, remodeling, and for protein turnover generally ranges from 1.2 to 2.0 g/kg/day (5). Laboratory studies show that muscle protein synthesis following exercise is enhanced with the consumption of higher biological value protein, providing approximately 10 g essential amino acids in the early recovery phase (zero to two hours after exercise). This can further be broken down to recommended protein servings of 0.25 to 0.3 g/kg BW or 15 to 25 g protein. This applies for the typical range of athlete body sizes, although the guidelines may need to be fine-tuned for athletes at extreme ends of the weight spectrum (5). Older references suggest goals for total protein intake over the day (grams/ kilogram BW), however, newer recommendations now highlight that these adaptations to training can be maximized by ingesting these targets when broken up into smaller more frequent amounts, such as 0.3 g/kg BW after key exercise sessions and every three to five hours over multiple meals.

Independent of type, dosing, and timing of protein consumption, a positive net protein balance is needed to prevent muscle breakdown and stimulate recovery.

# Just Protein, or Protein + Carbohydrate for Recovery?

As mentioned in the glycogen recovery section, the co-ingestion of carbohydrate with protein can further stimulate and enhance recovery to prevent injury. The combination of these two nutrients can raise insulin levels even higher than if the two nutrients were consumed independently of one another, in addition to providing amino acids as precursors for protein synthesis. With more insulin secreted, there are increased rates of absorption of both nutrients, thus protein synthesis is stimulated to a higher degree when consumed along with carbohydrate immediately after completion of exercise.

Muscle damage repair and skeletal muscle reconditioning are the reasons behind considering protein and amino acid intake during this sensitive recovery time frame. Carbohydrate may help to prevent muscle breakdown, as it can spare endogenous protein stores when in energy deficit, but it does not improve or increase muscle synthesis. For athletes looking for the benefits of strength training and conditioning to prevent injury, ingestion of protein can further benefit training. See Table 22-2 for carbohydrate and protein recovery snack ideas.

**Table 22-2** Carbohydrate and Protein Recovery Snack Options.

| Recovery Snack Ideas | | | |
|---|---|---|---|
| *Choose a food from protein column + food from carb column based on your training session!* | | | |
| Protein: 15–20 g | Protein: 20–25 g | Carbohydrates: 15–30 g | Carbohydrates: 45–60 g |
| • 2 c milk (cow or soy)<br>• ¾–1 c Greek yogurt<br>• ¾ c cottage cheese<br>• 2 string cheeses<br>• 1 c firm tofu<br>• 2–3 cooked eggs<br>• 2–3 oz deli meat<br>• 1½ c Kefir*<br>• 1½ oz jerky<br>• 2–3 oz fish<br>• ½ c nuts or seeds<br>• ½–¾ c edamame<br>• 4 Tbsp nut butter<br>• 1 c beans or lentils | • 3 c milk (cow or soy)<br>• 1½ c Greek yogurt<br>• 1½ c cottage cheese<br>• 3 string cheeses<br>• 1¼ c firm tofu<br>• 3–4 cooked eggs<br>• 3–4 oz deli meat<br>• 2–2¼ c Kefir<br>• 2–2½ oz jerky<br>• ¾–1 c nuts or seeds<br>• 1 c edamame<br>• 1–1½ c beans or lentils<br>• 1 scoop whey protein | • 1 piece or cup fresh fruit<br>• ¼–½ c dried fruit<br>• 1 c fruit juice<br>• 1 c chocolate milk<br>• ½ c oatmeal<br>• 1–2 slices sandwich bread<br>• ½ bagel<br>• 1 English muffin<br>• 1 granola or cereal bar<br>• 2 x 6" tortillas or wraps<br>• ½–¾ c rice or farro<br>• ½–1 c quinoa, beans, lentils<br>• ¾ c cooked pasta<br>• 4 Tbsp nut butter | • 2–3 piece or cups fresh fruit<br>• ¾–1 c dried fruit<br>• 2 c fruit juice<br>• 2 c chocolate milk<br>• 1–1½ c oatmeal<br>• 3–4 slices sandwich bread<br>• 1 bagel<br>• 2 English muffins<br>• 4 fig bar cookies<br>• 2 x 8" tortilla or wrap<br>• 1–1½ c rice or farro<br>• 1½–2 c quinoa, beans, lentils<br>• 1½ c pasta |

## Planning Protein Recovery

The timing of protein ingestion is of greatest priority for the highest degree of muscle damage prevention, especially when soreness prevention and improved recovery time are the focus. It is very easy to reach the recommended protein intakes through natural food, however, convenience of having these foods on hand can make it a bit more challenging. Here are a few tips to help make sure your recovery nutrition snack following training comes together when you need it:

- Throw all of the ingredients of your recovery smoothie together in the blender pitcher the night before, so that all you have to do is hit "blend" in the morning if you're running short on time.
- Have small chocolate milk boxes and/or Greek yogurts in the fridge to grab as soon as your workout is finished.
- Bring a small insulated lunch bag with your recovery items in it to keep in your car or office if access to a fridge/freezer is a problem.
- Work with a sport dietitian to find a safe and effective recovery protein powder that you can easily add to water or milk in shaker bottle for recovery on the go.

# Reinforce the Immune System

## Why Antioxidants for Recovery and Injury Prevention?

The body is placed under many forms of stress every day. Exogenous sources of reactive species or reactants are oxygen, radiation, air pollutants, xenobiotics, drugs, alcohol, heavy metals, bacteria, viruses, sunlight, food, and exercise. Exposure to these reactants is a normal part of life, and the ability to fight these off is vital for healthy, performance-ready athletes. Antioxidants play an important role in protecting the body from these stresses encountered on a daily basis.

Chronic training for athletes performing at a high level on a daily basis places a heavy load of stress on the body that can lead to injury and illness. Well-trained athletes may have a more developed endogenous antioxidant system than a less-active individuals and may not benefit from antioxidant supplementation, especially if they are already consuming a diet high in antioxidant-rich foods. There is little evidence that antioxidant supplements enhance athletic performance (6). Existing information and research is inconclusive due to flaws in study design. There is some evidence that antioxidant supplementation can actually negatively affect training adaptations and be pro-inflammatory.

It is common for athletes to use antioxidant supplements with the idea that these prevent the deleterious effects of exercise-induced oxidative stress, improve recovery, and can actually improve performance. None of these claims have been backed by research for efficacy and long-term safety. There has been quite a bit of research in this area, but there are essentially equal numbers of studies showing improvements as there are showing no effect of antioxidants on indices of cell damage or muscle soreness (6).

## How Many Antioxidants Are Needed for Recovery?

So if not antioxidant supplementation, why should antioxidants be factored into part of a recovery nutrition plan? Physically active individuals need to optimize their nutrition rather than use supplements. Diets rich in antioxidants can be attained by consuming a variety of fruits, vegetables, whole grains, and nuts (7). Whole foods, rather than capsules, contain antioxidants presented in beneficial ratios and numerous phytochemicals that may act in synergy with the former to optimize the antioxidant effect. Antioxidant supplementation may be warranted when individuals are exposed to high levels of oxidative stress and struggle to meet the dietary antioxidant requirements. Athletes who restrict their energy intake, use severe weight loss practices, and eliminate one or more food groups from their diet or consume unbalanced diets with low micronutrients densities, are at risk of suboptimal antioxidant status.

Numerous studies evaluating the effect of naturally found doses of antioxidants in food (vitamin C, vitamin E, beta-carotene, selenium, and zinc) suggest that consumption of fruits and vegetables is associated with a lower incidence of certain types of cancer, though the mechanism involved in such an association being largely unknown. These studies also suggested that supplementation is only effective in preventing cancer in subjects at higher risk for cancer and who have a particularly low baseline status of these nutrients. These studies also showed that high doses of antioxidant supplements may be deleterious in certain high risk subjects.

The application of this information to athletes and sport should focus on the high stress times of an athletes training schedule. After long runs and strenuous training sessions, natural doses of antioxidants found in whole grains, fruits, and vegetables can help to fight off free radicals produced during exercise. More research is needed to determine what the direct performance effects of these natural doses of antioxidants are.

---

## A Natural Antioxidant

Both pure Tart Cherry Juice and its concentrated form has increased in popularity for its natural dose of anthocyanins in helping fight off post-exercise stress and enhance recovery for subsequent training sessions. Results of a recent study revealed that short-term supplementation (ten days) of Tart Cherry Juice surrounding an endurance challenge (half marathon under two hours) attenuated markers of muscle catabolism, reduced immune, and inflammatory stress, better maintained redox balance, and increased performance in aerobically trained individuals (9). Redox balance refers to the degree to which stress markers are off-balanced by the intake of natural dietary and endogenously found antioxidants. Numerous other studies have suggested similar decreases in symptoms of muscle damage after exercise. These findings further suggest including natural levels of antioxidants found in foods can assist in recovery and injury prevent.

---

# Rehydrate

## Why is Rehydration an Important Part of Recovery to Prevent Injury?

High levels of dehydration or hypohydration (more than 3 percent of body mass loss), or more moderate levels combined with heat stress, may influence cognitive function, mood, and mental readiness. Leaner individuals with a higher percentage of their body weight in the form of muscle will have a larger total body water and a given weight reduction (body mass) from water loss compared to athletes with higher body fats.

Most athletes finish exercising with a fluid deficit and may need to restore ideal hydration status (euhydration) during the recovery period. Assuming that no more than 2 percent of total body weight was lost during training, the need for rehydration after training should only need to focus on replacing fluid losses. The replacement of sodium and restoration of sodium balance is a prerequisite for an effective restoration and maintenance of euhydration after training (5).

## How Much Hydration is Needed during this Recovery Phase?

Rehydration strategies should primarily involve the consumption of water and sodium at a modest rate that minimizes urinary losses (diuresis). Presence of dietary sodium/sodium chloride (from foods or fluids) helps to retain the ingested fluids, especially including circulating blood/plasma volume. Therefore, athletes should not be advised to restrict sodium in post-exercise nutrition, particularly when large sodium losses have been incurred.

It's important to consider that sweat losses and urine losses occur after the completion of exercise. Effective rehydration requires the intake of a greater volume of fluid (as high as 125 to 150 percent) of the final fluid deficit.

## Alcohol's Effect on Hydration

There is an increasing trend and visibility of beer tents after long races and competitions in the recreational race setting. It is important to consider that excessive alcohol in the recovery period is discouraged due to its diuretic effects. Only after full euhydration has been restored should moderate alcohol intake be considered to prevent detrimental effects on recovery and future performances.

### Figuring Out Personalized Ideal Hydration Plans

During hard/long training runs, measure body weight (without clothes) before and after the training session to monitor sweat losses during a training session. Divide total losses (add in how much fluid was consumed during the run) by the total number of hours run to determine the amount of fluid that should be consumed each hour of running.

[(Pre-run weight – Post-run weight) x 16 fl oz] + total # of ounces of fluid consumed = Max amount of fluid needing to be consumed during training session

Divide this number by the number of hours you plan to run to determine the rate of fluid consumption needed per hour during training sessions.

## How All of This Fits Together in a Performance-Enhancing Recovery Nutrition Plan

For high performing athletes, fueling the body before, during, and after training can improve the resilience of the body, while also helping it to recover quickly. When recovery time is limited, nutrition can help to prevent symptoms of exercise induced muscle soreness and breakdown, which can indirectly prevent injury. Training and competition induce several physiological changes that make the body fitter, faster, stronger, and/or improve skill level. A sound recovery nutrition protocol will ensure optimization in those training adaptations and can support performance to a higher potential in the next training bout or in preparation for competition. See Table 22-3 for guidelines to calculate recovery nutrient needs.

**Table 22-3** Calculating your Recovery Nutrient Needs

| First, you will need your weight calculated in kilograms: Weight in lbs: _____ / 2.2 = _____ kilograms | |
| --- | --- |
| **Carbohydrate Needs:**<br>Weight in kg x 1.0–1.2 g carbohydrate | _____ g carbohydrate |
| **Protein Needs:**<br>Weight in 0.25–0.30 g protein | _____ g protein |
| **Fluid Needs:**<br>[(Pre-run weight-Post-run weight) x 16 fl oz] x 150%<br>Max amount of fluid needing to be consumed post-training session to replace fluid losses and cool core temperature to baseline | _____ fluid ounces |
| **Dietary Fat Needs:**<br>Dietary fats should be consumed two hours outside of training (both before and after to prevent slowed digestion and absorption of key recovery nutrients) | |

## CHAPTER 23

# Recovery from Injury

BY ADAM S. TENFORDE AND KATE M. TENFORDE

## Key Points

1. Running injuries are very common and may persist if not properly treated.
2. The causes of most running injuries are multifactorial and require careful evaluation.
3. Proper initial management of the injury includes addressing pain and modifying activity level.
4. Return to running program can include a combination of addressing biomechanical deficits through physical therapy, optimizing nutrition, adequate sleep, and progressive training program.
5. One of the strongest risk factors for a running injury is history of the same injury; proper management may reduce injury recurrence.
6. Primary injury prevention is desirable. Evidence on methods to prevent development of running injuries is lacking, although common sense solutions include a guided progression and periodization of training, emphasis on nutrition and sleep quality, incorporation of cross-training to reduce impact loading and build aerobic endurance, and including strength/loading programs to enhance soft tissue and bone health.
7. Effective communication among physician, physical therapist, coach, and other members of the sports medicine team with the runner facilitates best outcomes for injury management and future injury prevention.

## Overview of Common Running Injuries

Overuse injuries of the bone, tendon, muscle, and connective tissue are common in runners. Therefore, the focus on this chapter will cover the management and prevention of these injuries. Although other forms of injury to skin and other organ systems are important to treat and prevent appropriately, these are outside the scope of this chapter and are covered elsewhere. For more information on specific musculoskeletal injuries, see Chapter 9.

Up to 79 percent of runners may sustain an injury in a given year (1), and a majority of teenage runners report history of one or more common overuse injuries (2). Similar to younger runners, medial tibial stress syndrome (commonly referred to as shin splints), Achilles tendinopathy, plantar fasciitis, and patellofemoral pain syndrome are common in adult runners (3). Additionally, bone stress injuries represent a common form of overuse injury in both sexes starting during adolescence (4). Given the high cumulative prevalence and rate of injury recurrence (4, 5), identifying effective methods to treat bone injuries is critically important for the overall health of the runner.

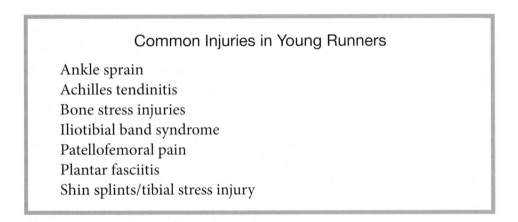

### Common Injuries in Young Runners

Ankle sprain
Achilles tendinitis
Bone stress injuries
Iliotibial band syndrome
Patellofemoral pain
Plantar fasciitis
Shin splints/tibial stress injury

In summary, the high prevalence of injuries involving bone, tendon, joints, and connective tissue is troubling and poses a challenge for enjoyment of the sport of running. Therefore, it is important to develop both effective treatment and prevention programs.

# Risk Factors for Injury

## Training Errors

Risk factors for running injuries are important to identify in order to guide effective management. The cause of most running injuries is multifactorial. Training errors can place a runner at risk for injury when the demands of cumulative training exceed the capacity of tissue to adapt. These risks may include changes in running volume, intensity, frequency, or running surface (such as running on uneven, slippery, or cambered surfaces).

## Training Factors that Can Contribute to Injury

- Sudden increases in training (increased running volume, frequency, and intensity)
- Training surfaces (uneven terrain, cambered surfaces, slippery surfaces)
- Change in footwear
- Running in old shoes

In addition to the repetitive loading encountered in running, some athletes choose to participate in other forms of activity that can also increase risk for injury. This can have both a negative and positive impact on running. For example, participating in additional sports, or adding group exercise and weight lifting programs to an exercise regimen, will challenge the musculoskeletal system. Adding in cross-training activities may also be beneficial for musculoskeletal adaptations, as these activities do not contribute to the same demands of running that cause overuse injuries. However, any additional forms of activity that a runner incorporates should be considered in the overall training plan to ensure that total exercise demand is not overwhelming and does not lead to overtraining.

In addition to training, changes in footwear may also result in altered biomechanics. For example, runners who make the change from cushioned shoes to shoes with minimal cushioning (minimalist footwear) may experience higher impact forces without appropriate preparation of the musculoskeletal system to adapt to the new demands. An initial reduction in overall training miles or a slow incorporation of minimalist footwear (gradually replacing time spent in traditional shoes to increased running in minimalist footwear) can allow for adaptation to the new footwear and foot strike forces, thus decreasing the risk of injury. Likewise, shoes typically need to be replaced every 350 to 500 miles, or when they begin to demonstrate excessive wear patterns. Use of old shoes that lack the original cushioning could result in failure of footwear to provide shock attenuation/absorption and lead to injury.

However, a focus on training factors or footwear alone is simplistic and often misses other important factors that contribute to running injuries. In addition, reducing running volume may result in undesirable decrement in running performance. Therefore, it would be inappropriate to broadly prescribe a specific volume of running without clear evidence or knowledge of an individual's training history to guide this recommendation (2).

# Female Athlete Triad and Nutrition Considerations

The Female Athlete Triad (Triad) is described as the interrelationship of three conditions: nutrition, menstrual function, and bone health. Each condition exists as a spectrum that ranges from optimal health to disease (6). Participation in sports while having received adequate nutrition may result in female runners experiencing adaptive benefits that greatly improve health in several mediums: optimal metabolic function, optimal reproductive function, bone mass accrual, and gains in lean tissue mass. Caloric intake that does not meet the needs for sports participation may result in low energy availability. Low energy availability often results in reduction or loss of menstrual cycles (oligomenorrhea/amenorrhea), alteration of hormones, and low bone density. The triad has been shown to contribute to overuse musculoskeletal injuries including bone stress injuries (4, 7).

Although research has primarily focused on female athletes, male athletes are also at risk for injury in the setting of inadequate nutrition. Malnutrition in male runners can cause reductions of sex hormones and bone mass (8). Major sports organizations are recognizing the negative influence of poor nutrition on overall health for both male and female athletes (9).

In addition to caloric intake, calcium, and vitamin D are two important aspects of nutrition that promote bone health. Calcium intake through food (as

---

### Female Athlete Triad and Nutrition Factors Contributing to Injury

Low energy availability (from a combination of inadequate caloric intake and/or excessive energy expenditure)

Poor calcium intake

Low vitamin D

Disordered eating/Eating disorder

Primary amenorrhea (first menstrual period age fifteen or older)

Secondary amenorrhea (three months without a menstrual period or having irregular menstrual periods for six months)

Low body mass index

Low bone mineral density

opposed to relying on supplements) is the preferable method to meet calcium needs as foods rich in calcium provide a source of calories and include other components that promote skeletal health including protein, phosphorus, and commonly are fortified with vitamin D. Additionally, one research study found that each cup (8 ounces) of skim milk consumed per day reduced risk for stress fractures by 62 percent (10). The Institute of Medicine recommends 600 IU of vitamin D for people ages nine and older (11). This number is challenging to reach from diet alone, so supplementation is often necessary. For further information on female athlete triad, see Chapter 10.

## Biomechanical Risk Factors

The biomechanics of running injuries is complex. Abdominal core and gluteal muscle weakness is common in most runners. One explanation for these weaknesses is that running is performed primarily in a front-to-back (sagittal) plane of movement. Without the multidirectional loading encountered in sports like soccer or basketball, there may be less opportunity for adaptive muscle development and promotion of core stability. In addition, strength deficits through the foot and ankle have been increasingly recognized as a target for more appropriate strengthening to decrease risk of lower extremity injuries (12). In addition to strength deficits, high rate of loading (described as impacts) can place increased demands on the lower extremities and contribute to injuries (13). See box below for a list of biomechanical risk factors for injury.

---

### Biomechanical risk factors for injury

- High impacts of loading
- Poor dynamic alignment during loading (including knee collapse, excessive pronation, or supination)
- Reduced hip abductor muscle strength
- Weak abdominal core strength
- Foot muscle weakness
- Flexibility impairments

---

## Injury Management

The guidelines for injury management depend on the type and severity of injury sustained. In general, the goal of effective treatment is to achieve pain control, address the contributors to injury, and develop a program to return to running safely. The classification of injuries and management are outlined by joint, tendon, ligament, and bone.

Anti-inflammatory medications can reduce pain and associated inflammation. They are reasonable for initial treatment, but their use should be limited to a maximum of two weeks due to concerns for side effects. Prescription of anti-inflammatory medications should not overlap with competition, due to risks associated with use during competition including gastrointestinal distress, and risk to damage of other vital organs including the kidney and heart. Additionally, it is not advisable to complete a competition using pain medications that mask symptoms, as this could contribute to worsening the injury by further exceeding the demand of the tissue. It is not uncommon to see runners who use over-the-counter anti-inflammatory medications without discussion with a medical provider. This is inadvisable due to the risks for harm including cardiac disease (including heart attack and stroke), gastrointestinal illness (including development of stomach ulcers), and injury to the kidney and liver. We advise discussion with a medical provider for use of these medications, especially in runners with any underlying medical condition (such as heart disease, kidney/liver disease, or conditions affecting the gastrointestinal tract) or in use with older runners (as vascular disease is more common with age).

In runners with pain that limits movement and participation in physical therapy, the use of an injection with steroid medication may help achieve pain control. Steroid use may have many side effects, including risks of damage to the targeted tissue and reducing bone health. The use of other forms of injections including use of orthobiological agents (stem cell treatment, platelet rich plasma, and other types of injections) is beyond the scope of this chapter, but these are reasonable options to discuss with physicians for chronic cases of injury that do not respond to earlier treatments.

Physical therapy is the mainstay of treatment. The goal of physical therapy is to guide a progressive program that initially restores range of motion, resolves swelling and local inflammation, relieves pain, and progresses to strengthening and full body alignment and movement (kinetic chain) assessment. A successful physical therapy program will include developing a home exercise program that runners can incorporate into their overall running program.

Traditional physical therapy may restore strength and function. However, abnormal movement patterns may persist despite strength gains. In cases of recurrent running injuries, gait evaluation and retraining can result in changes to movement patterns. The goal of gait retraining is to eventually achieve well-aligned, soft landings. Often, this involves a traditional strengthening and flexibility program to improve muscle, tendon, and bone loading capacity. Runners often are progressed to running in minimalist footwear to encourage forefoot strike running. Feedback (such as visualizing the new running pattern in a mirror) is gradually removed to help with learning a new movement pattern.

In general, cross-training exercises for the purposes of maintaining cardiovascular fitness can be instituted during the recovery from injury. The cross-training form of exercise should not provoke pain. Cross-training may be restricted for initial management of bone injuries, as weight bearing may be limited to help with healing. Common forms of exercise include an elliptical trainer, stationary bike, swimming, and deep-water running. In particular, deep-water running has been found to be very effective at maintaining fitness during injury recovery. The use of deep water running involves being in a pool that is deep enough that the runner's feet cannot strike the bottom of the pool. The runner maintains an upright position and brings the knees upward and hips into approximately 90 degrees of flexion. The arms can come slightly outward to help displace water, but should not be used to maintain the upright position. The use of a flotation device such as a foam belt can help to maintain upright posture.

As with all medical care, there is no "one size fits all" approach for cross-training. A runner should try out all cross-training options that are accessible. If one kind aggravates the injury, it should be avoided. Once the ideal form of exercise has been found, and a level of comfort with the new mode of exercise has been achieved, the runner can recreate a typical training week with an effort to build aerobic capacity. He or she can incorporate one long workout at a steady pace (mimicking the long run), one workout comprised of short intervals at a fast pace (mimicking a speed session on the track), and one workout comprised of a long, hard effort (mimicking a threshold workout). Other workouts throughout the week can be shorter and less intense (mimicking recovery runs). Adding in different workouts throughout the week will minimize boredom (boredom is common complaint from injured runners who are relegated to the gym or pool) and may allow the runner to maintain cardiovascular fitness and have added psychological benefits for the sense of developing a fitness routine.

Finally, the value of sleep and nutrition cannot be overemphasized for both injury management and prevention. Adequate sleep and rest will promote healing and recovery. In contrast, inadequate sleep and poor sleep quality may result in metabolic changes including elevated stress hormones and increased bone turnover (suggesting bone loss). In fact, one study demonstrated that three-days of impaired sleep resulted in elevated bone turnover and a 5 percent reduction in bone mass (14). In addition, nutrition should include sufficient calories with eating three meals and snacks to maintain good energy throughout the day. While exercise demand is reduced, sufficient caloric intake should be maintained in order for the injury to heal and for successful completion of a comprehensive rehabilitation program.

The return to running progression is based on the type of injury, competition schedule, and other factors. In general, a progression that gradually increases duration of running is recommended. Regular walking breaks should be included to monitor for pain response. The running progression should be completed in a controlled environment with level footing. This may include a track as long as running on the curves of the track does not provoke pain, a flat grass field, or a road without cambered surface or elevation changes. Running alternate days initially can help to ensure pain does not develop following each run progression.

## Developing an Effective Training Program

Runners often try to deconstruct the cause of injury, attributing it to a race, run, or workout. However, most running injuries reflect overuse and often reflect training errors. These training errors often occur in combination with other factors including sleep, nutrition, strength, flexibility, and faulty running mechanics. An effective training program encompasses more than just the time spent running. By developing greater body awareness, runners can gain insight into training and lifestyle choices that help or hinder training and races. A common way of developing this body awareness is through a training log. The log should contain more than just mileage and splits. There should be notes on how the runner felt during and after workouts, sleep quality, pre-workout fueling, etc. This level of detail will allow the runner to evaluate for patterns in fitness gains or injury risk. For example, if a runner is routinely sore for numerous days after a certain workout, the runner can schedule extra recovery time or avoid this workout leading up to a race. If a runner finds that when training mileage reaches a certain level, it results in poor sleep quality or if heart rate increases too easily in workouts, the runner can bring the mileage down to a more manageable range and maximize training without the same risk of injury.

---

### Elements to Consider for a Training Log

Dates (day of week, date, month and year)

Type of workout (run versus cross-training or day off)

Volume of workout

Details on intensity (including running pace and recovery between efforts)

Races and performance

Effort (including heart rate or perceived exertion)

Sleep (number of hours, quality of sleep)

Notes (for entries such as when an injury occurred and time off)

Components for a training log can include a variety of components to keep track of changes in effort and identify patterns with training including recovery for injury prevention.

---

In addition to looking for negative patterns, runners should watch for positive patterns as well. For example, if a runner finds that replacing one easy run with a bike ride consistently yields a terrific long run, this type of cross-training should be incorporated into the workout routine. Or if an athlete runs best when getting nine hours of sleep, it should be a priority to get to bed at a regular time every night.

If the runner has a coach, positive or negative patterns in training should be discussed. Together, the pair can develop a solution. If running with a team, the individual runner's needs must be protected, despite group team training sessions, in order to remain healthy and perform best in both training and in races.

The recommendations for injury management are general and meant for healthy runners without chronic injury. Consultation with a medical provider who commonly treats athletes with running injuries is advisable. Some specific considerations for different classes of injuries are discussed other specific chapters, but an overview is provided below.

## Joint Injury

Management for a joint injury depends on the location and underlying condition. The goal of treatment for joint injury is to eliminate pain and reduce risk for injury recurrence. These goals can be accomplished through medication (including possible injection), restoration of joint range of motion, improvement of overall movement pattern and muscle strength, and reduction of impact through the joint. Runners with continued pain after initial treatment should consult their medical provider to ensure they have clear guidelines for advancing activity. For more information, refer to Chapter 9.

## Tendon Injury

The goals for treatment of tendon injury depend on many factors including the total time of injury. An acute tendon injury (injury lasting days to weeks) is typically managed with activity modification to avoid painful activities, and a short course of anti-inflammatory medications to resolve inflammation and swelling. The physical therapy program initially starts with restoring motion of the tendon and surrounding tissues along with a progressive strengthening program. In acute tendon injuries, the progression is typically performed and guided by maintaining pain-free status.

More chronic forms of tendon disease (tendon pain lasting months to years) is managed differently. The term tendinopathy is the more common term used to describe a failed healing response of the tendon. This distinction is important to understand as chronic tendon disease and related pain may result from both inflammatory and non-inflammatory causes (15). For more information, refer to Chapter 9.

## Ligament and Soft Tissue Injuries

Common forms of ligament and non-tendon soft tissue injury sustained by runners include lateral ankle sprains and plantar fasciitis. When there is significant pain with both running and basic daily tasks such as walking, initial immobilization with a walking boot may be prescribed to allow the soft tissue to be offloaded and for initial tissue healing. The progression following immobilization is weaning from use of the boot or other supportive devices, restoring range of motion of the immobilized region, and progressive strengthening and proprioception program. Without restoring strength and balance and addressing the full kinetic chain, ankle sprains and other soft tissue injuries are likely to persist or recur.

## Bone Injuries

As described earlier, bone stress injuries are a common overuse injury in runners. In contrast to other forms of injury, no form of activity that causes pain is acceptable when training through recovery of a bone stress injury. High risk injuries, particularly involving the pelvis, hip, anterior leg, and key locations in the foot (including the inner ankle bone/medial malleolus, tarsal navicular bone, talus, second, and fifth metatarsals) require medical attention to ensure healing occurs. Initial treatment for this condition should not include anti-inflammatory medications, as this may impair rate of bone healing. Also, pain is an important aspect of understanding the stage of healing for the bone. Pain localized to the site of bone injury represents excess demand to the tissue and will further delay healing of the bone. For more information, refer to Chapter 10.

## Injury Prevention

The goal of effective management for a running injury is to address the underlying contributor(s) to the injury. Without addressing the underlying contributors, the injury will likely recur. Ideally, each runner would be equipped with knowledge for strategies to prevent injury. Evidence-based medical practice on methods to prevent running injuries is lacking. Practical recommendations are as follows:

Proper training: Most successful runners are not identified as stars in youth running. Participating in a variety of sports during childhood and adolescence promotes cross-over benefits of athletic development. These cross-over benefits contribute to future success. For example, participation in high impact multidirectional loading and jumping activities such as ball sports participation (basketball and soccer) during childhood and adolescence may reduce risk for future bone stress injuries (16). The higher impact multidirectional loading may promote adaptive bone remodeling. Additionally, participating in multidirectional sports may develop other muscle groups that are not normally developed in runners, given that running is done in a primarily front-to-back (sagittal) plane with low variability in direction of landing. After skeletal maturation, following training principles as outlined above including periodization of training may allow the body to recover and provide a helpful mental break prior to training for the next running event

Nutrition: Proper nutrition includes adequate caloric intake spaced throughout the day to maintain consistent fueling for running and recovery. This includes not skipping meals, proper hydration (urine should be light yellow), and eating foods that contain both calcium and vitamin D. Runners who have dietary restrictions may benefit from speaking with a sports nutritionist to ensure their diet contains enough calories and nutrients to meet the demands for skeletal health and muscle recovery.

Sleep: The value of adequate sleep cannot be overemphasized. Short duration and poor sleep have been associated with loss of bone mass (14). Associated elevated stress hormones (including cortisol) promote a destructive (catabolic) state in the body that makes gains in training difficult to sustain due to suboptimal recovery. While sleep cannot always be optimized due to stressors of life, making practical decisions to modify training plan or effort is prudent to ensure that demand is lowered during a time of increased susceptibility to injury.

Strength training: There is little evidence that strength training and specific stretches prevent injury. However, incorporating a rehabilitation program for a prior injury into a maintenance and strengthening program is reasonable to reduce risk for re-injury. Additionally, basic exercises to improve abdominal, core and foot strength are excellent to improve properly aligned movement (kinetic chain).

Gait retraining: in cases of runners with difficult-to-treat injuries or history of multiple prior overuse injuries, the use of gait retraining can be an effective strategy to modify running mechanics. Current recommended gait retraining principles include a progressive program designed to facilitate soft and well-aligned landing patterns (17). Such a program requires supervision from a trained provider to ensure the appropriate cues are translating to proper changes in running form. Additionally, the transition of running mechanics to a new foot strike pattern requires fortifying the musculoskeletal system and strengthening the feet so that the runner can tolerate a new running pattern. Concepts of gait retraining represent the exciting new frontier in better treatment and prevention of running injuries.

## Summary

In conclusion, running injuries are very common and are often multifactorial. Initial treatment for an injury includes efforts to resolve pain through activity modification followed by a customized rehabilitation program to optimize strength, flexibility, and mechanics. Addressing both nutrition and sleep during injury management and for future injury prevention is critical. Effective communication between the runner and the sports medicine team is crucial toward ensuring a successful return to running program. Running training requires periodization and variability to allow for adequate recovery and injury reduction. Having a running coach can be helpful to ensure appropriate training and active modification of the program to reduce injury. Injury prevention includes optimizing sleep, nutrition, variation in sport activity, proper training, and gait retraining, especially in runners with recurrent or persistent conditions.

# REFERENCE LIST

## Chapter 1

1. van Gent RN, Siem D, van Middelkoop M, et al. Incidence and determinants of lower extremity running injuries in long distance runners: a systematic review. Br J Sports Med 2007; 41: 469–80.
2. Eijsvogels TM, Fernandez AB, Thompson PD. Are There Deleterious Cardiac Effects of Acute and Chronic Endurance Exercise? Physiol Rev 2016; 96: 99–125.
3. Alexander, RM. Exploring Biomechanics: Animals in Motion, 2nd Ed. New York: Scientific American Library; 1992.
4. Bortz WM. Physical exercise as an evolutionary force. J Hum Evol 1985; 14: 145–155.
5. Carrier DR. The energetic paradox of human running and hominid evolution. Curr Anthropol 1984; 24: 483–495.
6. Bramble DM, Lieberman DE. Endurance running and the evolution of Homo. Nature 2004; 432: 345–352.
7. Smith RJ, Jungers WL. Body mass in comparative primatology. J Hum Evol 1997; 32: 523–59.
8. Aiello L, Dean MC. An Introduction to Human Evolutionary Anatomy. London: Academic Press; 1990.
9. Taylor CR, Rowntree VJ. Running on two or on four legs: which consumes more energy? Science. 1973; 179: 186–7.
10. Sockol MD, Raichlen DA, Pontzer H. Chimpanzee locomotor energetics and the origin of human bipedalism. Proc Natl Acad Sci U S A. 2007; 104: 12265–9.
11. Pontzer H, Wrangham RW. Climbing and the daily energy cost of locomotion in wild chimpanzees: implications for hominoid locomotor evolution. J Hum Evol. 2004; 46: 317–35.
12. Yamagiwa J, Mwanza N, Yumoto T, Maruhashi T. Seasonal change in the composition of the diet of eastern lowland gorillas. Primates. 1994; 35: 1–14.
13. Zachos J, Pagani M, Sloan L, Thomas E, Billups K. Trends, rhythms, and aberrations in global climate 65 Ma to present. Science. 2001; 292: 686–93.
14. Carey TS, Crompton RH. The metabolic costs of 'bent-hip, bent-knee' walking in humans. J Hum Evol. 2005; 48: 25–44.
15. Hunt KD. Positional behavior of Pan troglodytes in the Mahale Mountains and Gombe Stream National Parks, Tanzania. Am J Phys Anthropol. 1992; 87: 83–105.
16. Thorpe SK, Holder RL, Crompton RH. Origin of human bipedalism as an adaptation for locomotion on flexible branches. Science. 2007; 316: 1328–31.
17. Lieberman DE. The Story of the Human Body: Evolution, Health and Disease. New York: Pantheon; 2013.
18. Rolian C, Lieberman DE, Hamill J, Scott JW, Werbel W. Walking, running and the evolution of short toes in humans. J Exp Biol. 2009; 212: 713–21.
19. Fleagle JG, Lieberman DE. Major transformations in the evolution of primate locomotion. In: Dial KP, Shubin N, Brainerd EL, editors. Great Transformations in Vertebrate Evolution. Chicago, IL: University of Chicago Press; 2015. p. 257–278.

20. Cerling TE, Wynn JG, Andanje SA, et al. Woody cover and hominin environments in the past 6 million years. Nature. 2011; 476: 51–6.

21. Wood BW, Constantino P. Paranthropus boisei: fifty years of evidence and analysis. Ybk Phys Anthropol. 2007; 45: 106–32.

22. Villmoare B, Kimbel WH, Seyoum C, et al. Early Homo at 2.8 Ma from Ledi-Geraru, Afar, Ethiopia. Science. 2015; 347: 1352–5.

23. Leakey MG, Spoor F, Dean MC, et al. New fossils from Koobi Fora in northern Kenya confirm taxonomic diversity in early Homo. Nature. 2012; 488: 201–4.

24. Harmand S, Lewis JE, Feibel CS, et al. 3.3-million-year-old stone tools from Lomekwi 3, West Turkana, Kenya. Nature. 2015; 521: 310–5.

25. Semaw S, Renne P, Harris JW, et al. 2.5-million-year-old stone tools from Gona, Ethiopia. Nature. 1997; 385: 333–6.

26. Domínguez-Rodrigo, M. Hunting and Scavenging by Early Humans: The State of the Debate. J World Prehistory 2002; 16: 1–54.

27. Diez-Martín F, Sánchez Yustos P, Uribelarrea D, et al. The Origin of The Acheulean: The 1.7 Million-Year-Old Site of FLK West, Olduvai Gorge (Tanzania). Sci Rep. 2015; 5: 17839.

28. Zink KD, Lieberman DE. Impact of meat and Lower Palaeolithic food processing techniques on chewing in humans. Nature. 2016; 531: 500–3.

29. Van Valkenburgh B. The dog-eat-dog world of carnivores: a review of past and present carnivore community dynamics. In: Stanford CB, Bunn HT, editors. Meat-Eating and Human Evolution. Oxford: Oxford University Press; 2001. p 101–121.

30. Garland T. The relation between maximal running speed and body mass in terrestrial mammals. J Zoology 1983; 199: 1557–1570.

31. Wilkins J, Schoville BJ, Brown KS, Chazan M. Evidence for early hafted hunting technology. Science. 2012; 338: 942–6.

32. Shea JJ. Stone Tools in Human Evolution: Behavioral Differences among Technological Primates. Cambridge University Press; 2016.

33. Churchill SE. Weapon technology, prey size selection and hunting methods in modern hunter-gatherers: implications for hunting in the Palaeolithic and Mesolithic. Arch Papers Am Anthropol Assoc 1993; 4: 11–24.

34. Liebenberg L. Persistence Hunting by Modern Hunter-Gatherers. Curr Anthropol 1996; 47: 1017–1025.

35. Lieberman DE, Bramble DM, Raichlen DA, Shea JJ. The evolution of endurance running and the tyranny of ethnography. J Hum Evol. 2007; 53: 439–42.

36. Montagna W. The skin of nonhuman primates. Am Zool 1972; 12: 109–124.

37. Folk GE Jr, Semken HA Jr. The evolution of sweat glands. Int J Biometereology 1991; 35: 181–186.

38. Schultz AA. The density of hair in primates. Hum Biol 1931; 3: 303–317.

39. Lieberman DE. Human locomotion and heat loss: an evolutionary perspective. Comprehensive Physiology 2015; 5: 99–117.

40. Bramble DM, Jenkins FA Jr. Mammalian locomotor-respiratory integration: Implications for diaphragmatic and pulmonary design. Science 1993; 262: 235–240.

41. Kamberov YG, Wang S, Tan J, et al. Modeling Recent Human Evolution in Mice by Expression of a Selected EDAR Variant. Cell 2013; 152: 691–702.

42. Dill DB, Edwards HT, Talbott JH. Studies in muscular activity: VII. Factors limiting the capacity for work. J Physiol 1932; 77: 49–62.

43. Pontzer H. Predicting the energy cost of terrestrial locomotion: A test of the LiMb model in humans and quadrupeds. J Exp Biol 2007; 210: 484–494.

44. Lieberman DE, Raichlen DA, Pontzer H, et al. The human gluteus maximus and its role in running. 2006; J Exp Biol. 209: 2143–215.

45. Thompson NE, Demes B, O'Neill MC, Holowka NB, Larson SG. Surprising trunk rotational capabilities in chimpanzees and implications for bipedal walking proficiency in early hominins. Nat Commun. 2015; 6: 8416.

46. Lieberman DE. The Evolution of the Human Head. Cambridge: Harvard University Press; 2011.

47. Spoor F, Wood BA, Zonneveld F. Implications of early hominid labyrinthine morphology for the evolution of human bipedal locomotion. Nature 1994; 369: 645–648.

48. Jungers WL. Relative joint size and hominid locomotor adaptations with implications for the evolution of hominid bipedalism. J Hum Evol 1988; 17: 247–265.

49. Liebenberg L. The Art of Tracking: The Origin of Science. Claremont, South Africa: David Philip Publishers; 2001.

50. Raichlen DA, Polk JD. Linking brains and brawn: exercise and the evolution of human neurobiology. Proc Biol Sci. 2013; 280: 20122250.

51. Raichlen DA, Foster AD, Seillier A, Giuffrida A, Gerdeman GL. Exercise-induced endocannabinoid signaling is modulated by intensity. Eur J Appl Physiol. 2013; 113: 869–75.

52. Pickering TR, Bunn HT. The endurance running hypothesis and hunting and scavenging in savanna-woodlands. J Hum Evol. 2007; 53: 434–8.

53. Kroeber AL. Handbook of the Indians of California. Washington, DC: Bureau of American Ethnology; 1925.

54. Nabokov P. Native American Running. Santa Fe (NM): Ancient City Press; 1981.

55. Garber CE, Blissmer B, Deschenes MR, et al. American College of Sports Medicine position stand. Quantity and quality of exercise for developing and maintaining cardiorespiratory, musculoskeletal, and neuromotor fitness in apparently healthy adults: guidance for prescribing exercise. Med Sci Sports Exerc. 2011; 43: 1334–59.

56. Lieberman DE. Is Exercise Really Medicine? An Evolutionary Perspective. Curr Sports Med Rev. 14: 313–19.

57. Wen DY. Risk factors for overuse injuries in runners. Curr Sports Med Rep. 2007; 6: 307–13.

58. Lavie CJ, O'Keefe JH, Sallis RE. Exercise and the heart—the harm of too little and too much. Curr Sports Med Rep. 2015; 14: 104–9.

59. McDougall C. Born to Run: A Hidden Tribe, Superathletes, and the Greatest Race the World Has Never Seen. New York (NY): Knopf; 2009.

60. Lieberman DE. Strike type variation among Tarahumara Indians in minimal sandals versus conventional running shoes. J Sport Health Sci 2014; 3: 86–94.

61. Lieberman DE, Castillo ER, Otarola-Castillo E, et al. Variation in Foot Strike Patterns among Habitually Barefoot and Shod Runners in Kenya. PLoS One. 2015; 10: e0131354.

62. Hreljac A. Etiology, prevention, and early intervention of overuse injuries in runners: a biomechanical perspective. Phys Med Rehabil Clin N Am. 2005; 16: 651–667.

63. Ferris DP, Liang K, Farley CT. Runners adjust leg stiffness for their 1st step on a new running surface. Journal of Biomechanics 1999; 32: 787–794.

64. Lieberman DE, Venkadesan M, Werbel W, et al. Foot strike patterns and collision forces in habitually barefoot versus shod runners. 2010; Nature 463: 531–5.

65. Butler RJ, Crowell HP, Davis IM. Lower extremity stiffness: implications for performance and injury. Clinical Biomechanics 2003; 18 (6): 511–517.

67. Nigg BM, Wakeling JM. Impact forces and muscle tuning: a new paradigm. Exerc Sport Sci Rev. 2001; 29: 37–41.

68. Lieberman DE. What we can learn about running from barefoot running: an evolutionary medical perspective. Exerc. Sci Sports Review 2012; 40: 63–72.

69. Nigg BM. Biomechanics of Sports Shoes. Calgary: Benno Nigg; 2011.

70. Perl DP, Daoud AI, Lieberman DE. Effects of footwear and strike type on running economy. Med Sci Sports Exerc. 2012; 44: 1335–43.

71. Franz JR, Wierzbinski CM, Kram R. Metabolic cost of running barefoot versus shod: is lighter better? Med Sci Sports Exerc. 2012; 44: 1519–25.

72. Kelly LA, Lichtwark GA, Farris DJ, Cresswell A. Shoes alter the spring-like function of the human foot during running. J R Soc Interface. 2016; 13: 20160174.

73. Larson P. Comparison of foot strike patterns of barefoot and minimally shod runners in a recreational road race. J Sport Health Sci 2014; 3: 137–42.

74. Daoud AI, Geissler GJ, Wang F, et al. Foot Strike and Injury Rates in Endurance Runners: a retrospective study. 2012; Med Sci Sports Exerc. 2012; 44: 1325–34.

75. Davis IS, Bowser BJ, Mullineaux DR. Greater vertical impact loading in female runners with medically diagnosed injuries: a prospective investigation. Br J Sports Med. 2016; 50: 887–92.

76. Kerrigan DC, Franz JR, Keenan GS, et al. The effect of running shoes on lower extremity joint torques. Physiol. Med. Rehabil. 2009; 1: 1058–63.

77. Bruggemann GP, Potthast W, Braunstein B, Niehoff A. Effect of increased mechanical stimuli on foot muscles functional capacity. Proceedings ISB XXth Congress, American Society of Biomechanics, Cleveland 2005, p. 553.

78. Miller EE, Whitcome KK, Lieberman DE, Norton HL, Dyer RE. The effect of minimal shoes on arch structure and intrinsic foot muscle strength. J Sport Health Sci 2014; 3: 74–85.

79. Squadrone R, Gallozi C. Biomechanical and physiological comparison of barefoot and two shod conditions in experienced barefoot runners. J Sports Med Phys Fitness. 2009; 49: 6–13.

80. Lieberman DE, Warrener AG, Wang J, Castillo ER. Effects of stride frequency and foot position at landing on braking force, hip torque, impact peak force and the metabolic cost of running in humans. J Exp Biol. 2015; 218: 3406–14.

81. Schubert AG, Kempf J, Heiderscheit BC. Influence of stride frequency and length on running mechanics: a systematic review. Sports Health. 2014; 6: 210–7.

82. Lox C, Ginis KAM; Petruzzello SJ. The Psychology of Exercise: Integrating Theory and Practice, 4th ed. Scottsdale (AZ) Holcomb, Hathaway; 2014.

## Chapter 2

1. Bramble DM, Lieberman DE. Endurance running and the evolution of Homo. Nature. 2004; 432(7015): 345–352.

2. Lieberman DE, Bramble DM. The evolution of marathon running: capabilities in humans. Sports Med. 2007; 37(4–5): 288–290.

3.  Running USA. http://www.running.usa.org/statistics. Accessed 14 Oct 2016.

4.  Ultra Running. https://www.ultrarunning.com/featured/2013-ultrarunning-partici-pation-by-the-numbers/. Accessed 14 Oct 2016.

5.  Krabak BJ, Waite B, Lipman G. Injury and illnesses prevention for ultramarathoners. Curr Sports Med Rep. 2013; 12(3): 183–189.

6.  Jakobsen BW, Krøner K, Schmidt SA, Jensen J. [Running injuries sustained in a marathon race. Registration of the occurrence and types of injuries in the 1986 Arhus Marathon]. Ugeskr Laeger. 1989; 151(35): 2189–2192.

7.  Maughan RJ, Miller JD. Incidence of training-related injuries among marathon runners. Br J Sports Med. 1983; 17(3): 162–165.

8.  Kim JH, Malhotra R, Chiampas G, et al. Cardiac arrest during long-distance running races. N Engl J Med. 2012; 366(2): 130–140.

9.  Jokl P, Sethi PM, Cooper AJ. Master's performance in the New York City Marathon 1983–1999. Br J Sports Med. 2004; 38(4): 408–412.

10. Hoffman MD, Fogard K. Factors related to successful completion of a 161-km ultramarathon. Int J Sports Physiol Perform. 2011; 6(1): 25–37.

11. Hoffman MD, Krishnan E. Health and exercise-related medical issues among 1,212 ultramarathon runners: baseline findings from the Ultrarunners Longitudinal TRAcking (ULTRA) Study. PLoS One. 2014; 9(1): e83867.

12. Knoth C, Knechtle B, Rüst CA, Rosemann T, Lepers R. Participation and performance trends in multistage ultramarathons-the 'Marathon des Sables' 2003–2012. Extrem Physiol Med. 2012; 1(1): 13.

13. Scheer BV, Murray A. Al Andalus Ultra Trail: an observation of medical interventions during a 219-km, 5-day ultramarathon stage race. Clin J Sport Med. 2011; 21(5): 444–446.

14. Cosca DD, Navazio F. Common problems in endurance athletes. Am Fam Physician. 2007; 76(2): 237–244.

15. Krabak BJ, Waite B, Schiff MA. Study of injury and illness rates in multiday ultramarathon runners. Med Sci Sports Exerc. 2011; 43(12): 2314–2320.

16. Fallon KE. Musculoskeletal injuries in the ultramarathon: the 1990 Westfield Sydney to Melbourne run. Br J Sports Med. 1996; 30(4): 319–323.

17. Crouse B, Beattie K. Marathon medical services: strategies to reduce runner morbidity. Med Sci Sports Exerc. 1996; 28(9): 1093–1096.

18. Skenderi KP, Kavouras SA, Anastasiou CA, Yiannakouris N, Matalas AL. Exertional Rhabdomyolysis during a 246-km continuous running race. Med Sci Sports Exerc. 2006; 38(6): 1054–1057.

19. Roberts WO. Heat and cold: what does the environment do to marathon injury? Sports Med. 2007; 37(4–5): 400–403.

20. Trapasso LM, Cooper JD. Record performances at the Boston Marathon: biometeorological factors. Int J Biometeorol. 1989; 33(4): 233–237.

21. Schwabe K, Schwellnus M, Derman W, Swanevelder S, Jordaan E. Medical complications and deaths in 21 and 56 km road race runners: a 4-year prospective study in 65 865 runners—SAFER study I. Br J Sports Med. 2014; 48(11): 912–918.

22. Getzin AR, Milner C, LaFace KM. Nutrition update for the ultraendurance athlete. Curr Sports Med Rep. 2011; 10(6): 330–339.

23. Kluitenberg B, van Middelkoop M, Diercks R, van der Worp H. What are the Differences in Injury Proportions Between Different Populations of Runners? A Systematic Review and Meta-Analysis. Sports Med. 2015; 45(8): 1143–1161.

24. Satterthwaite P, Norton R, Larmer P, Robinson E. Risk factors for injuries and other health problems sustained in a marathon. Br J Sports Med. 1999; 33(1): 22–26.

25. Wilder RP, Sethi S. Overuse injuries: tendinopathies, stress fractures, compartment syndrome, and shin splints. Clin Sports Med. 2004; 23(1): 55–81, vi.

26. van Gent RN, Siem D, van Middelkoop M, van Os AG, Bierma-Zeinstra SM, Koes BW. Incidence and determinants of lower extremity running injuries in long distance runners: a systematic review. Br J Sports Med. 2007; 41(8): 469–480; discussion 480.

27. Pasquina PF, Griffin SC, Anderson-Barnes VC, Tsao JW, O'Connor FG. Analysis of injuries from the Army Ten Miler: A 6-year retrospective review. Mil Med. 2013; 178(1): 55–60.

28. Hutson MA. Medical implications of ultra marathon running: observations on a six day track race. Br J Sports Med. 1984; 18(1): 44–45.

29. Saragiotto BT, Yamato TP, Hespanhol Junior LC, Rainbow MJ, Davis IS, Lopes AD. What are the main risk factors for running-related injuries? Sports Med. 2014; 44(8): 1153–1163.

30. Nicholl JP, Williams BT. Medical problems before and after a popular marathon. Br Med J (Clin Res Ed). 1982; 285(6353): 1465–1466.

31. Caselli MA, Longobardi SJ. Lower extremity injuries at the New York City Marathon. J Am Podiatr Med Assoc. 1997; 87(1): 34–37.

32. Macera CA, Pate RR, Woods J, Davis DR, Jackson KL. Postrace morbidity among runners. Am J Prev Med. 1991; 7(4): 194–198.

33. Kretsch A, Grogan R, Duras P, Allen F, Sumner J, Gillam I. 1980 Melbourne marathon study. Med J Aust. 1984; 141(12–13): 809–814.

34. Roberts WO, Nicholson WG. Youth marathon runners and race day medical risk over 26 years. Clin J Sport Med. 2010; 20(4): 318–321.

35. Taunton JE, Ryan MB, Clement DB, McKenzie DC, Lloyd-Smith DR, Zumbo BD. A retrospective case-control analysis of 2002 running injuries. Br J Sports Med. 2002; 36(2): 95–101.

36. McKean KA, Manson NA, Stanish WD. Musculoskeletal injury in the masters runners. Clin J Sport Med. 2006; 16(2): 149–154.

37. Jakobsen BW, Krøner K, Schmidt SA, Kjeldsen A. Prevention of injuries in long-distance runners. Knee Surg Sports Traumatol Arthrosc. 1994; 2(4): 245–249.

38. Roberts WO. A 12-yr profile of medical injury and illness for the Twin Cities Marathon. Med Sci Sports Exerc. 2000; 32(9): 1549–1555.

39. Bishop GW, Fallon KE. Musculoskeletal injuries in a six-day track race: ultramarathoner's ankle. Clin J Sport Med. 1999; 9(4): 216–220.

40. Khodaee M, Ansari M. Common ultramarathon injuries and illnesses: race day management. Curr Sports Med Rep. 2012; 11(6): 290–297.

41. Fredericson M, Wolf C. Iliotibial band syndrome in runners: innovations in treatment. Sports Med. 2005; 35(5): 451–459.

42. Lopes AD, Hespanhol Júnior LC, Yeung SS, Costa LO. What are the main running-related musculoskeletal injuries? A Systematic Review. Sports Med. 2012; 42(10): 891–905.

43. Tenforde AS, Sayres LC, McCurdy ML, Collado H, Sainani KL, Fredericson M. Overuse injuries in high school runners: lifetime prevalence and prevention strategies. PM R. 2011; 3(2): 125–131; quiz 131.

44. Simpson MR, Howard TM. Tendinopathies of the foot and ankle. Am Fam Physician. 2009; 80(10): 1107–1114.

45. Schwellnus MP, Allie S, Derman W, Collins M. Increased running speed and pre-race muscle damage as risk factors for exercise-associated muscle cramps in a 56 km ultramarathon: a prospective cohort study. Br J Sports Med 2011; 45(14): 1132–1136.

46. Edouard, P. Exercise associated muscle cramps: Discussion on causes, prevention and treatment. Science & Sports 2014; 29(6): 299–305.

47. Holtzhausen LM, Noakes TD, Kroning B, de Klerk M, Roberts M, Emsley R. Clinical and biochemical characteristics of collapsed ultra-marathon runners. Med Sci Sports Exerc. 1994; 26(9): 1095–1101.

48. Sanchez LD, Corwell B, Berkoff D. Medical problems of marathon runners. Am J Emerg Med. 2006; 24(5): 608–615.

49. Wyndham CH, Strydom NB. The danger of an inadequate water intake during marathon running. S Afr Med J. 1969; 43(29): 893–896.

50. Mohseni M, Silvers S, McNeil R, et al. Prevalence of hyponatremia, renal dysfunction, and other electrolyte abnormalities among runners before and after completing a marathon or half marathon. Sports Health. 2011; 3(2): 145–151.

51. Almond CS, Shin AY, Fortescue EB, et al. Hyponatremia among runners in the Boston Marathon. N Engl J Med. 2005; 352(15): 1550–1556.

52. Knechtle B, Gnädinger M, Knechtle P, et al. Prevalence of exercise-associated hyponatremia in male ultraendurance athletes. Clin J Sport Med. 2011; 21(3): 226–232.

53. Hew-Butler T, Ayus JC, Kipps C, et al. Statement of the Second International Exercise-Associated Hyponatremia Consensus Development Conference, New Zealand, 2007. Clin J Sport Med. 2008; 18(2): 111–121.

54. Hoffman MD, Hew-Butler T, Stuempfle KJ. Exercise-associated hyponatremia and hydration status in 161-km ultramarathoners. Med Sci Sports Exerc. 2013; 45(4): 784–791.

55. Robach P, Boisson RC, Vincent L, et al. Hemolysis induced by an extreme mountain ultra-marathon is not associated with a decrease in total red blood cell volume. Scand J Med Sci Sports. 2014; 24(1): 18–27.

56. Lipman GS, Krabak BJ, Waite BL, Logan SB, Menon A, Chan GK. A prospective cohort study of acute kidney injury in multi-stage ultramarathon runners: the Biochemistry in Endurance Runner Study (BIERS). Res Sports Med. 2014; 22(2): 185–192.

57. Lipman, GS Shea K, et al. Ibuprofen versus placebo effect on acute kidney injury in ultramarathon runners. Annals of Emergency Medicine. 2016; 68(4s): s130.

58. McCullough PA, Chinnaiyan KM, Gallagher MJ, et al. Changes in renal markers and acute kidney injury after marathon running. Nephrology (Carlton). 2011; 16(2): 194–199.

59. Page AJ, Reid SA, Speedy DB, Mulligan GP, Thompson J. Exercise-associated hyponatremia, renal function, and nonsteroidal antiinflammatory drug use in an ultraendurance mountain run. Clin J Sport Med. 2007; 17(1): 43–48.

60. Elers J, Pedersen L, Backer V. Asthma in elite athletes. Expert Rev Respir Med. 2011; 5(3): 343–351.

61. Robson-Ansley P, Howatson G, Tallent J, et al. Prevalence of allergy and upper respiratory tract symptoms in runners of the London marathon. Med Sci Sports Exerc. 2012; 44(6): 999–1004.
62. Mahler DA, Loke J. Pulmonary dysfunction in ultramarathon runners. Yale J Biol Med. 1981; 54(4): 243–248.
63. Green GA. Gastrointestinal disorders in the athlete. Clin Sports Med. 1992; 11(2): 453–470.
64. Baska RS, Moses FM, Deuster PA. Cimetidine reduces running-associated gastrointestinal bleeding. A prospective observation. Dig Dis Sci. 1990; 35(8): 956–960.
65. Morton DP, Callister R. Factors influencing exercise-related transient abdominal pain. Med Sci Sports Exerc. 2002; 34(5): 745–749.
66. ter Steege RW, Van der Palen J, Kolkman JJ. Prevalence of gastrointestinal complaints in runners competing in a long-distance run: an internet-based observational study in 1281 subjects. Scand J Gastroenterol. 2008; 43(12): 1477–1482.
67. Riddoch C, Trinick T. Gastrointestinal disturbances in marathon runners. Br J Sports Med. 1988; 22(2): 71–74.
68. Keeffe EB, Lowe DK, Goss JR, Wayne R. Gastrointestinal symptoms of marathon runners. West J Med. 1984; 141(4): 481–484.
69. Peters HP, Bos M, Seebregts L, et al. Gastrointestinal symptoms in long-distance runners, cyclists, and triathletes: prevalence, medication, and etiology. Am J Gastroenterol. 1999; 94(6): 1570–1581.
70. Glace B, Murphy C, McHugh M. Food and fluid intake and disturbances in gastrointestinal and mental function during an ultramarathon. Int J Sport Nutr Exerc Metab. 2002; 12(4): 414–427.
71. Stuempfle KJ, Hoffman MD. Gastrointestinal distress is common during a 161-km ultramarathon. J Sports Sci. 2015; 33(17): 1814–1821.
72. Pfeiffer B, Stellingwerff T, Hodgson AB, et al. Nutritional intake and gastrointestinal problems during competitive endurance events. Med Sci Sports Exerc. 2012; 44(2): 344–351.
73. Simons SM, Kennedy RG. Gastrointestinal problems in runners. Curr Sports Med Rep. 2004; 3(2): 112–116.
74. Ryan AJ, Chang RT, Gisolfi CV. Gastrointestinal permeability following aspirin intake and prolonged running. Med Sci Sports Exerc. 1996; 28(6): 698–705.
75. Mailler EA, Adams BB. The wear and tear of 26.2: dermatological injuries reported on marathon day. Br J Sports Med. 2004; 38(4): 498–501.

## Chapter 3

1. Bramble DM, Lieberman DE. Endurance running and the evolution of Homo. Nature. 2004;432:345–352.
2. Davis IS. The re-emergence of the minimal running shoe. J Orthop Sports Phys Ther. 2014;44:775–784.
3. Lilley K, Stiles V, Dixon S. The influence of motion control shoes on the running gait of mature and young females. Gait Posture. 2013;37:331–335.
4. Clarke TE, Frederick EC, Hamill CL. The effects of shoe design parameters on rearfoot control in running. Med Sci Sports Exerc. 1983;15:376–381.

5. Hamill J, Freedson PS, Boda W, Reichsman F. Effects of shoe type on cardiorespiratory responses and rearfoot motion during treadmill running. Med Sci Sports Exerc. 1988;20:515–521.
6. Milani T, Schnabel G, Hennig E. Rearfoot motion and pressure distribution patterns during running in shoes with varus and valgus wedges. J Appl Biomech. 1995;11:177–187.
7. Cheung RTH, Ng GYF. Efficacy of motion control shoes for reducing excessive rearfoot motion in fatigued runners. Phys Ther Sport. 2007;8:75–81.
8. Perry SD, Lafortune MA. Influences of inversion/eversion of the foot upon impact loading during locomotion. Clin Biomech Bristol Avon. 1995;10:253–257.
9. Butler RJ, Davis IS, Hamill J. Interaction of arch type and footwear on running mechanics. Am J Sports Med. 2006;34:1998–2005.
10. Butler RJ, Hamill J, Davis I. Effect of footwear on high and low arched runners' mechanics during a prolonged run. Gait Posture. 2007;26:219–225.
11. Knapik JJ, Trone DW, Tchandja J, Jones BH. Injury-reduction effectiveness of prescribing running shoes on the basis of foot arch height: summary of military investigations. J Orthop Sports Phys Ther. 2014;44:805–812.
12. Ryan MB, Valiant GA, McDonald K, Taunton JE. The effect of three different levels of footwear stability on pain outcomes in women runners: a randomised control trial. Br J Sports Med. 2011;45:715–721.
13. Malisoux L, Chambon N, Delattre N, Gueguen N, Urhausen A, Theisen D. Injury risk in runners using standard or motion control shoes: a randomised controlled trial with participant and assessor blinding. Br J Sports Med. 2016;50:481–487.
14. Theisen D, Malisoux L, Genin J, Delattre N, Seil R, Urhausen A. Influence of midsole hardness of standard cushioned shoes on running-related injury risk. Br J Sports Med. 2014;48:371–376.
15. Hasegawa H, Yamauchi T, Kraemer WJ. Foot strike patterns of runners at the 15-km point during an elite-level half marathon. J Strength Cond Res. 2007;21:888–893.
16. Milner CE, Ferber R, Pollard CD, Hamill J, Davis IS. Biomechanical factors associated with tibial stress fracture in female runners. Med Sci Sports Exerc. 2006;38:323–328.
17. Rice HM, Jamison ST, Davis IS. Footwear matters: influence of footwear and foot strike on load rates during running. Med Sci Sports Exerc. 2016;48:2462–2468.
18. Lieberman DE, Venkadesan M, Werbel WA, et al. Foot strike patterns and collision forces in habitually barefoot versus shod runners. Nature. 2010;463:531–535.
19. Lieberman DE, Castillo ER, Otarola-Castillo E, et al. Variation in foot strike patterns among habitually barefoot and shod runners in Kenya. PloS One. 2015;10:e0131354.
20. Wearing SC, Hooper SL, Dubois P, Smeathers JE, Dietze A. Force-deformation properties of the human heel pad during barefoot walking. Med Sci Sports Exerc. 2014;46:1588–1594.
21. Samaan CD, Rainbow MJ, Davis IS. Reduction in ground reaction force variables with instructed barefoot running. J Sport Health Sci. 2014;3:143–151.
22. Bonacci J, Saunders PU, Hicks A, Rantalainen T, Vicenzino BGT, Spratford W. Running in a minimalist and lightweight shoe is not the same as running barefoot: a biomechanical study. Br J Sports Med. 2013;47:387–392.
23. Almonroeder T, Willson JD, Kernozek TW. The effect of foot strike pattern on achilles tendon load during running. Ann Biomed Eng. 2013;41:1758–1766.

24. Komi PV. Relevance of in vivo force measurements to human biomechanics. J Biomech. 1990;23:23–34.
25. Bayliss AJ, Weatherholt AM, Crandall TT, et al. Achilles tendon material properties are greater in the jump leg of jumping athletes. J Musculoskelet Neuronal Interact. 2016;16:105–112.
26. Kubo K, Miyazaki D, Tanaka S, Shimoju S, Tsunoda N. Relationship between Achilles tendon properties and foot strike patterns in long-distance runners. J Sports Sci. 2015;33:665–669.
27. Histen K, Arntsen J, L'Hereux L, et al. Achilles tendon properties in minimalist and traditionally shod runners. J Sport Rehabil. August 2016:1–16.
28. Squadrone R, Gallozzi C. Biomechanical and physiological comparison of barefoot and two shod conditions in experienced barefoot runners. J Sports Med Phys Fitness. 2009;49:6–13.
29. Joseph MF, Histen K, Arntsen J, et al. Achilles tendon adaptation during transition to a minimalist running style. J Sport Rehabil. September 2016:1–17.
30. de Jonge S, van den Berg C, de Vos RJ, et al. Incidence of midportion Achilles tendinopathy in the general population. Br J Sports Med. 2011;45:1026–1028.
31. Bonacci J, Vicenzino B, Spratford W, Collins P. Take your shoes off to reduce patellofemoral joint stress during running. Br J Sports Med. 2014;48:425–428.
32. Shinohara J, Gribble P. Wearing five-toed socks improves static postural control in individuals with and without chronic ankle instability. J Athl Train. 2010;45:S-65.
33. Bishop M, Fiolkowski P, Conrad B, Brunt D, Horodyski M. Athletic footwear, leg stiffness, and running kinematics. J Athl Train. 2006;41:387–392.
34. Robbins SE, Hanna AM. Running-related injury prevention through barefoot adaptations. Med Sci Sports Exerc. 1987;19:148–156.
35. Rao UB, Joseph B. The influence of footwear on the prevalence of flat foot. A survey of 2300 children. J Bone Joint Surg Br. 1992;74:525–527.
36. Warne JP, Smyth BP, Fagan JO, et al. Kinetic changes during a six-week minimal footwear and gait-retraining intervention in runners. J Sports Sci. August 2016:1–9.
37. Esculier J-F, Dubois B, Dionne CE, Leblond J, Roy J-S. A consensus definition and rating scale for minimalist shoes. J Foot Ankle Res. 2015;8:42.
38. Squadrone R, Rodano R, Hamill J, Preatoni E. Acute effect of different minimalist shoes on foot strike pattern and kinematics in rearfoot strikers during running. J Sports Sci. 2015;33:1196–1204.
39. Fyhrie DP, Milgrom C, Hoshaw SJ, et al. Effect of fatiguing exercise on longitudinal bone strain as related to stress fracture in humans. Ann Biomed Eng. 1998;26:660–665.
40. Ridge ST, Johnson AW, Mitchell UH, et al. Foot bone marrow edema after a 10-wk transition to minimalist running shoes. Med Sci Sports Exerc. 2013;45:1363–1368.
41. Salzler MJ, Bluman EM, Noonan S, Chiodo CP, de Asla RJ. Injuries observed in minimalist runners. Foot Ankle Int. 2012;33:262–266.
42. Warne JP, Kilduff SM, Gregan BC, Nevill AM, Moran KA, Warrington GD. A 4-week instructed minimalist running transition and gait-retraining changes plantar pressure and force. Scand J Med Sci Sports. 2014;24:964–973.
43. Chen TL-W, Sze LKY, Davis IS, Cheung RTH. Effects of training in minimalist shoes on the intrinsic and extrinsic foot muscle volume. Clin Biomech Bristol Avon. 2016;36:8–13.

44. Ryan M, Elashi M, Newsham-West R, Taunton J. Examining injury risk and pain perception in runners using minimalist footwear. Br J Sports Med. 2014;48:1257–1262.

45. McKeon PO, Hertel J, Bramble D, Davis I. The foot core system: a new paradigm for understanding intrinsic foot muscle function. Br J Sports Med. 2015;49:290.

46. Moore IS, Jones A, Dixon S. The pursuit of improved running performance: Can changes in cushioning and somatosensory feedback influence running economy and injury risk? Footwear Sci. 2014;6:1–11.

47. Perl DP, Daoud AI, Lieberman DE. Effects of footwear and strike type on running economy. Med Sci Sports Exerc. 2012;44:1335–1343.

48. Warne JP, Warrington GD. Four-week habituation to simulated barefoot running improves running economy when compared with shod running. Scand J Med Sci Sports. 2014;24:563–568.

49. Cheung RT, Ngai SP. Effects of footwear on running economy in distance runners: A meta-analytical review. J Sci Med Sport. 2016;19:260–266.

50. Fuller JT, Thewlis D, Tsiros MD, Brown NAT, Buckley JD. Effects of a minimalist shoe on running economy and 5-km running performance. J Sports Sci. 2016;34:1740–1745.

51. Sinclair J, Fau-Goodwin J, Richards J, Shore H. The influence of minimalist and maximalist footwear on the kinetics and kinematics of running. Footwear Sci. 2016;8:33–39.

52. Ferris DP, Louie M, Farley CT. Running in the real world: adjusting leg stiffness for different surfaces. Proc Biol Sci. 1998;265:989–994.

## Chapter 4

1. Borresen, J., & Lambert, M. I. (2007). Changes in heart rate recovery in response to acute changes in training load. (4), 503–511. doi: 10.1007/s00421-007-0516-6.

2. Coutts, A. J., Slattery, K. M., & Wallace, L. K. (2007). Practical tests for monitoring performance, fatigue and recovery in triathletes. (6), 372–381. doi: 10.1016/j.jsams.2007.02.007.

3. Gibala, M. J., Little, J. P., Macdonald, M. J., & Hawley, J. A. (2012). Physiological adaptations to low-volume, high-intensity interval training in health and disease. (5), 1077–1084. doi: 10.1113/jphysiol.2011.224725.

4. Holloszy, J. O., & Coyle, E. F. (1984). Adaptations of skeletal muscle to endurance exercise and their metabolic consequences. (4), 831–838.

5. Kreher, J. B., & Schwartz, J. B. (2012). Overtraining syndrome: a practical guide. (2), 128–138. doi: 10.1177/1941738111434406.

6. Kubukeli, Z. N., Noakes, T. D., & Dennis, S. C. (2002). Training techniques to improve endurance exercise performances. (8), 489–509.

7. Lamberts, R. P., Lemmink, K. A., Durandt, J. J., & Lambert, M. I. (2004). Variation in heart rate during submaximal exercise: implications for monitoring training. (3), 641–645. doi: 10.1519/1533-4287(2004)18<641: VIHRDS>2.0.CO; 2.

8. Magrini, D., Khodaee, M., San-Millan, I., Hew-Butler, T., & Provance, A. J. (2017). Serum creatine kinase elevations in ultramarathon runners at high altitude. 1–5. doi: 10.1080/00913847.2017.1280371.

8. McNair, D. M., Lorr, M., Droppelmann L.F. (1971). San Diego, CA: Educational and Industrial Testing Service.

9. Meeusen, R., Duclos, M., Foster, C., Fry, A., Gleeson, M., Nieman, D., . . . American College of Sports, M. (2013). Prevention, diagnosis, and treatment of the over-training syndrome: joint consensus statement of the European College of Sport Science and the American College of Sports Medicine. (1), 186–205. doi: 10.1249/MSS.0b013e318279a10a.

10. Meeusen, R., Duclos, M., Gleeson, M., Rietjens, G., Steinacker, J., & Urhausen, A. (2006). Prevention, diagnosis and treatment of the Overtraining Syndrome. (1), 1–14. doi: 10.1080/17461390600617717.

11. Noakes, T. D., Myburgh, K. H., & Schall, R. (1990). Peak treadmill running veloc-ity during the VO2 max test predicts running performance. (1), 35–45. doi: 10.1080/02640419008732129.

12. Selye, H. (1998). A syndrome produced by diverse nocuous agents. 1936. (2), 230–231. doi: 10.1176/jnp.10.2.230a.

## Chapter 5

1. Verbalis JG. Disorders of body water homeostasis. Best Pract Res Clin Endocrinol Metab 2003; 17(4): 471–503.

2. McKinley MJ, Johnson AK. The physiological regulation of thirst and fluid intake. News Physiol Sci 2004; 19: 1–6.

3. Bourque CW. Central mechanisms of osmosensation and systemic osmoregulation. Nat Rev Neurosci 2008; 9(7): 519–531.

4. Fitzsimons JT. Angiotensin, thirst, and sodium appetite. Physiol Rev 1998; 78(3): 583–686.

5. Hurley SW, Johnson AK. The biopsychology of salt hunger and sodium deficiency. Pflugers Arch 2015; 467(3): 445–456.

6. Stricker EM, Verbalis JG. Hormones and Behavior. American Scientist 1988; 76: 261–267.

7. Takamata A, Mack GW, Gillen CM, Nadel ER. Sodium appetite, thirst, and body fluid regulation in humans during rehydration without sodium replacement. Am J Physiol 1994; 266(5 Pt 2): R1493-R1502.

8. Convertino VA, Armstrong LE, Coyle EF, et al. American College of Sports Medicine position stand. Exercise and fluid replacement. Med Sci Sports Exerc 1996; 28(1): i-vii.

9. Sharwood K, Collins M, Goedecke J, Wilson G, Noakes T. Weight changes, sodium levels, and performance in the South African Ironman Triathlon. Clin J Sport Med 2002; 12(6): 391–399.

10. Goulet ED. Effect of exercise-induced dehydration on endurance performance: eval-uating the impact of exercise protocols on outcomes using a meta-analytic proce-dure. Br J Sports Med 2013; 47(11): 679–686.

11. Knechtle B, Knechtle P, Rosemann T. Do male 100-km ultra-marathoners overdrink? Int J Sports Physiol Perform 2011; 6(2): 195–207.

12. Hew-Butler T, Rosner MH, Fowkes-Godek S, et al. Statement of the Third International Exercise-Associated Hyponatremia Consensus Development Conference, Carlsbad, California, 2015. Clin J Sport Med 2015; 25(4): 303–320.

13. Beltrami F, Hew-Butler T, Noakes TD. Drinking policies and exercise-associated hyponatremia: is anyone still promoting overdrinking? Br J Sports Med 2008; 42(10): 496–501.

14. Winger JM, Dugas JP, Dugas LR. Beliefs about hydration and physiology drive drinking behaviours in runners. Br J Sports Med 2011; 45(8): 646–649.

15. Sawka MN, Noakes TD. Does dehydration impair exercise performance? Med Sci Sports Exerc 2007; 39(8): 1209–1217.

16. Sawka MN, Burke LM, Eichner ER, Maughan RJ, Montain SJ, Stachenfeld NS. American College of Sports Medicine position stand. Exercise and fluid replacement. Med Sci Sports Exerc 2007; 39(2): 377–390.

17. Montain SJ, Coyle EF. Influence of graded dehydration on hyperthermia and cardiovascular drift during exercise. J Appl Physiol 1992; 73(4): 1340–1350.

18. Beis LY, Wright-Whyte M, Fudge B, Noakes T, Pitsiladis YP. Drinking behaviors of elite male runners during marathon competition. Clin J Sport Med 2012; 22(3): 254–261.

19. Fudge BW, Easton C, Kingsmore D, et al. Elite Kenyan endurance runners are hydrated day-to-day with ad libitum fluid intake. Med Sci Sports Exerc 2008; 40(6): 1171–1179.

20. Lee JK, Nio AQ, Lim CL, Teo EY, Byrne C. Thermoregulation, pacing and fluid balance during mass participation distance running in a warm and humid environment. Eur J Appl Physiol 2010; 109(5): 887–898.

21. Byrne C, Lee JK, Chew SA, Lim CL, Tan EY. Continuous thermoregulatory responses to mass-participation distance running in heat. Med Sci Sports Exerc 2006; 38(5): 803–810.

22. Davis BA, O'Neal EK, Johnson SL, Pribyslavska V, Farley RS. Ad Libitum Fluid Replacement Threshold Evidenced in Runners at 12-h Post-run in Hot Environment: 638 Board #1 June 1, 1: 00 PM - 3: 00 PM. Med Sci Sports Exerc 2016; 48(5 Suppl 1): 166.

23. Saunders CJ, de ML, Hew-Butler T, et al. Dipsogenic genes associated with weight changes during Ironman Triathlons. Hum Mol Genet 2006; 15(20): 2980–2987.

24. Yau AM, Moss AD, James LJ, Gilmore W, Ashworth JJ, Evans GH. The influence of angiotensin converting enzyme and bradykinin receptor B2 gene variants on voluntary fluid intake and fluid balance in healthy men during moderate-intensity exercise in the heat. Appl Physiol Nutr Metab 2015; 40(2): 184–190.

25. Davis BA, Thigpen LK, Hornsby JH, Green JM, Coates TE, O'Neal EK. Hydration kinetics and 10-km outdoor running performance following 75 percent versus 150 percent between bout fluid replacement. Eur J Sport Sci 2014; 14(7): 703–710.

26. Institute of Medicine of the National Academies. Dietary Reference Intakes for Water, Potassium, Sodium, Chloride, and Sulfate. Washington D.C.: The National Academies Press, 2004.

27. Thompson CJ, Bland J, Burd J, Baylis PH. The osmotic thresholds for thirst and vasopressin release are similar in healthy man. Clin Sci (Lond) 1986; 71(6): 651–656.

28. McKenna K, Thompson C. Osmoregulation in clinical disorders of thirst appreciation. Clin Endocrinol (Oxf) 1998; 49(2): 139–152.

29. Maughan RJ, Shirreffs SM, Leiper JB. Errors in the estimation of hydration status from changes in body mass. J Sports Sci 2007; 25(7): 797–804.

30. O'Neal EK, Wingo JE, Richardson MT, Leeper JD, Neggers YH, Bishop PA. Half-marathon and full-marathon runners' hydration practices and perceptions. J Athl Train 2011; 46(6): 581–591.

31. Passe D, Horn M, Stofan J, Horswill C, Murray R. Voluntary dehydration in runners despite favorable conditions for fluid intake. Int J Sport Nutr Exerc Metab 2007; 17(3): 284–295.

32. O'Neal EK, Caufield CR, Lowe JB, Stevenson MC, Davis BA, Thigpen LK. 24-h fluid kinetics and perception of sweat losses following a 1-h run in a temperate environment. Nutrients 2014; 6(1): 37–49.

33. O'Neal EK, Davis BA, Thigpen LK, Caufield CR, Horton AD, McIntosh JR. Runners greatly underestimate sweat losses before and after a 1-hr summer run. Int J Sport Nutr Exerc Metab 2012; 22(5): 353–362.

34. Cheuvront SN, Kenefick RW, Zambraski EJ. Spot Urine Concentrations Should Not be Used for Hydration Assessment: A Methodology Review. Int J Sport Nutr Exerc Metab 2015; 25(3): 293–297.

35. Armstrong LE. Performing in Extreme Environments. Champaign, IL: Human Kinetics Publishers, 2000.

36. Hooper L, Bunn DK, Abdelhamid A, et al. Water-loss (intracellular) dehydration assessed using urinary tests: how well do they work? Diagnostic accuracy in older people. Am J Clin Nutr 2016; 104(1): 121–131.

37. Beets I, Temmerman L, Janssen T, Schoofs L. Ancient neuromodulation by vasopressin/oxytocin-related peptides. Worm 2013; 2(2): e24246.

38. Dion T, Savoie FA, Asselin A, Gariepy C, Goulet ED. Half-marathon running performance is not improved by a rate of fluid intake above that dictated by thirst sensation in trained runners. Eur J Appl Physiol. 2013 Dec; 113 (12): 3011–20.

39. Casa DJ, Stearns RL, Lopez RM, Ganio MS, McDermott BP, Walker Yeargin S, Maresh CM. Influence of hydration on physiological function and performance during trail running in the heat. J Athl Train. 2010 Mar-Apr; 45 (2): 147–56.

40. Lopez RM, Casa DJ, Jense JA, Sterns RL, DeMartini JK, Pagnotta KD, Maresh CM. Comparison of two fluid replacement protocols during a 20 km trail running race in the heat. J Strength Cond Res 2016 Sep; 30 (9): 2609–2616.

## Chapter 6

1. Kruseman M, Bucher S, Bovard M, Kayer B, Bovier PA. Nutrient intake and perfomance during a mountain marathon: an observational study. Eur J Appl Physiol. 2005; 94: 151–7.

2. Rowell LB, Backmon JR, Bruce RA. Indocyanine-green clearance and estimated hepatic blood flow during mild exercise in upright men. J Clin Invest. 1984; 43: 1677–80.

3. World Health Organization. Energy and Protein Requirements. Report of a Joint FAO/WHO/UNU expert Consultation. Technical Report Series. 724. Geneva, Switzerland. World Health Organization; 1985: 206.

4. Bergstrom J, Hermansen L, Holtman E, Saltin B. Diet, muscle glycogen and physical performance. Acta Physiol. Scand, 1967; 71: 140.

5.  Costill DL, Bowers R, Branam G, Sparks K. Muscle glycogen utilization during prolonged exercise on successive days. J Appl Physiol. 1971; 31: 834–8.

6.  Coyle EF, Coggan AR, Hemmert MK, Ivy J. Muscle glycogen utilization during prolonged exercise when fed carbohydrate. J Appl Physiol. 1986; 21: 670–4.

7.  Hargreaves M, Costill DL, Coggan A, Fink WJ, Nishibata I. Effect of carbohydrate feedings on muscle glycogen utilization and exercise performance. Med Sci Sports Exerc. 1984; 16: 219–22.

8.  Karlsson J, Saltin B. Diet, muscle glycogen and endurance performance. J Appl Physiol. 1971; 31: 203–6.

9.  IOC consensus statement on sports nutrition 2010. Journal of Sports Sciences, 29(sup1), pp. S3–S4.

10. Burke LM, Hawley JA, Wong SH, Jeudenfrup AE. Carbohydrates for training and competition. J Sports Sci. 2011; 29 Suppl 1: S17–27.

11. Jentgens RLPG, Moseley L, Waring RH. Oxidation of combined ingestion of glucose and fructose during exercise. J Appl Physiol. 2004; 96: 1277–84.

12. Jentgens RLPG, Achten J, Jeudenkrup AE. High oxidation rates from combined carbohydrates ingested during exercise. Med Sci Sports Exerc. 2004; 36: 1551–8.

13. Getzin AR, Milner C, LaFace KM. Nutrition update for the Ultraendurance athlete. Curr Sport Med Rep. 2011; Nov-Dec; 10(6): 330–9.

14. Hawley JA, Bueke LM. Carbohydrate availability and training adaptation: effects on cell metabolism. Exerc Sport Sci Rev 2010; 38(4): 152–60.

15. Burke LM, Angus DJ, Cox GR, Cummings NK, Febbraio MA, Gawthorn K, Hawley JA, Minehan M, Martin DT, Hargreaves M. Effect of fat adaptation and carbohydrate restoration on metabolism and performance during prolonged cycling. Journal of Applied Physiology 2000; 89(6): 2413–2421.

16. Phillips SM, Moore DR, Tang JE. A Critical Examination of Dietary Protein Requirements, Benefits, and Excesses in Athletes. IJSNEM 2007; 17(suppl): S58-S76.

17. Tarnopolsky M, Atkinson S, MacDougall JD, Seonr BB, Lemon P, Schwarcz H. Whole body leucine metabolism during and after resistance exercise in fed humans. Med Sci Sports Exerc. 1991; 23: 326–33.

18. Febbraio MA, Stewart KL. CHO feeding before prolonged exercise: effect of glycemic index on muscle glycogenolysis and exercise performance. J Appl Physiol. 1996; 81: 1115–20.

19. Helge JW, Wulff B, Kiens B. Impact of a fat-rich diet on endurance in man: role of the dietary period. Med Sci Sport Exerc. 1998; 30: 456–61.

20. Jeudenjrup AE, Thielens JJ, Wagenmakers AJ, Brouns F, Saris WH. Effect of medium-chain triacylglycerol and carbohydrate ingestion during exercise on substrate utilization and subsequent cycling performance. Am J Clin Nutr. 1998: 67: 397–404.

21. Noakes T. Fluid replacement during marathon running. Clin J Sport Med. 2003; 13: 309–18.

22. Schwellnus MP, Nicol J, Laubscher R , Noakes T. Serum electrolyte concentrations and hydration status are not associated with exercise associated muscle cramping (WAMC) in distance runners. Br J Sports Med. 2004; 38: 488–92.

23. Dietary Reference Intakes for Calcium, Phosphorous, Magnesium, Vitamin D, and Fluoride (1997); Dietary Reference Intakes for Thiamin, Riboflavin, Niacin, Vitamin

B6, Folate, Vitamin B12, Pantothenic Acid, Biotin, and Choline (1998); Dietary Reference Intakes for Vitamin C, Vitamine E, Selenium, and Carotenoids (2000); Dietary Reference Intakes for Vitamin A, Vitamin K, Arsenic, Boron, Chromium, Copper, Iodine, Iron, Manganese, Molybdenum, Nickel, Silicon, Vanadium, and Zinc (2001); and Dietary Reference Intakes for Calcium and Vitamin D (2011), Food and Nutrition Board, National Academies of Science, Institute of Medicine.

24. Mountjoy M, Sundgot-Borgen J, Burke L, Carter S, Constantini N, Lebrun C, Meyer N, Sherman R, Steffen K, Budgett R, Ljungqvist A. The IOC consensus statement: beyond the Female Athlete Triad—Relative Energy Deficiency in Sport (RED-S) ll. Br J Sports Med 2014; 48: 491–497.

## *Chapter 7*

1. International Association for the Study of Pain (IASP). Part III: Pain terms, a current list with definitions and notes on usage. In: Merskey H, Bogduk N, eds. Classification of chronic pain. 2nd ed. Seattle, WA: IASP Press; 1994: 209–214.

2. Melzack R, Wall PD. Pain mechanisms: a new theory. Science. 1965; 150(3699): 971–979.

3. Engel GL. The need for a new medical model: a challenge for biomedicine. Science. 1977; 196(4286): 129–136.

4. Kerns RD, Turk DC, Rudy TE. The West Haven-Yale Multidimensional Pain Inventory (WHYMPI). Pain. 1985; 23(4): 345–356.

5. Wiese-Bjornstal DM, Smith AM, Shaffer SM, Morrey MA. An integrated model of response to sport injury: Psychological and sociological dynamics. Journal of Applied Sport Psychology. 1998; 10(1): 46–69.

6. Wiese-Bjornstal DM. Psychology and socioculture affect injury risk, response, and recovery in high-intensity athletes: a consensus statement. Scandinavian Journal of Medicine & Science in Sports. 2010; 20(s2): 103–111.

7. Nippert AH, Smith AM. Psychologic stress related to injury and impact on sport performance. Phys Med Rehabil Clin N Am. 2008; 19(2): 399–418, x.

8. Junge A. The influence of psychological factors on sports injuries. Review of the literature. Am J Sports Med. 2000; 28(5 Suppl): S10–15.

9. Smith AM, Stuart MJ, Wiese-Bjornstal DM, Milliner EK, O'Fallon WM, Crowson CS. Competitive athletes: preinjury and postinjury mood state and self-esteem. Mayo Clin Proc. 1993; 68(10): 939–947.

10. Brewer BW, Cornelius AE, Sklar JH, et al. Pain and negative mood during rehabilitation after anterior cruciate ligament reconstruction: a daily process analysis. Scand J Med Sci Sports. 2007; 17(5): 520–529.

11. Leddy MH, Lambert MJ, Ogles BM. Psychological consequences of athletic injury among high-level competitors. Res Q Exerc Sport. 1994; 65(4): 347–354.

12. Brewer BW, Linder DE, Phelps CM. Situational correlates of emotional adjustment to athletic injury. Clin J Sport Med. 1995; 5(4): 241–245.

13. Bonanno GA. Loss, trauma, and human resilience: have we underestimated the human capacity to thrive after extremely aversive events? Am Psychol. 2004; 59(1): 20–28.

14. Silverman AM, Verrall AM, Alschuler KN, Smith AE, Ehde DM. Bouncing back again, and again: a qualitative study of resilience in people with multiple sclerosis. Disabil Rehabil. 2016: 1–9.

15. Silverman AM, Molton IR, Alschuler KN, Ehde DM, Jensen MP. Resilience predicts functional outcomes in people aging with disability: a longitudinal investigation. Arch Phys Med Rehabil. 2015; 96(7): 1262–1268.

16. Tan-Kristanto S, Kiropoulos LA. Resilience, self-efficacy, coping styles and depressive and anxiety symptoms in those newly diagnosed with multiple sclerosis. Psychol Health Med. 2015; 20(6): 635–645.

17. Senders A, Bourdette D, Hanes D, Yadav V, Shinto L. Perceived stress in multiple sclerosis: the potential role of mindfulness in health and well-being. J Evid Based Complementary Altern Med. 2014; 19(2): 104–111.

18. Vlaeyen JW, Kole-Snijders AM, Boeren RG, van Eek H. Fear of movement/(re)injury in chronic low back pain and its relation to behavioral performance. Pain. 1995; 62(3): 363–372.

19. Vlaeyen J, KoleSnijders A, Rotteveel A, Ruesink R, Heuts P. The role of fear of movement (re)injury in pain disability. Journal of Occupational Rehabilitation. 1995; 5(4): 235–252.

20. Crombez G, Vlaeyen JW, Heuts PH, Lysens R. Pain-related fear is more disabling than pain itself: evidence on the role of pain-related fear in chronic back pain disability. Pain. 1999; 80(1–2): 329–339.

21. Vlaeyen JW, Linton SJ. Fear-avoidance and its consequences in chronic musculoskeletal pain: a state of the art. Pain. 2000; 85(3): 317–332.

22. Leeuw M, Goossens ME, Linton SJ, Crombez G, Boersma K, Vlaeyen JW. The fear-avoidance model of musculoskeletal pain: current state of scientific evidence. J Behav Med. 2007; 30(1): 77–94.

23. Tripp DA, Stanish W, Ebel-Lam A, Brewer BW, Birchard J. Fear of reinjury, negative affect, and catastrophizing predicting return to sport in recreational athletes with anterior cruciate ligament injuries at 1 year postsurgery. Rehabilitation Psychology. 2007; 52(1): 74–81.

24. Hermesdorf M, Berger K, Baune BT, Wellmann J, Ruscheweyh R, Wersching H. Pain Sensitivity in Patients With Major Depression: Differential Effect of Pain Sensitivity Measures, Somatic Cofactors, and Disease Characteristics. J Pain. 2016; 17(5): 606–616.

25. Evans L, Hardy L. Injury rehabilitation: a goal-setting intervention study. Res Q Exerc Sport. 2002; 73(3): 310–319.

26. Linton SJ, Nicholas MK, MacDonald S, et al. The role of depression and catastrophizing in musculoskeletal pain. Eur J Pain. 2011; 15(4): 416–422.

27. Spetch LA, Kolt GS. Adherence to sport injury rehabilitation: implications for sports medicine providers and researchers. Physical Therapy in Sport. 2001; 2(2): 80–90.

28. Brown C. Injuries: The Psychology of Recovery and Rehab. In: Murphy S, ed. The Sport Psych Handbook. Champaign, IL: Human Kinetics; 2005: 215–236.

29. Smith AM. Psychological Impact of Injuries in Athletes. Sports Medicine. 1996; 22(6): 391–405.

## Chapter 8

1.  Akers WA, Sulzberger MB. The friction blister. Mil Med. 1972; 137(1): 1–7.
2.  Hoeffler DF. Friction blisters and cellulitis in a navy recruit population. Mil Med. 1975; 140(5): 333–337.
3.  Twombly SE, Schussman LC. Gender differences in injury and illness rates on wilderness backpacking trips. Wilderness and Environmental Medicine. 1995; 4: 363–376.
4.  Boulware DR, Forgey WW, Martin WJ, 2nd. Medical risks of wilderness hiking. The American Journal of Medicine. 2003; 114(4): 288–293.
5.  Mailler EA, Adams BB. The wear and tear of 26.2: dermatological injuries reported on marathon day. Br J Sports Med. 2004; 38(4): 498–501.
6.  Scheer BV, Reljic D, Murray A, Costa RJ. The enemy of the feet blisters in ultraendurance runners. J Am Podiatr Med Assoc. 2014; 104(5): 473–478.
7.  Lipman GS, Ellis MA, Lewis EJ, et al. A Prospective Randomized Blister Prevention Trial Assessing Paper Tape in Endurance Distances (Pre-TAPED). Wilderness & Environmental Medicine.
8.  Lipman GS, Sharp LJ, Christensen M, et al. Paper Tape Prevents Foot Blisters: Randomized Prevention Trial Assessing Paper Tape in Endurance Distance II (Pre-TAPED II). Paper presented at: Wilderness Medical Society Winter Meeting; February 15, 2015, 2015; Park City, UT.
9.  Lipman GS, Sharp LJ, Christensen M, et al. Paper Tape Prevents Foot Blisters: A Randomized Prevention Trial Assessing Paper Tape in Endurance Distances II (Pre-TAPED II). Clin J Sport Med. 2016.
10. Hoffman MD, Fogard K. Factors related to successful completion of a 161-km ultramarathon. International journal of sports physiology and performance. 2011; 6(1): 25–37.
11. Krabak BJ, Waite B, Schiff MA. Study of injury and illness rates in multiday ultramarathon runners. Med Sci Sports Exerc. 2011; 43(12): 2314–2320.
12. McLaughlin KA, Townes DA, Wedmore IS, Billingsley RT, Listrom CD, Iverson LD. Pattern of injury and illness during expedition-length adventure races. Wilderness Environ Med. 2006; 17(3): 158–161.
13. Townes DA, Talbot TS, Wedmore IS, Billingsly R. Event medicine: injury and illness during an expedition-length adventure race. J Emerg Med. 2004; 27(2): 161–165.
14. In: Mish FC, ed. Merriam-Webster's Collegiate Dictionary 11th ed.: Library of Congress; 2003.
15. Naylor P. The skin surface and friction. Br J Dermatol. 1955; 67: 239–248.
16. Akers WA. Measurements of friction injuries in man. Am J Ind Med. 1985; 8(4–5): 473–481.
17. Comaish JS. Epidermal fatigue as a cause of friction blisters. Lancet. 1973; 1: 81–83.
18. Comaish S, Bottoms E. The skin and friction: deviations from amonton's laws and the effect of hydration and lubrication. Br J Dermatol. 1971; 84: 37–43.
19. Knapik JJ, Reynolds KL, Duplantis KL, Jones BH. Friction blisters. Pathophysiology, prevention and treatment. Sports medicine (Auckland, N.Z.). 1995; 20(3): 136–147.
20. Zhang M, Mak AFT. In vivo friction properties of human skin. Prosthet Orthot Int. 1999; 23: 125–141.
21. Sulzberger MB, Cortese TA, Fishman L, Wiley HS. Studies on blisters produced by friction. I. Results of linear rubbing and twisting technics. J Invest Dermatol. 1966; 47(5): 456–465 contd.

22. Cortese TA, Jr., Sams WM, Jr., Sulzberger MB. Studies on blisters produced by friction. II. The blister fluid. J Invest Dermatol. 1968; 50(1): 47–53.
23. Epstein WL, Fukuyama K, Cortese TA. Autographic study of friction blisters. RNA, DNA, and protein synthesis. Arch Derm. 1969; 99: 94–106.
24. Knapik J, Harman E, Reynolds K. Load carriage using packs: a review of physiological, biomechanical and medical aspects. Appl Ergon. 1996; 27(3): 207–216.
25. Quatrale RP, Coble DW, Stoner KL, Felger CB. Mechanism of anti-perspirant action on aluminium salts. III. Histological observations of human sweat glands inhibited by aluminium zirconium chlorohy-drate glycine complex. J Soc Cosmet Chem. 1981; 32: 195–222.
26. Quatrale RP, Coble DW, Stoner KL, Felger CB. The mechanism of antiperspirant action of aluminium salts. II. Histological observations of human eccrine sweat glands inhibited by aluminium chlorhydrate. J Soc Cosmet Chem. 1997; 19: 271–280.
27. Quijano VJJ, Palamarchuk H, et al. Field Efficacy of Blist-O-Ban bandage in 100 MS walk participants. Am Prof Wound Care Assoc Meeting; 2006, April 6–8; Philadelphia, PA.
28. Sian-Wei Tan S, Kok SK, Lim JK. Efficacy of a new blister prevention plaster under tropical conditions. Wilderness Environ Med. 2008; 19(2): 77–81.
29. Polliack AA, Scheinberg S. A new technology for reducing shear and friction forces on the skin: implications for blister care in the wilderness setting. Wilderness Environ Med. 2006; 17(2): 109–119.
30. Darrigrand A, Reynolds K, Jackson R, Hamlet M, Roberts D. Efficacy of antiperspirants on feet. Mil Med. 1992; 157(5): 256–259.
31. Knapik JJ, Reynolds K, Barson J. Influence of an antiperspirant on foot blister incidence during cross-country hiking. J Am Acad Dermatol. 1998; 39(2 Pt 1): 202–206.
32. Brennan FH, Jr. Managing blisters in competitive athletes. Curr Sports Med Rep. 2002; 1(6): 319–322.
33. Nacht S, Close J, Yeung D, Gans EH. Skin friction coefficient: changes induced by skin hydration and emollient application and correlation with perceived skin feel. J Soc Cosmet Chem. 1981; 32: 55–65.
34. Cortese TA, Jr., Fukuyama K, Epstein W, Sulzberger MB. Treatment of friction blisters. An experimental study. Arch Dermatol. 1968; 97(6): 717–721.
35. Levy PD, Hile DC, Hile LM, Miller MA. A prospective analysis of the treatment of friction blisters with 2-octylcyanoacrylate. J Am Podiatr Med Assoc. 2006; 96(3): 232–237.
36. Wikipedia. Merbromin. 2010; http://en.wikipedia.org/wiki/Merbromin.

## Chapter 9

1. Krabak BJ, Waite, B, Schiff MA. Study of injury and illness rates in multiday ultra-marathon runners. Med Sci Sports Exerc. 2011; 43(12): 2314–20.
2. Lysholm J, Wiklander J. Injuries in runners. Am J Sports Med. 1987; 15: 168–71.
3. Lopes AD, Hespanhol Júnior LC, Yeung SS, Costa LO. What are the main running-related musculoskeletal injuries? A Systematic Review. Sports Med. 2012 Oct 1; 42(10): 891–905.

4.  Fallon KE. Musculoskeletal injuries in the ultramarathon: The 1990 Westfield Sydney to Melbourne run. Br J Sports Med 1996; 30(4): 319–23.

5.  Scheer BV, Murray A. Al Andalus Ultra Trail: An observation of medical interventions during a 219km, 5-day ultramarathon stage race. Clin J Sport Med 2011; 21(5): 444–6.

6.  Fields KB, Running injuries: changing trends and demographics. Curr Sports Med Rep 2011; 10(5): 299–303.

7.  Marti B, Vader JP, Minder CE, et al. On the epidemiology of running injuries: the 1984 Bern Grand-Prix study. Am J Sports Med 1988; 16: 285–94.

8.  Saragiotto BT, Yamato TP, Hespanhol Junior LC, et al. Sports Med 2014; 44: 1153–63.

9.  Nielsen R, Parner E, Nohr E, et al. Excessive progression in weekly running distance and risk of running-related injuries: an association which varies according to type of injury. J Orthop Sports Phys Ther 2014; 44(10): 739–47.

10. van Poppel D, de Koning J, Verhagen AP, Scholten-Peeters GG. Risk factors for lower extremity injuries among half marathon and marathon runners of the Lage Landen Marathon Eindhoven 2012: A prospective cohort study in the Netherlands. Scand J Med Sci Sports. 2016; 26: 226–34.

11. Taunton JE, Ryan MB, Clement DB, et al. A retrospective case-control analysis of 2002 running injuries. Br J Sports Medicine 2002; 2: 95–101.

12. Krabak BJ, Waite BW, Lipman G. Injury and Illnesses Prevention for Ultramarathoners. Curr Sports Med Rep 2013; 12(3): 183–9.

13. Wilson JJ, Best TM. Common Overuse Tendon Problems: A review and recommendation for treatment. Am Fam Physician. 2005; 72(5): 811–18.

14. Hoffman MD, Krishnan E. Health and exercise-related medical issues among 1,212 ultramarathon runners: baseline findings from the ultrarunners longitudinal tracking (ULTRA) study. PLoS One 2014; 9(1): e83867.

15. Vaishya R, Pariyo GB, Agarwal AK, et al. Non-operative management of osteoarthritis of the knee joint. J Clinical Orthopaedics and Trauma. 2016; 7(3): 170–76.

16. Hansen P, English M, Willick SE. Does running cause osteoarthritis in the hip or knee? PM&R 2012; 4(5): S117-S21.

17. Mallow M, Nazarian LN. Greater trochanteric pain syndrome diagnosis and treatment. Phys Med Rehabil Clin N Am. 2014; 25(2): 279–89.

18. Taunton JE, Ryan MB, Clement DB, et al. A Prospective study of running injuries: the Vancouver Sun Run "In Training" clinics. Br J Sports Med 2003; 37: 239–44.

19. DeHaven KE, Lintner DM. Athletic Injuries: comparison by age sport, and gender. Am J Sports Med 1986; 14(3): 218–24.

20. Boling M, Padua D, Marshall S, et al. Gender differences in the incidence and prevalence of patellofemoral pain syndrome. Scand J Med Sci Sports 2010; 20(5): 725–30.

21. Stracciolini A. Casciano R, Levey Friedman H, et al. Pediatric sports injuries: a comparison of males versus females. Am J Sports Med 2014; 42(4): 965–72.

22. Dutton RA, Khadavi MJ, Fredericson M. Patellofemoral Pain. Phys Med Rehabil Clin N Am. 2016; 27(1): 31–52.

23. Fredericson M, Yoon K. Physical examination and patellofemoral pain syndrome. Am J Phys Med Rehabil 2006; 85(3): 234–43.

24. Moyano FR, Valenza MC, Martin LM, et al. Effectiveness of different exercises and stretching physiotherapy on pain and movement in patellofemoral pain syndrome: a randomized controlled trial. Clin Rehabil 2013; 27(5): 409–17.

25. Crossley K, Cowan SM, Bennell KL, et al. Patellar taping: is clinical success supported by scientific evidence? Man Ther 2000; 5(3): 142–50.

26. Stecco A, Gilliar W, Hill R, et al. The anatomical and functional relation between gluteus maximus and fasica lata. J Body Mov Ther 2013; 4: 512–517.

27. Fairclough J, Hayashi K, Toumi H, et al. The functional anatomy of the iliotibial band during flexion and extension of the knee: implications for understanding iliotibial band syndrome. J Anat 2006; 3: 309–16.

28. Orchard JW, Fricker PA, Abud AT, el al. Biomechanics of iliotibial band friction syndrome in runners. Am J Sports Med 1996; 3: 375–9.

29. Baker RL, Fredericson M. Iliotibial Band Syndrome in Runners Biomechanical Implications and Exercise intervention. Phys Med Rehabil Clin N Am. 2016 Feb; 27(1): 53–77.

30. Fredericson M, Cookingham CL, Chaudhari AM, et al. Hip abductor weakness in distance runners with iliotibial band syndrome. Clin J Sport Med 2000; 3: 169–75.

31. Distefano LJ, Blackburn JT, Marshall SW, et al. Gluteal muscle activation during common therapeutic exercises. J Orthop Sports Phys Ther 2009; 7: 532–40.

32. Gunter P, Schwellnus MP. Local corticosteroid injection in the iliotibial band friction syndrome in runners: a randomized controlled trial. Br J Sports Med 2004; 3: 269–72.

33. Carr AJ, Norris SH. The blood supply of the calcaneal tendon. J Bone Joint Surg Br 1989; 71(1): 100–1.

34. Kane TP, Ismail M, Calder JD. Topical glyceryl trinitrate and noninsertional Achilles tendinopathy: a clinical and cellular investigation. Am J Sports Med 2008; 36(6): 1160–3.

35. Alfredson H, Pietila T, Jonsson P, et al. Heavy-load eccentric calf muscle training for the treatment of chronic Achilles tendinosis. Am J Sports Med 1998; 26(3): 360–6.

36. Holmes GB Jr, Mann RA. Possible epidemiological factors associated with rupture of the posterior tibial tendon. Foot Ankle 1992; 13(2): 70–9.

37. Alvarez RG, Marini A, Schimitt C, et al. Stage I and II posterior tibial tendon dysfunction treated by a structured non-operative management protocol: an orthosis and exercise program. Foot Ankle Int 2006; 27(1): 2–8.

38. Deben SE, Pomeroy GC. Subtle cavus foot diagnosis and management. J Am Acad Ortho Surg 2014; 22(8): 512–20.

39. Hicks JH. The mechanics of the foot. The planter aponeurosis of the arch. J Ant 1954; 88(1): 25–30.

40. DiGiovanni BF, Nawoczenski DA, Malay DP, et al. Plantar fascia-specific stretching exercise improves outcomes in patients with chronic plantar fasciitis. A prospective clinical trial with two-year follow up. J Bone Joint Surg Am 2006; 88(8): 1775–81.

41. DiGiovanni BF, Nawoczenski DA, Lintal ME, et al. Tissue-specific plantar fascia-stretching exercise enhances outcomes in patients with chronic heel pain. A prospective, randomized study. J Bone Joint Surg Am 2003; 85-A(7): 1270–7.

42. Stiell IG, Greenberg GH, McKinght RD, et al. A study to develop the clinical decision rules for the use of radiography in acute ankle injuries. Ann Emert Med 1992; 21(4): 384–90.

43. Warden SJ. Cyclo-oxygenase-2 inhibitors: beneficial or detrimental for athletes with acute musculoskeletal injuries? Sports Med 2005; 35(4): 271–83.

44. Wikstrom EA, Naik S, Lodha N, et al. Balance capabilities after lateral ankle trauma and intervention: a meta-analysis. Med Sci Sports Exerc 2009; 41(6): 1287–95.

## Chapter 10

1. Tenforde AS, Nattiv A, Barrack MT, et al. Distribution of Bone Stress Injuries in Elite Male and Female Collegiate Endurance Runners. Med Sci Sports Exerc 2015; 47(5S).

2. Warden SJ, Davis IS, Fredericson M. Management and prevention of bone stress injuries in long-distance runners. J Orthop Sports Phys Ther 2014; 44(10): 749–765.

3. Boden BP, Osbahr DC. High-risk stress fractures: evaluation and treatment. J Am Acad Orthop Surg 2000; 8(6): 344–353.

4. Nattiv A, Kennedy G, Barrack MT, et al. Correlation of MRI grading of bone stress injuries with clinical risk factors and return to play: a 5-year prospective study in collegiate track and field athletes. Am J Sports Med 2013; 41(8): 1930–1941.

5. Wentz L, Liu PY, Haymes E, et al. Females have a greater incidence of stress fractures than males in both military and athletic populations: a systemic review. Mil Med 2011; 176(4): 420–430.

6. De Souza MJ, Nattiv A, Joy E, Misra M, Williams NI, Mallinson RJ, Gibbs JC, Olmsted M, Goolsby M, Matheson G. 2014 Female Athlete Triad Coalition consensus statement on treatment and return to play of the female athlete triad: 1st International Conference held in San Francisco, CA, May 2012, and 2nd International Conference held in Indianapolis, IN, May 2013. Clinical Journal of Sport Medicine 2014; 24 (2): 96–119.

7. Barrack MT, Gibbs JC, De Souza MJ, et al. Higher incidence of bone stress injuries with increasing female athlete triad-related risk factors: a prospective multisite study of exercising girls and women. Am J Sports Med 2014; 42(4): 949–958.

8. Tenforde AS, Barrack MT, Nattiv A, Fredericson M. Parallels with the Female Athlete Triad in Male Athletes. Sports Medicine 2016; 46(2): 171–182.

9. Hackney AC, Sinning WE, Bruot BC. Hypothalamic-pituitarytesticular axis function in endurance-trained males. Int J Sports Med 1990; 11(4): 298–303.

10. Kelsey JL, Bachrach LK, Procter-Gray E, et al. Risk factors for stress fracture among young female cross-country runners. Med Sci Sports Exerc 2007; 39: 1457–1463.

11. Nieves JW, Melsop K, Curtis M, et al. Nutritional factors that influence change in bone density and stress fracture risk among young female cross-country runners. PM R 2010; 2(8): 740–750; quiz 794.

12. Ruohola JP, Laaksi I, Ylikomi T, et al. Association between serum 25(OH)D concentrations and bone stress fractures in Finnish young men. J Bone Miner Res 2006; 21(9): 1483–1488.

13. Bennell KL, Malcolm SA, Thomas SA, et al. Risk factors for stress fractures in track and field athletes. A twelve-month prospective study. Am J Sports Med 1996; 24(6): 810–818.

14. Korpelainen R, Orava S, Karpakka J, et al. Risk factors for recurrent stress fractures in athletes. Am J Sports Med 2001; 29(3): 304–310.

15. Friberg O. Leg length asymmetry in stress fractures. A clinical and radiological study. J Sports Med Phys Fitness 1982; 22(4): 485–488.

16. Simkin A, Leichter I, Giladi M, et al. Combined effect of foot arch structure and an orthotic device on stress fractures. Foot Ankle 1989; 10(1): 25–29.

17. Sullivan D, Warren RF, Pavlov H, et al. Stress fractures in 51 runners. Clin Orthop Relat Res 1984; (187): 188–192.

18. Tenforde AS, Kraus E, Fredericson M. Bone Stress Injuries in Runners. Physical Medicine and Rehabilitation Clinics of North America 2016; 27(1): 139–149.

19. Nattiv A, Kennedy G, Barrack MT, et al. Correlation of MRI grading of bone stress injuries with clinical risk factors and return to play: a 5-year prospective study in collegiate track and field athletes. Am J Sports Med 2013; 41(8): 1930–1941.

20. Fredericson M, Bergman AG, Hoffman KL, et al. Tibial stress reaction in runners. Correlation of clinical symptoms and scintigraphy with a new magnetic resonance imaging grading system. Am J Sports Med 1995; 23(4): 472–481.

21. Tenforde AS, Watanabe LM, Moreno TJ, Fredericson M. Use of an antigravity treadmill for rehabilitation of a pelvic stress injury. PMR. 2012; 4: 629–31.

22. Ihle R, Loucks AB. Dose-response relationships between energy availability and bone turnover in young exercising women. Journal of Bone and Mineral Research 2004; 19(8): 1231–1240.

23. Institute of Medicine. Dietary reference intakes for calcium and vitamin D. National Academy of Sciences; November 2010, Report Brief. https: //www.nationalacademies. org/hmd/~/media/Files/Report   percent20Files/2010/Dietary-Reference-Intakes-for-Calcium-and-Vitamin-D/Vitamin percent20D percent20and percent20Calcium percent202010 percent20Report percent20Brief.pdf. Accessed August 1, 2016.

24. Buist I, Bredeweg SW, van Mechelen W, Lemmink KA, Pepping GJ, Diercks RL. No effect of a graded training program on the number of running-related injuries in novice runners: a randomized controlled trial. Am J Sports Med. 2008; 36: 33–39.

25. Nigg B M, Baltich J, Hoerzer S, Enders H. Running shoes and running injuries: mythbusting and a proposal for two new paradigms: 'preferred movement path' and 'comfort filter'. British Journal of Sports Medicine 2015; 49(20): 1290–1294.

26. Tenforde AS, Fredericson M. Influence of sports participation on bone health in the young athlete: a review of the literature. PM R 2011; 3(9): 861–867.

27. Specker BL, Wey HE, Smith EP. Rates of bone loss in young adult males. Int J Clin Rheumtol 2010; 5(2): 215–228.

28. Valdimarsson O, Alborg HG, Duppe H, et al. Reduced training is associated with increased loss of BMD. J Bone Miner Res 2005; 20(6): 906–912.

29. Kudlac J, Nichols DL, Sanborn CF, et al. Impact of detraining on bone loss in former collegiate female gymnasts. Calcif Tissue Int 2004; 75(6): 482–487.

30. Edwards WB, Taylor D, Rudolphi TJ, Gillette JC, Derrick TR. Effects of stride length and running mileage on a probabilistic stress fracture model. Med Sci Sports Exerc. 2009; 41: 2177–2184.

31. Lieberman DE, Venkadesan M, Werbel WA, et al. Foot strike patterns and collision forces in habitually barefoot versus shod runners. Nature. 2010; 463: 531–535.

32. Ridge ST, Johnson AW, Mitchell UH, et al. Foot bone marrow edema after a 10-wk transition to minimalist running shoes. Med Sci Sports Exerc. 2013; 45: 1363–1368.

33. Altman AR, Davis IS. Barefoot running: biomechanics and implications for running injuries. Curr Sports Med Rep. 2012; 11: 244–250.

## Chapter 11

1. Hew-Butler T, Rosner MH, Fowkes-Godek S, et al. Statement of the Third International Exercise-Associated Hyponatremia Consensus Development Conference, Carlsbad, California, 2015. Clin J Sport Med 2015; 25: 303–320.
2. Verbalis JG. Brain volume regulation in response to changes in osmolality. Neuroscience 2010; 168: 862–870.
3. Helwig FC, Schutz CB, Curry DE. Water Intoxication: Report of a fatal human case with clinical, pathologic and experimental studies. JAMA 1935; 104: 1569–1575.
4. Friedman B, Cirulli J. Hyponatremia in critical care patients: frequency, outcome, characteristics, and treatment with the vasopressin V2-receptor antagonist tolvaptan. J Crit Care 2013; 28: 219–12.
5. Hennrikus E, Ou G, Kinney B et al. Prevalence, Timing, Causes, and Outcomes of Hyponatremia in Hospitalized Orthopaedic Surgery Patients. J Bone Joint Surg Am 2015; 97: 1824–1832.
6. Mortelmans LJ, Van LM, De Cauwer HG, Merlevede K. Seizures and hyponatremia after excessive intake of diet coke. Eur J Emerg Med 2008; 15: 51.
7. Kamijo Y, Soma K, Asari Y, Ohwada T. Severe rhabdomyolysis following massive ingestion of oolong tea: caffeine intoxication with coexisting hyponatremia. Vet Hum Toxicol 1999; 41: 381–383.
8. Kamijo Y, Soma K, Asari Y, Ohwada T. Severe rhabdomyolysis following massive ingestion of oolong tea: caffeine intoxication with coexisting hyponatremia. Vet Hum Toxicol 1999; 41: 381–383.
9. Noakes TD, Goodwin N, Rayner BL, Branken T, Taylor RK. Water intoxication: a possible complication during endurance exercise. Med Sci Sports Exerc 1985; 17: 370–375.
10. Renneboog B, Musch W, Vandemergel X, Manto M, Decaux G. Mild Chronic Hyponatremia is Associated with Falls, Unsteadiness, and Attention Deficits. Am J Med 2006; 119 (1): 71.e1–71.e8e.
11. Speedy DB, Noakes TD, Boswell T, Thompson JM, Rehrer N, Boswell DR. Response to a fluid load in athletes with a history of exercise induced hyponatremia. Med Sci Sports Exerc 2001; 33: 1434–1442.
12. Noakes TD, Wilson G, Gray DA, Lambert MI, Dennis SC. Peak rates of diuresis in healthy humans during oral fluid overload. S Afr Med J 2001; 91: 852–857.
13. Godek SF, Bartolozzi AR, Burkholder R, Sugarman E, Peduzzi C. Sweat rates and fluid turnover in professional football players: a comparison of National Football League linemen and backs. J Athl Train 2008; 43: 184–189.
14. Hew-Butler T. Arginine vasopressin, fluid balance and exercise: is exercise-associated hyponatraemia a disorder of arginine vasopressin secretion? Sports Med 2010; 40: 459–479.
15. Owen BE, Rogers IR, Hoffman MD, et al. Efficacy of oral versus intravenous hypertonic saline in runners with hyponatremia. J Sci Med Sport 2014; 17: 457–462.
16. Brown MB, McCarty NA, Millard-Stafford M. High-sweat Na+ in cystic fibrosis and healthy individuals does not diminish thirst during exercise in the heat. Am J Physiol Regul Integr Comp Physiol 2011; 301: R1177-R1185.
17. Fitzsimons JT. Angiotensin, thirst, and sodium appetite. Physiol Rev 1998; 78: 583–686.

18. Verbalis JG. Disorders of body water homeostasis. Best Pract Res Clin Endocrinol Metab 2003; 17: 471–503.
19. Walker SH. Dangers of Hydra-Lyte. Pediatrics 1981; 68: 463–464.
20. Sawka MN, Burke LM, Eichner ER, Maughan RJ, Montain SJ, Stachenfeld NS. American College of Sports Medicine position stand. Exercise and fluid replacement. Med Sci Sports Exerc 2007; 39: 377–390.
21. Siegel AJ, d'Hemecourt P, Adner MM, Shirey T, Brown JL, Lewandrowski KB. Exertional dysnatremia in collapsed marathon runners: a critical role for point-of-care testing to guide appropriate therapy. Am J Clin Pathol 2009; 132: 336–340.
22. Rogers IR, Hook G, Stuempfle KJ, Hoffman MD, Hew-Butler T. An Intervention Study of Oral versus Intravenous Hypertonic Saline Administration in Runners with Exercise-Associated Hyponatremia. Clin.J Sport Med 2011; 21(3): 200–203.
23. Thompson CJ, Bland J, Burd J, Baylis PH. The osmotic thresholds for thirst and vasopressin release are similar in healthy man. Clin Sci (Lond) 1986; 71: 651–656.
24. Bourque CW. Central mechanisms of osmosensation and systemic osmoregulation. Nat Rev Neurosci 2008; 9: 519–531.
25. Twerenbold R, Knechtle B, Kakebeeke TH, et al. Effects of different sodium concentrations in replacement fluids during prolonged exercise in women. Br J Sports Med 2003; 37: 300–303.
26. Davis JM, Bailey SP. Possible mechanisms of central nervous system fatigue during exercise. Med Sci Sports Exerc 1997; 29: 45–57.
27. Hew-Butler TD, Sharwood K, Collins M, Speedy D, Noakes T. Sodium supplementation is not required to maintain serum sodium concentrations during an Ironman triathlon. Br J Sports Med 2006; 40: 255–259.
28. Speedy DB, Thompson JM, Rodgers I, Collins M, Sharwood K, Noakes TD. Oral salt supplementation during ultradistance exercise. Clin J Sport Med 2002; 12: 279–284.

## Chapter 12

1. Bracker M. Hyperthermia: man's adaptation to a warm climate. Sports Med Dig 1991; 13: 1–2.
2. Brewster SJ, O'Connor FG, Lillegard WA. Exercise-induced heat injury: diagnosis and management. Sports Med Arthrosc Rev 1995; 3: 260–6.
3. Haymes E, Wells C. Environment and Human Performance. Champaign, IL: Human Kinetics 1986.
4. Castellani J. Physiology of Heat Stress. In: Armstrong L, ed. Exertional Heat Illnesses. Champaign, IL: Human Kinetics 2003. 1–15.
5. Shirreffs SM. The importance of good hydration for work and exercise performance. Nutr Rev 2005; 63: S14–21.
6. Kenney W. Thermoregulation during exercise in the heat. Athl Ther Today 1996; 1: 13–6.
7. Casa DJ, DeMartini JK, Bergeron MF, et al. National Athletic Trainers' Association Position Statement: Exertional Heat Illnesses. J Athl Train 2015; 50: 986–1000. doi: 10.4085/1062-6050-50.9.07

8.  González-Alonso J, Mora-Rodríguez R, Below PR, et al. Dehydration markedly impairs cardiovascular function in hyperthermic endurance athletes during exercise. J Appl Physiol Bethesda Md 1985 1997; 82: 1229–36.

9.  Casa DJ, Stearns RL, Lopez RM, et al. Influence of hydration on physiological function and performance during trail running in the heat. J Athl Train 2010; 45: 147–56. doi: 10.4085/1062–6050–45.2.147

10. Ebert TR, Martin DT, Bullock N, et al. Influence of hydration status on thermoregulation and cycling hill climbing. Med Sci Sports Exerc 2007; 39: 323–9. doi: 10.1249/01.mss.0000247000.86847.de

11. González-Alonso J, Mora-Rodríguez R, Below PR, et al. Dehydration reduces cardiac output and increases systemic and cutaneous vascular resistance during exercise. J Appl Physiol Bethesda Md 1985 1995; 79: 1487–96.

12. González-Alonso J, Mora-Rodríguez R, Coyle EF. Stroke volume during exercise: interaction of environment and hydration. Am J Physiol Heart Circ Physiol 2000; 278: H321–30.

13. Montain SJ, Coyle EF. Influence of graded dehydration on hyperthermia and cardiovascular drift during exercise. J Appl Physiol Bethesda Md 1985 1992; 73: 1340–50.

14. Buono MJ, Wall AJ. Effect of hypohydration on core temperature during exercise in temperate and hot environments. Pflüg Arch Eur J Physiol 2000; 440: 476–80.

15. Montain SJ, Sawka MN, Latzka WA, et al. Thermal and cardiovascular strain from hypohydration: influence of exercise intensity. Int J Sports Med 1998; 19: 87–91. doi: 10.1055/s-2007–971887

16. Sawka MN, Young AJ, Francesconi RP, et al. Thermoregulatory and blood responses during exercise at graded hypohydration levels. J Appl Physiol Bethesda Md 1985 1985; 59: 1394–401.

17. Adams WM, Ferraro EM, Huggins RA, et al. Influence of body mass loss on changes in heart rate during exercise in the heat: a systematic review. J Strength Cond Res 2014; 28: 2380–9. doi: 10.1519/JSC.0000000000000501

18. Huggins R, Martschinske J, Applegate K, et al. Influence of Dehydration on Internal Body Temperature Changes During Exercise in the Heat: A Meta-Analysis. Med Sci Sports Exerc 2012; 44: 791.

19. Cheuvront SN, Kenefick RW, Montain SJ, et al. Mechanisms of aerobic performance impairment with heat stress and dehydration. J Appl Physiol Bethesda Md 1985 2010; 109: 1989–95. doi: 10.1152/japplphysiol.00367.2010

20. Cheuvront SN, Kenefick RW. Dehydration: physiology, assessment, and performance effects. Compr Physiol 2014; 4: 257–85. doi: 10.1002/cphy.c130017

21. Sawka MN, Burke LM, Eichner ER, et al. American College of Sports Medicine position stand. Exercise and fluid replacement. Med Sci Sports Exerc 2007; 39: 377–90. doi: 10.1249/mss.0b013e31802ca597

22. Armstrong LE, Maresh CM. The Induction and Decay of Heat Acclimatisation in Trained Athletes. Sports Med 1991; 12: 302–12. doi: 10.2165/00007256–199112050–00003

23. Périard JD, Racinais S, Sawka MN. Adaptations and mechanisms of human heat acclimation: Applications for competitive athletes and sports. Scand J Med Sci Sports 2015; 25 Suppl 1: 20–38. doi: 10.1111/sms.12408

24. Shapiro Y, Moran D, Epstein Y. Acclimatization strategies—preparing for exercise in the heat. Int J Sports Med 1998; 19 Suppl 2: S161–3. doi: 10.1055/s-2007–971986

25. Pandolf KB. Time course of heat acclimation and its decay. Int J Sports Med 1998; 19 Suppl 2: S157–60. doi: 10.1055/s-2007–971985

26. Chalmers S, Esterman A, Eston R, et al. Short-term heat acclimation training improves physical performance: a systematic review, and exploration of physiological adaptations and application for team sports. Sports Med Auckl NZ 2014; 44: 971–88. doi: 10.1007/s40279–014–0178–6

27. Garrett AT, Rehrer NJ, Patterson MJ. Induction and decay of short-term heat acclimation in moderately and highly trained athletes. Sports Med Auckl NZ 2011; 41: 757–71. doi: 10.2165/11587320–000000000–00000

28. Garrett AT, Goosens NG, Rehrer NJ, et al. Induction and decay of short-term heat acclimation. Eur J Appl Physiol 2009; 107: 659–70. doi: 10.1007/s00421–009–1182–7

29. Taylor NAS. Principles and Practices of Heat Adaptation. J Hum-Environ Syst 2000; 4: 11–22. doi: 10.1618/jhes.4.11

30. Myllymäki T, Kyröläinen H, Savolainen K, et al. Effects of vigorous late-night exercise on sleep quality and cardiac autonomic activity. J Sleep Res 2011; 20: 146–53. doi: 10.1111/j.1365–2869.2010.00874.x

31. Samuels C. Sleep, recovery, and performance: the new frontier in high-performance athletics. Neurol Clin 2008; 26: 169–80; ix – x. doi: 10.1016/j.ncl.2007.11.012

32. Adam K. Sleep as a Restorative Process and a Theory to Explain Why. In: P.S. McConnell GJB, H. J. Romijn, N. E. Van De Poll and M. A. Corner, ed. Progress in Brain Research. Elsevier 1980. 289–305. http: //www.sciencedirect.com/science/article/pii/S0079612308600709 (accessed 28 May 2016).

33. Knutson KL, Spiegel K, Penev P, et al. The metabolic consequences of sleep deprivation. Sleep Med Rev 2007; 11: 163–78. doi: 10.1016/j.smrv.2007.01.002

34. Arnal PJ, Drogou C, Sauvet F, et al. Effect of Sleep Extension on the Subsequent Testosterone, Cortisol and Prolactin Responses to Total Sleep Deprivation and Recovery. J Neuroendocrinol 2016; 28. doi: 10.1111/jne.12346

35. Porkka-Heiskanen T. Sleep homeostasis. Curr Opin Neurobiol 2013; 23: 799–805. doi: 10.1016/j.conb.2013.02.010

36. Taylor SR, Rogers GG, Driver HS. Effects of training volume on sleep, psychological, and selected physiological profiles of elite female swimmers. Med Sci Sports Exerc 1997; 29: 688–93.

37. Driver HS, Rogers GG, Mitchell D, et al. Prolonged endurance exercise and sleep disruption. Med Sci Sports Exerc 1994; 26: 903–7.

38. Martin BJ. Sleep loss and subsequent exercise performance. Acta Physiol Scand Suppl 1988; 574: 28–32.

39. VanHelder T, Radomski MW. Sleep deprivation and the effect on exercise performance. Sports Med Auckl NZ 1989; 7: 235–47.

40. Kubitz KA, Landers DM, Petruzzello SJ, et al. The effects of acute and chronic exercise on sleep. A meta-analytic review. Sports Med Auckl NZ 1996; 21: 277–91.

41. Youngstedt SD, O'Connor PJ, Dishman RK. The effects of acute exercise on sleep: a quantitative synthesis. Sleep 1997; 20: 203–14.

42. Flausino NH, Da Silva Prado JM, de Queiroz SS, et al. Physical exercise performed before bedtime improves the sleep pattern of healthy young good sleepers. Psychophysiology 2012; 49: 186–92. doi: 10.1111/j.1469–8986.2011.01300.x

43. O'Connor PJ, Breus MJ, Youngstedt SD. Exercise-induced increase in core temperature does not disrupt a behavioral measure of sleep. Physiol Behav 1998; 64: 213–7.

44. Vuori I, Urponen H, Hasan J, et al. Epidemiology of exercise effects on sleep. Acta Physiol Scand Suppl 1988; 574: 3–7.

45. Alvarez GG, Ayas NT. The impact of daily sleep duration on health: a review of the literature. Prog Cardiovasc Nurs 2004; 19: 56–9.

46. Irwin M. Effects of sleep and sleep loss on immunity and cytokines. Brain Behav Immun 2002; 16: 503–12. doi: 10.1016/S0889–1591(02)00003-X

47. Pilcher JJ, Huffcutt AI. Effects of sleep deprivation on performance: a meta-analysis. Sleep 1996; 19: 318–26.

48. Walker MP. Cognitive consequences of sleep and sleep loss. Sleep Med 2008; 9, Supplement 1: S29–34. doi: 10.1016/S1389–9457(08)70014–5

49. Whitney P, Hinson JM, Jackson ML, et al. Feedback Blunting: Total Sleep Deprivation Impairs Decision Making that Requires Updating Based on Feedback. Sleep 2015; 38: 745–54. doi: 10.5665/sleep.4668

50. Lim J, Dinges DF. Sleep deprivation and vigilant attention. Ann N Y Acad Sci 2008; 1129: 305–22. doi: 10.1196/annals.1417.002

51. Tokizawa K, Sawada S-I, Tai T, et al. Effects of partial sleep restriction and subsequent daytime napping on prolonged exertional heat strain. Occup Environ Med 2015; 72: 521–8. doi: 10.1136/oemed-2014–102548

52. Sawka MN, Gonzalez RR, Pandolf KB. Effects of sleep deprivation on thermoregulation during exercise. Am J Physiol 1984; 246: R72–7.

53. Dewasmes G, Bothorel B, Hoeft A, et al. Regulation of local sweating in sleep-deprived exercising humans. Eur J Appl Physiol 1993; 66: 542–6.

54. Oliver SJ, Costa RJS, Laing SJ, et al. One night of sleep deprivation decreases treadmill endurance performance. Eur J Appl Physiol 2009; 107: 155–61. doi: 10.1007/s00421–009–1103–9

55. Driver HS, Taylor SR. Exercise and sleep. Sleep Med Rev 2000; 4: 387–402. doi: 10.1053/smrv.2000.0110

56. Killer SC, Svendsen IS, Jeukendrup AE, et al. Evidence of disturbed sleep and mood state in well-trained athletes during short-term intensified training with and without a high carbohydrate nutritional intervention. J Sports Sci 2015: 1–9. doi: 10.1080/02640414.2015.1085589

57. Adams W. Rehydration on Subsequent Performance and Recovery Following Exercise-Induced Dehydration: Ad Libitum Versus Prescribed Fluid Replacement. Dr Diss Published Online First: 21 June 2016. http://digitalcommons.uconn.edu/dissertations/1184

58. National Center for Health Statistics. International Classification of Diseases, Ninth Revision, Clinical Modification (ICD-9-CM). Hyattsville, MD.

59. Bergeron MF. Muscle Cramps during Exercise-Is It Fatigue or Electrolyte Deficit?: Curr Sports Med Rep 2008; 7: S50–5. doi: 10.1249/JSR.0b013e31817f476a

60. Eichner ER. The role of sodium in "heat cramping." Sports Med Auckl NZ 2007; 37: 368–70.

61. Schwellnus MP, Derman EW, Noakes TD. Aetiology of skeletal muscle "cramps" during exercise: a novel hypothesis. J Sports Sci 1997; 15: 277–85. doi: 10.1080/026404197367281

62. Jung AP, Bishop PA, Al-Nawwas A, et al. Influence of Hydration and Electrolyte Supplementation on Incidence and Time to Onset of Exercise-Associated Muscle Cramps. J Athl Train 2005; 40: 71–5.

63. Schwellnus MP, Drew N, Collins M. Increased running speed and previous cramps rather than dehydration or serum sodium changes predict exercise-associated muscle cramping: a prospective cohort study in 210 Ironman triathletes. Br J Sports Med 2011; 45: 650–6. doi: 10.1136/bjsm.2010.078535

64. Casa D, Roberts W. Considerations for the medical staff in preventing, identifying and treating exertional heat illnesses. In: Armstrong L, ed. Exertional Heat Illnesses. Champaign, IL: Human Kinetics 2003.

65. Poh PYS, Armstrong LE, Casa DJ, et al. Orthostatic hypotension after 10 days of exercise-heat acclimation and 28 hours of sleep loss. Aviat Space Environ Med 2012; 83: 403–11.

66. Armstrong LE, Casa DJ, Millard-Stafford M, et al. American College of Sports Medicine position stand. Exertional heat illness during training and competition. Med Sci Sports Exerc 2007; 39: 556–72. doi: 10.1249/MSS.0b013e31802fa199

67. Armstrong L, Anderson J. Heat Exhaustion, Exercise-Associated Collapse, and Heat Syncope. In: Armstrong L, ed. Exertional Heat Illnesses. Champaign, IL: Human Kinetics 2003.

68. Knochel JP. Environmental heat illness. An eclectic review. Arch Intern Med 1974; 133: 841–64.

69. McCance R. Medical problems in mineral metabolism III: Experimental human salt deficiency. Lancet 1936; 1: 823–34.

70. Marriott H. Water and salt-depletion. Springfield, IL: Charles C Thomas Publisher 1950.

71. Backer HD, Shopes E, Collins SL, et al. Exertional heat illness and hyponatremia in hikers. Am J Emerg Med 1999; 17: 532–9.

72. Lipman G, Ellis M, Gaudio F, et al. Wilderness Medical Society practice guidelines for the prevention and treatment of heat-related illness: 2014 updated. Wilderness Environ Med 2014; 25: S55–65.

73. Bouchama A, Knochel JP. Heat stroke. N Engl J Med 2002; 346: 1978–88. doi: 10.1056/NEJMra011089

74. Epstein Y, Roberts WO. The pathopysiology of heat stroke: an integrative view of the final common pathway. Scand J Med Sci Sports 2011; 21: 742–8. doi: 10.1111/j.1600–0838.2011.01333.x

75. Epstein Y, Hadad E, Shapiro Y. Pathological factors underlying hyperthermia. J Therm Biol 2004; 29: 487–94. doi: 10.1016/j.jtherbio.2004.08.018

76. Rav-Acha M, Hadad E, Epstein Y, et al. Fatal exertional heat stroke: a case series. Am J Med Sci 2004; 328: 84–7.

77. Adams WM, Hosokawa Y, Casa DJ. The Timing of Exertional Heat Stroke Survival Starts prior to Collapse. Curr Sports Med Rep 2015; 14: 273–4. doi: 10.1249/JSR.0000000000000166

78. McDermott BP, Casa DJ, Ganio MS, et al. Acute Whole-Body Cooling for Exercise-Induced Hyperthermia: A Systematic Review. J Athl Train 2009; 44: 84–93.

79. Luhring K, Butts C, Smith C, et al. Cooling Effectiveness of Modified Cold-Water Immersion Method Following Exercise-Induced Hyperthermia. J Athl Train; 50: S – 1.

80. Hosokawa Y, Adams W, Belval L, et al. Tarp-assisted cooling as a method of whole body cooling in hyperthermic individuals. Ann Emerg Med.

81. Casa DJ, Armstrong LE, Kenny GP, et al. Exertional heat stroke: new concepts regarding cause and care. Curr Sports Med Rep 2012; 11: 115–23. doi: 10.1249/JSR.0b013e31825615cc

## Chapter 13

1. Castellani JW, Young AJ, Ducharme MB et al. American College of Sports Medicine. American College of Sports Medicine Position Stand: Prevention of Cold Injuries during Exercise. Med Sci Sports Exerc. 2006; 38(11): 2012–2029.

2. Fudge J. Exercise in the Cold: Preventing and Managing Hypothermia and Frostbite Injury. Sports Health. 2016; 8(2): 133–139.

3. Fudge JR, Bennet BL, Simanis JP, et al. Medical Evaluation for Exposure Extremes: Cold. Clin J Sport Med. 2015; 25(5): 432–436.

4. McMahon JA, Howe A. Cold Weather issues in Sideline and Event Management. Curr Sports Med Rep. 2012; 11(3): 135–141.

5. NOAA. National Weather Service. Office of Climate, Water and Weather Services. 2013. Available at: http: //www.nws.noaa.gov/om/winter/windchill.shtml. Accessed August 30, 2016.

6. Keatinge WR. Freezing-point of human skin. Lancet. 1960; 1(7114): 11–14.

7. Molnar GW, Hughes AL, Wilson O, et al. Effect of skin wetting on finger cooling and freezing. J Appl Physiol. 1973; 35(2): 205–207.

8. Kenefick RW, Hazzard MP, Mahood NV, et al. Thirst Sensations and AVP Response at Rest and during Exercise-Cold Exposure. Med Sci Sports Exerc. 2004; 36(9): 1528–1534.

9. Lehmuskallio E. Cold Protecting Ointments and Frostbite: A Questionnaire Study of 830 Conscripts in Finland. Acta Derm Venereol. 1999; 79: 67–70.

10. Lehmuskallio E, Rintamaki H, Anttonen H. Thermal Effects of Emollients on Facial Skin in the Cold. Acta Derm Venereol. 2000; 80: 203–207.

11. Brown DJ, Brugger H, Boyd J, et al. Accidental Hypothermia. N Engl J Med. 2012. 367: 1930–1938.

12. American Heart Association. 2005 American Heart Association (AHA) guidelines for cardiopulmonary resuscitation and emergency cardiovascular care Part 10.4: Hypothermia. Circulation. 2005; 112: IV-136-IV-138.

13. McIntosh SE, Opacic M, Freer L, et al. Wilderness Medical Society Practice Guidelines for the Prevention and Treatment of Frostbite: 2014 Update. Wilderness Environ Med. 2014; 25: S43-S54.

## Chapter 14

1. Luks AM, Schoene RB, Swenson ER. High Altitude. In: Murray and Nadel's Textbook of Respiratory Medicine. 6th Ed. Philadelphia, PA: Elsevier; 2016.

2. Luks AM. Physiology in Medicine: A physiologic approach to prevention and treatment of acute high-altitude illnesses. J Appl Physiol. 2015; 118(5): 509–519.

3. Luks AM, McIntosh SE, Grissom CK, et al. Wilderness Medical Society practice guidelines for the prevention and treatment of acute altitude illness: 2014 update. Wilderness and Environ Med. 2014; 25(4 Suppl): S4–S14.
4. Bärtsch P, Swenson ER. Clinical practice: Acute high-altitude illnesses. N Engl J Med. 2013; 368(24): 2294–2302.
5. Luks AM. Clinician's corner: What do we know about safe ascent rates at high altitude? High Alt Med Biol. 2012; 13(3): 147–152.
6. Beidleman BA, Fulco CS, Muza SR, et al. Effect of six days of staging on physiologic adjustments and acute mountain sickness during ascent to 4300 meters. High Alt Med Biol. 2009; 10(3): 253–260.
7. Beidleman BA, Muza SR, Fulco CS, et al. Intermittent altitude exposures reduce acute mountain sickness at 4300 m. Clin Sci. 2004; 106(3): 321–328.
8. Schommer K, Wiesegart N, Menold E, et al. Training in normobaric hypoxia and its effects on acute mountain sickness after rapid ascent to 4559 m. High Alt Med Biol. 2010; 11(1): 19–25.
9. Fulco CS, Muza SR, Beidleman BA, et al. Effect of repeated normobaric hypoxia exposures during sleep on acute mountain sickness, exercise performance, and sleep during exposure to terrestrial altitude. Am J Physiol Regul Integr Comp Physiol. 2011; 300(2): R428–R436.
10. Dehnert C, Böhm A, Grigoriev I, Menold E, Bärtsch P. Sleeping in moderate hypoxia at home for prevention of acute mountain sickness (AMS): a placebo-controlled, randomized double-blind study. Wilderness and Environ Med. 2014; 25(3): 263–271.
11. Gonzales JU, Scheuermann BW. Effect of acetazolamide on respiratory muscle fatigue in humans. Respir Physiol Neurobiol. 2013; 185(2): 386–392.
12. Bradwell AR, Myers SD, Beazley M, et al. Exercise limitation of acetazolamide at altitude (3459 m). Wilderness and Environ Med. 2014; 25(3): 272–277.
13. Lipman GS, Kanaan NC, Holck PS, Constance BB, Gertsch JH, PAINS Group. Ibuprofen prevents altitude illness: a randomized controlled trial for prevention of altitude illness with nonsteroidal anti-inflammatories. Ann Emerg Med. 2012; 59(6): 484–490.
14. Calbet JAL, Lundby C. Air to muscle O2 delivery during exercise at altitude. High Alt Med Biol. 2009; 10(2): 123–134.
15. Calbet JAL, Boushel R, Rådegran G, Søndergaard H, Wagner PD, Saltin B. Why is VO2 max after altitude acclimatization still reduced despite normalization of arterial O2 content? Am J Physiol Regul Integr Comp Physiol. 2003; 284(2): R304–R316.
16. Chapman RF, Laymon AS, Levine BD. Timing of arrival and pre-acclimatization strategies for the endurance athlete competing at moderate to high altitudes. High Alt Med Biol. 2013; 14(4): 319–324.
17. Gore CJ, McSharry PE, Hewitt AJ, Saunders PU. Preparation for football competition at moderate to high altitude. Scand J Med Sci Sports. 2008; 18 Suppl 1: 85–95.
18. Levine BD, Stray-Gundersen J. "Living high-training low": effect of moderate-altitude acclimatization with low-altitude training on performance. J Appl Physiol. 1997; 83(1): 102–112.

19. Siebenmann C, Robach P, Jacobs RA, et al. "Live high-train low" using normobaric hypoxia: a double-blinded, placebo-controlled study. J Appl Physiol. 2012; 112(1): 106–117.

20. Sinex JA, Chapman RF. Hypoxic training methods for improving endurance exercise performance. J Sport Health Sci. 2015.

21. Chapman RF, Karlsen T, Resaland GK, et al. Defining the "dose" of altitude training: how high to live for optimal sea level performance enhancement. J Appl Physiol. 2014; 116(6): 595–603.

22. Chapman RF, Laymon Stickford AS, Lundby C, Levine BD. Timing of return from altitude training for optimal sea level performance. J Appl Physiol. 2014; 116(7): 837–843.

23. Bonetti DL, Hopkins WG. Sea-level exercise performance following adaptation to hypoxia: a meta-analysis. Sports Med. 2009; 39(2): 107–127.

24. Porcari JP, Probst L, Forrester K, et al. Effect of Wearing the Elevation Training Mask on Aerobic Capacity, Lung Function, and Hematological Variables. J Sports Sci Med. 2016; 15(2): 379–386.

25. Granados J, Gillum TL, Castillo W, Christmas KM, Kuennen MR. "Functional" Respiratory Muscle Training During Endurance Exercise Causes Modest Hypoxemia but Overall is Well Tolerated. J Strength Cond Res. 2016; 30(3): 755–762.

26. Levine BD. Should "artificial" high altitude environments be considered doping? Scand J Med Sci Sports. 2006; 16(5): 297–301.

27. Athlete Guide to the 2016 Prohibited List. US Anti Doping Agency Website. http:// www.usada.org/substances/prohibited-list/athlete-guide/. Accessed September 9, 2016

28. Sanchis-Gomar F, Pareja-Galeano H, Brioche T, Martinez-Bello V, Lippi G. Altitude exposure in sports: the Athlete Biological Passport standpoint. Drug Test Anal. 2014; 6(3): 190–193.

## Chapter 15

1. 2015 Running USA Annual Marathon Report. 2015; http: //www.runningusa.org/ marathon-report-2016?returnTo=main. Accessed November 27, 2016.

2. Jose AD, Collison D. The normal range and determinants of the intrinsic heart rate in man. Cardiovasc Res. 1970; 4(2): 160–167.

3. Uusitalo AL, Uusitalo AJ, Rusko HK. Exhaustive endurance training for 6–9 weeks did not induce changes in intrinsic heart rate and cardiac autonomic modulation in female athletes. Int J Sports Med. 1998; 19(8): 532–540.

4. Wasfy MM, Weiner RB, Wang F, et al. Endurance Exercise-Induced Cardiac Remodeling: Not All Sports Are Created Equal. J Am Soc Echocardiogr. 2015; 28(12): 1434–1440.

5. Levine BD. VO$_2$ max: what do we know, and what do we still need to know? J Physiol. 2008; 586(1): 25–34.

6. Fletcher GF, Balady GJ, Amsterdam EA, et al. Exercise standards for testing and training: a statement for healthcare professionals from the American Heart Association. Circulation. 2001; 104(14): 1694–1740.

7. Gulati M, Black HR, Shaw LJ, et al. The prognostic value of a nomogram for exercise capacity in women. N Engl J Med. 2005; 353(5): 468–475.

8. Forman DE, Myers J, Lavie CJ, Guazzi M, Celli B, Arena R. Cardiopulmonary exercise testing: relevant but underused. Postgrad Med. 2010; 122(6): 68–86.

9. Thompson PD, Funk EJ, Carleton RA, Sturner WQ. Incidence of death during jogging in Rhode Island from 1975 through 1980. JAMA. 1982; 247(18): 2535–2538.

10. Siscovick DS, Weiss NS, Fletcher RH, Lasky T. The incidence of primary cardiac arrest during vigorous exercise. N Engl J Med. 1984; 311(14): 874–877.

11. Mittleman MA, Maclure M, Tofler GH, Sherwood JB, Goldberg RJ, Muller JE. Triggering of acute myocardial infarction by heavy physical exertion. Protection against triggering by regular exertion. Determinants of Myocardial Infarction Onset Study Investigators. N Engl J Med. 1993; 329(23): 1677–1683.

12. Albert CM, Mittleman MA, Chae CU, Lee IM, Hennekens CH, Manson JE. Triggering of sudden death from cardiac causes by vigorous exertion. N Engl J Med. 2000; 343(19): 1355–1361.

13. Kim JH, Malhotra R, Chiampas G, et al. Cardiac arrest during long-distance running races. N Engl J Med. 2012; 366(2): 130–140.

14. Webner D, DuPrey KM, Drezner JA, Cronholm P, Roberts WO. Sudden cardiac arrest and death in United States marathons. Med Sci Sports Exerc. 2012; 44(10): 1843–1845.

15. Harmon KG, Asif IM, Klossner D, Drezner JA. Incidence of sudden cardiac death in National Collegiate Athletic Association athletes. Circulation. 2011; 123(15): 1594–1600.

16. Harris KM, Henry JT, Rohman E, Haas TS, Maron BJ. Sudden death during the triathlon. JAMA. 2010; 303(13): 1255–1257.

17. Maron BJ, Friedman RA, Kligfield P, et al. Assessment of the 12-lead electrocardiogram as a screening test for detection of cardiovascular disease in healthy general populations of young people (12–25 years of age): a scientific statement from the American Heart Association and the American College of Cardiology. J Am Coll Cardiol. 2014; 64(14): 1479–1514.

18. Maron BJ, Haas TS, Murphy CJ, Ahluwalia A, Rutten-Ramos S. Incidence and causes of sudden death in U.S. college athletes. J Am Coll Cardiol. 2014; 63(16): 1636–1643.

19. Maron BJ. Counterpoint/Mandatory ECG screening of young competitive athletes. Heart Rhythm. 2012; 9(11): 1897.

20. Maron BJ, Haas TS, Ahluwalia A, Rutten-Ramos SC. Incidence of cardiovascular sudden deaths in Minnesota high school athletes. Heart Rhythm. 2013; 10(3): 374–377.

21. Corrado D, Basso C, Pavei A, Michieli P, Schiavon M, Thiene G. Trends in sudden cardiovascular death in young competitive athletes after implementation of a preparticipation screening program. JAMA. 2006; 296(13): 1593–1601.

22. Corrado D, Pelliccia A, Bjornstad HH, et al. Cardiovascular pre-participation screening of young competitive athletes for prevention of sudden death: proposal for a common European protocol. Consensus Statement of the Study Group of Sport Cardiology of the Working Group of Cardiac Rehabilitation and Exercise Physiology and the Working Group of Myocardial and Pericardial Diseases of the European Society of Cardiology. Eur Heart J. 2005; 26(5): 516–524.

23. Steinvil A, Chundadze T, Zeltser D, et al. Mandatory electrocardiographic screening of athletes to reduce their risk for sudden death proven fact or wishful thinking? J Am Coll Cardiol. 2011; 57(11): 1291–1296.

24. Maron BJ, Levine BD, Washington RL, Baggish AL, Kovacs RJ, Maron MS. Eligibility and Disqualification Recommendations for Competitive Athletes With Cardiovascular Abnormalities: Task Force 2: Preparticipation Screening for Cardiovascular Disease in Competitive Athletes: A Scientific Statement From the American Heart Association and American College of Cardiology. J Am Coll Cardiol. 2015; 66(21): 2356–2361.

25. Maron BJ, Haas TS, Doerer JJ, Thompson PD, Hodges JS. Comparison of U.S. and Italian experiences with sudden cardiac deaths in young competitive athletes and implications for preparticipation screening strategies. Am J Cardiol. 2009; 104(2): 276–280.

26. Sattelmair J, Pertman J, Ding EL, Kohl HW, 3rd, Haskell W, Lee IM. Dose response between physical activity and risk of coronary heart disease: a meta-analysis. Circulation. 2011; 124(7): 789–795.

27. Sofi F, Capalbo A, Cesari F, Abbate R, Gensini GF. Physical activity during leisure time and primary prevention of coronary heart disease: an updated meta-analysis of cohort studies. Eur J Cardiovasc Prev Rehabil. 2008; 15(3): 247–257.

28. Wen CP, Wai JP, Tsai MK, et al. Minimum amount of physical activity for reduced mortality and extended life expectancy: a prospective cohort study. Lancet. 2011; 378(9798): 1244–1253.

29. Paffenbarger RS, Jr., Hyde RT, Wing AL, Lee IM, Jung DL, Kampert JB. The association of changes in physical-activity level and other lifestyle characteristics with mortality among men. N Engl J Med. 1993; 328(8): 538–545.

30. Wasfy MM, Baggish AL. Exercise Dose in Clinical Practice. Circulation. 2016; 133(23): 2297–2313.

31. Kodama S, Tanaka S, Saito K, et al. Effect of aerobic exercise training on serum levels of high-density lipoprotein cholesterol: a meta-analysis. Arch Intern Med. 2007; 167(10): 999–1008.

32. Zilinski JL, Contursi ME, Isaacs SK, et al. Myocardial adaptations to recreational marathon training among middle-aged men. Circ Cardiovasc Imaging. 2015; 8(2): e002487.

33. Kelley GA, Kelley KS, Vu Tran Z. Aerobic exercise, lipids and lipoproteins in overweight and obese adults: a meta-analysis of randomized controlled trials. Int J Obes (Lond). 2005; 29(8): 881–893.

34. Law MR, Wald NJ, Thompson SG. By how much and how quickly does reduction in serum cholesterol concentration lower risk of ischaemic heart disease? BMJ. 1994; 308(6925): 367–372.

35. Eckel RH, Jakicic JM, Ard JD, et al. 2013 AHA/ACC guideline on lifestyle management to reduce cardiovascular risk: a report of the American College of Cardiology/American Heart Association Task Force on Practice Guidelines. Circulation. 2014; 129(25 Suppl 2): S76–99.

36. Fagard RH. Exercise characteristics and the blood pressure response to dynamic physical training. Med Sci Sports Exerc. 2001; 33(6 Suppl): S484–492; discussion S493–484.

37. Cornelissen VA, Fagard RH. Effects of endurance training on blood pressure, blood pressure-regulating mechanisms, and cardiovascular risk factors. Hypertension. 2005; 46(4): 667–675.

38. Whelton SP, Chin A, Xin X, He J. Effect of aerobic exercise on blood pressure: a meta-analysis of randomized, controlled trials. Ann Intern Med. 2002; 136(7): 493–503.

39. Halbert JA, Silagy CA, Finucane P, Withers RT, Hamdorf PA, Andrews GR. The effectiveness of exercise training in lowering blood pressure: a meta-analysis of randomised controlled trials of 4 weeks or longer. J Hum Hypertens. 1997; 11(10): 641–649.

40. Kelley G, Tran ZV. Aerobic exercise and normotensive adults: a meta-analysis. Med Sci Sports Exerc. 1995; 27(10): 1371–1377.

41. Kelley GA, Kelley KA, Tran ZV. Aerobic exercise and resting blood pressure: a meta-analytic review of randomized, controlled trials. Prev Cardiol. 2001; 4(2): 73–80.

42. Irwin ML, Yasui Y, Ulrich CM, et al. Effect of exercise on total and intra-abdominal body fat in postmenopausal women: a randomized controlled trial. JAMA. 2003; 289(3): 323–330.

43. Slentz CA, Aiken LB, Houmard JA, et al. Inactivity, exercise, and visceral fat. STRRIDE: a randomized, controlled study of exercise intensity and amount. J Appl Physiol (1985). 2005; 99(4): 1613–1618.

44. McTiernan A, Sorensen B, Irwin ML, et al. Exercise effect on weight and body fat in men and women. Obesity (Silver Spring). 2007; 15(6): 1496–1512.

45. Donnelly JE, Hill JO, Jacobsen DJ, et al. Effects of a 16-month randomized controlled exercise trial on body weight and composition in young, overweight men and women: the Midwest Exercise Trial. Arch Intern Med. 2003; 163(11): 1343–1350.

46. Goodyear LJ, Kahn BB. Exercise, glucose transport, and insulin sensitivity. Annu Rev Med. 1998; 49: 235–261.

47. Henriksen EJ. Invited review: Effects of acute exercise and exercise training on insulin resistance. J Appl Physiol (1985). 2002; 93(2): 788–796.

48. Johnson JL, Slentz CA, Houmard JA, et al. Exercise training amount and intensity effects on metabolic syndrome (from Studies of a Targeted Risk Reduction Intervention through Defined Exercise). Am J Cardiol. 2007; 100(12): 1759–1766.

49. Dube JJ, Allison KF, Rousson V, Goodpaster BH, Amati F. Exercise dose and insulin sensitivity: relevance for diabetes prevention. Med Sci Sports Exerc. 2012; 44(5): 793–799.

50. Tuomilehto J, Lindstrom J, Eriksson JG, et al. Prevention of type 2 diabetes mellitus by changes in lifestyle among subjects with impaired glucose tolerance. N Engl J Med. 2001; 344(18): 1343–1350.

51. Knowler WC, Barrett-Connor E, Fowler SE, et al. Reduction in the incidence of type 2 diabetes with lifestyle intervention or metformin. N Engl J Med. 2002; 346(6): 393–403.

52. Blair SN, Kohl HW, 3rd, Paffenbarger RS, Jr., Clark DG, Cooper KH, Gibbons LW. Physical fitness and all-cause mortality. A prospective study of healthy men and women. JAMA. 1989; 262(17): 2395–2401.

53. Blair SN, Kampert JB, Kohl HW, 3rd, et al. Influences of cardiorespiratory fitness and other precursors on cardiovascular disease and all-cause mortality in men and women. JAMA. 1996; 276(3): 205–210.

54. Kokkinos P, Myers J, Faselis C, et al. Exercise capacity and mortality in older men: a 20-year follow-up study. Circulation. 2010; 122(8): 790–797.

55. Spina RJ. Cardiovascular adaptations to endurance exercise training in older men and women. Exerc Sport Sci Rev. 1999; 27: 317–332.
56. Seals DR, Hurley BF, Schultz J, Hagberg JM. Endurance training in older men and women II. Blood lactate response to submaximal exercise. J Appl Physiol Respir Environ Exerc Physiol. 1984; 57(4): 1030–1033.
57. Bouchard C, Rankinen T. Individual differences in response to regular physical activity. Med Sci Sports Exerc. 2001; 33(6 Suppl): S446–451; discussion S452–443.
58. Colivicchi F, Ammirati F, Santini M. Epidemiology and prognostic implications of syncope in young competing athletes. Eur Heart J. 2004; 25(19): 1749–1753.
59. Biffi A, Pelliccia A, Verdile L, et al. Long-term clinical significance of frequent and complex ventricular tachyarrhythmias in trained athletes. J Am Coll Cardiol. 2002; 40(3): 446–452.
60. Biffi A, Maron BJ, Verdile L, et al. Impact of physical deconditioning on ventricular tachyarrhythmias in trained athletes. J Am Coll Cardiol. 2004; 44(5): 1053–1058.
61. Sorokin AV, Araujo CG, Zweibel S, Thompson PD. Atrial fibrillation in endurance-trained athletes. Br J Sports Med. 2011; 45(3): 185–188.
62. Mont L, Sambola A, Brugada J, et al. Long-lasting sport practice and lone atrial fibrillation. Eur Heart J. 2002; 23(6): 477–482.
63. Molina L, Mont L, Marrugat J, et al. Long-term endurance sport practice increases the incidence of lone atrial fibrillation in men: a follow-up study. Europace. 2008; 10(5): 618–623.
64. Stein R, Medeiros CM, Rosito GA, Zimerman LI, Ribeiro JP. Intrinsic sinus and atrioventricular node electrophysiologic adaptations in endurance athletes. J Am Coll Cardiol. 2002; 39(6): 1033–1038.
65. Mont L, Tamborero D, Elosua R, et al. Physical activity, height, and left atrial size are independent risk factors for lone atrial fibrillation in middle-aged healthy individuals. Europace. 2008; 10(1): 15–20.
66. Coumel P. Paroxysmal atrial fibrillation: a disorder of autonomic tone? Eur Heart J. 1994; 15 Suppl A: 9–16.
67. Yesil M, Bayata S, Postaci N, Yucel O, Aslan O. Cardioversion with sotalol in selected patients with vagally and adrenergically mediated paroxysmal atrial fibrillation. Angiology. 1999; 50(9): 729–733.
68. Hoogsteen J, Schep G, Van Hemel NM, Van Der Wall EE. Paroxysmal atrial fibrillation in male endurance athletes. A 9-year follow up. Europace. 2004; 6(3): 222–228.
69. Andersen K, Farahmand B, Ahlbom A, et al. Risk of arrhythmias in 52 755 long-distance cross-country skiers: a cohort study. Eur Heart J. 2013; 34(47): 3624–3631.
70. Mohlenkamp S, Lehmann N, Breuckmann F, et al. Running: the risk of coronary events: Prevalence and prognostic relevance of coronary atherosclerosis in marathon runners. Eur Heart J. 2008; 29(15): 1903–1910.
71. Kim JH, Baggish AL. Physical Activity, Endurance Exercise, and Excess-Can One Overdose? Curr Treat Options Cardiovasc Med. 2016; 18(11): 68.
72. Schnohr P, O'Keefe JH, Marott JL, Lange P, Jensen GB. Dose of jogging and long-term mortality: the Copenhagen City Heart Study. J Am Coll Cardiol. 2015; 65(5): 411–419.
73. Arem H, Moore SC, Patel A, et al. Leisure time physical activity and mortality: a detailed pooled analysis of the dose-response relationship. JAMA Intern Med. 2015; 175(6): 959–967.

74. Marijon E, Tafflet M, Antero-Jacquemin J, et al. Mortality of French participants in the Tour de France (1947–2012). Eur Heart J. 2013; 34(40): 3145–3150.
75. Sarna S, Sahi T, Koskenvuo M, Kaprio J. Increased life expectancy of world class male athletes. Med Sci Sports Exerc. 1993; 25(2): 237–244.
76. Chakravarty EF, Hubert HB, Lingala VB, Fries JF. Reduced disability and mortality among aging runners: a 21-year longitudinal study. Arch Intern Med. 2008; 168(15): 1638–1646.

## Chapter 16

1.  Gisolfi CV. Is the GI System Built For Exercise? News Physiol Sci 2000; 15: 114–119.
2.  Sanchez LD, Corwell B, Berkoff D. Medical problems of marathon runners. Am J Emerg Med 2006; 24(5): 608–615.
3.  Stellingwerff T, Jeukendrup AE. Don't forget the gut- it is an important athletic organ! J Appl Physiol 2011; 110(1): 278.
4.  Hoffman MD, Fogard K. Factors related to successful completion of a 161-km ultra-marathon. Int J Sports Physiol Perform 2011; 6(1): 25–37.
5.  Jeukendrup AE, Vet-Joop K, Sturk A, et al. Relationship between gastro-intestinal complaints and endotoxaemia, cytokine release and the acute-phase reaction during and after a long-distance triathlon in highly trained men. Clin Sci 2000; 98: 47–55.
6.  Stuempfle KJ, Hoffman MD. Gastrointestinal distress is common during a 161-km ultramarathon. J Sports Sci 2015; 33(17): 1814–1821.
7.  Gill SK, Hankey J, Wright A, et al. The Impact of a 24-hour Ultra-Marathon on Circulatory Endotoxin and Cytokine Profile. Int J Sports Med 2015; 36: 688–695.
8.  Gill SK, Teixeira A, Rama L, et al. Circulatory endotoxin concentration and cytokine profile in response to exertional-heat stress during a multi-stage ultra-marathon competition. Exerc Immunol Rev 2015; 21: 114–128.
9.  Hoffman MD, Pasternak A, Rogers IR, et al. Medical services at ultra-endurance food races in remote environments: medical issues and consensus guidelines. Sports Med. 2014; 44(8): 105–1069.
10. Murray R. Training the gut for competition. Curr Sports Med Rep 2006; 5(3): 161–164.
11. ter Steege RW, Van der Palen J, Kolkman JJ. Prevalence of gastrointestinal complaints in runners competing in a long-distance run: an internet-based observational study in 1281 subjects. Scand J Gastroenterol 2008; 43(12): 1477–1482.
12. Leiper JB. Fate of ingested fluids: factors affecting gastric emptying and intestinal absorption of beverages in humans. Nutr Rev 2015; 73(S2): 57–72.
13. ter Steege RW, Kolkman JJ. The pathophysiology and management of gastrointestinal symptoms during physical exercise, and the role of splanchnic blood flow. Aliment Pharmacol Ther 2012; 35: 516–528.
14. van Wijck K, Lenaerts K, van Loon LJ, Peters WH, Buurman WA, Dejong CH. Exercise-induced splanchnic hypoperfusion results in gut dysfunction in healthy men. PLoS One 2011; 6(7): e22366.
15. van Wijck K, Lenaerts K, Grootjans J, et al. Physiology and pathophysiology of splanchnic hypoperfusion and intestinal injury during exercise: strategies for evaluation and preventions. Am J Physiol 2012; 303: G155-G168.

16. Pfeiffer B, Stellingwerff T, Hodgson AB, et al. Nutritional intake and gastrointesti-nal problems during competitive endurance events. Med Sci Sports Exerc 2012; 44: 344–351.

17. van Nieuwenhoven MA, Brouns F, Brummer RJ. Gastrointestinal profile of symp-tomatic athletes at rest and during physical exercise. Eur J Appl Physiol 2004; 91(4): 429–434.

18. Stuempfle KJ, Hoffman MD, Hew-Butler T. Association of gastrointestinal distress in ultramarathoners with race diet. Int J Sport Nutr Exerc Metab 2013; 23: 103–109.

19. Costa RJS, Snipe R, Camões-Costa V, Scheer BV, Murray A. The impact of gastro-intestinal symptoms and dermatological injuries on nutritional intake and hydra-tion status during ultramarathon events. Sports Medicine-Open 2016; 2(16): 1–14.

20. Miall A, Khoo A, Rauch C, Gibson P, Costa RJS. Repetitive gut challenge reduces gastrointestinal symptoms and malabsorption of carbohydrates during exertional stress. J Nutr Intermediary Metab 2014; 1: 31–32 abstract.

21. Miall A, Khoo A, Rauch C, Gibson P, Costa RJS. Does gut-training reduce gastro-intestinal symptom and carbohydrate malabsorption during endurance running? Sports Dietitians Australian 2015; abstract.

22. Costa RJS, Swancott A, Gill S, et al. Compromised energy and nutritional intake of ultra-endurance runners during a multi-stage ultra-marathon conducted in a hot ambient environment. Int J Sports Sci 2013; 3(2): 51–61.

23. Costa RJS, Gill SK, Hankey J, Wright A, Marczak S. Perturbed energy balance and hydration status in ultra-endurance runners during a 24 h ultra-marathon. Br J Nutri 2014; 112: 428–437.

24. van Wijck K, Pennings B, van Bijnen AA, et al. Dietary protein digestion and absorp-tion are impaired during acute postexercise recovery in young men. Am J Phyiol Regul Integr Comp Physiol 2013; 304(5): R356-R361.

25. ter Steege RW, Geelkerken RH, Huisman AB, Kolkman JJ. Abdominal symptoms during physical exercise and the role of gastrointestinal ischaemia: a study in 12 symptomatic athletes. Br J Sports Med 2012; 46(13): 931–935.

26. Rehrer NJ, Smets A, Reynaert H, Goes E, De Meirleir K. Effect of exercise on portal vein blood flow in man. Med Sci Sports Exerc 2001; 33(9): 1533–1537.

27. Grootjans J, Lenaerts K, Buurman WA, Dejong CH, Derikx JP. Life and death at the mucosal-luminal interface: New perspectives on human intestinal ischemia-reperfu-sion. World J Gastroenterol 2016; 22(9): 2760–2770.

28. Zuhl M, Schneider S, Lanphere K, Conn C, Dokladny K, Moseley P. Exercise regula-tion of intestinal tight junction proteins. Br J Sports Med 2014; 48(12): 980–986.

29. Dokladny K, Zuhl MN, Moseley PL. Intestinal epithelial barrier function and tight junction proteins with heat and exercise. J Appl Physiol 2016; 120(6): 692–701.

30. Bosenberg AT, Brock-Utne JG, Gaffin SL, Wells MT, Blake GT. Strenuous exercise causes systemic endotoxemia. J Appl Physiol 1988; 65: 106–108.

31. Camus G, Poortmans J, Nys M, et al. Mild endotoxaemia and the inflammatory response induced by a marathon race. Clin Sci 1997; 92: 415–422.

32. Lim CL, Pyne D, Horn P, et al. The effects of increased endurance training load on biomarkers of heat intolerance during intense exercise in the heat. Appl Physiol Nutr Metab 2009; 34(4): 616–624.

33. Walsh NP, Gleeson M, Shephard RJ, et al. Position statement. Part one: immune function and exercise. Exerc Immunol Rev 2011; 17: 6–63.
34. Walsh NP, Gleeson M, Pyne DB, et al. Position statement. Part two: maintaining immune health. Exerc Immunol Rev 2011; 17: 64–103.
35. Peake JM, Della Gatta P, Suzuki K, Nieman DC. Cytokine expression and secretion by skeletal muscle cells: regulatory mechanisms and exercise effects. Exerc Immunol Rev 2015; 21: 8–25.
36. Selkirk GA, McLellan TM, Wright HE, Rhind SG. Mild endotoxemia, NF-kB translocation, and cytokine increase during exertional heat stress in trained and untrained individuals. Am J Physiol Regul Integr Comp Physiol 2008; 295: 611–623.
37. Capaldo CT, Nusrat A. Cytokine regulation of tight junctions. Biochim Biophys Acta 2009; 1788(4): 864–871.
38. Lang JA, Gisolfi CV, Lambert GP. Effect of exercise intensity on active and passive glucose absorption. Int J Sport Nutr Exerc Metab 2006; 16(5): 485–493.
39. Putkonen L, Yao CK, Gibson PR. Fructose malabsorption syndrome. Curr Opin Clin Nutr Metab Care 2013; 6(4): 473–477.
40. Yao CK, Muir JG, Gibson PR. Review article: insights into colonic protein fermentation, its modulation and potential health implications. Aliment Pharmacol Ther 2016; 43(2): 181–196.
41. Layer P, Peschel S, Schlesinger T, Goebell H. Human pancreatic secretion and intestinal motility: effects of ileal nutrient perfusion. Am J Physiol Gastrointest Liver Physiol 1990; 258: G196–201.
42. Shin HS, Ingram JR, McGill AT, Poppitt SD. Lipids, CHOs, proteins: can all macronutrients put a 'brake' on eating? Physiol. Behav. 2013; 120: 114–123.
43. Derikx JP, Matthijsen RA, de Bruïne AP, et al. Rapid reversal of human intestinal ischemia-reperfusion induced damage by shedding of injured enterocytes and reepithelialisation. PLoS One 2008; 3(10): e3428.
44. Grames C, Berry-Cabán CS. Ischemic colitis in an endurance runner. Case Rep. Gastrointest Med 2012; 2012: 356895.
45. Lucas W, Schroy PC. Reversible ischemic colitis in a high endurance athlete. Am J Gastroenterol 1998; 93(11): 2231–2234.
46. Caradonna L, Amati L, Magrone T, Pellegrino NM, Jirillo E, Caccavo D. Enteric bacteria, lipopolysaccharides and related cytokines in inflammatory bowel disease: biological and clinical significance. J Endotoxin Res 2000; 6(3): 205–214.
47. Morris G, Berk M, Galecki P, Maes M. The Emerging Role of Autoimmunity in Myalgic Encephalomyelitis/Chronic Fatigue Syndrome (ME/cfs). Mol Neurobiol 2014; 49: 741–756.
48. Robson P. Elucidating the unexplained underperformance syndrome in endurance athletes: the interleukin-6 hypothesis. Sports Med 2003; 33(10): 771–781.
49. Marchbank T, Davison G, Oakes JR, et al. The nutriceutical bovine colostrum truncates the increase in gut permeability caused by heavy exercise in athletes. Am J Physiol Gastrointest Liver Physiol 2011; 300(3): G477-G484.
50. Shing CM, Peake JM, Lim CL, et al. Effects of probiotics supplementation on gastrointestinal permeability, inflammation and exercise performance in the heat. Eur J Appl Physiol 2014; 114: 93–103.

51. Rehrer NJ, Brouns F, Beckers EJ, ten Hoor F, Saris WH. Gastric emptying with repeated drinking during running and bicycling. Int J Sports Med 1990; 11(3): 238–243.

52. Snipe R, Kitic C, Gibson P, Costa RJS. Heat stress during prolonged running results in exacerbated intestinal epithelial injury and gastrointestinal symptoms. Exercise and Sports Science Australia 2016; abstract.

53. Rehrer NJ, Meijer GA. Biomechanical vibration of the abdominal region during running and bicycling. J Sports Med Phys Fitness 1991; 31: 231–234.

54. O'Connor FG, Casa DJ, Bergeron MF, et al. American College of Sports Medicine round table on exertional heat stroke. Return to duty/return to play: Conference Proceedings. Curr Sports Med Rep 2010; 9: 314–321.

55. Rav-Acha M, Hadad E, Epstein Y, Heled Y, Moran DS. Fatal exertional heat stroke: a case series. Am J Med Sci 2004; 328: 84–87.

56. Lambert GP, Boylan M, Laventure JP, Bull A, Lanspa S. Effect of aspirin and ibuprofen on GI permeability during exercise. Int J Sports Med 2007; 28(9): 722–726.

57. Ryan AJ, Chang RT, Gisolfi CV. Gastrointestinal permeability following aspirin intake and prolonged running. Med Sci Sports Exerc 1996; 28(6): 698–705.

58. Warden SJ. Prophylactic use of NSAIDs by athletes: a risk/benefit assessment. Phys Sportsmed 2010; 38(1): 132–138.

59. Shephard RJ. The case for increased physical activity in chronic inflammatory bowel disease: a brief review. Int J Sports Med 2016; 37: 505–515.

60. Brown K, DeCoffe D, Molcan E, Gibson DL. Diet-induced dysbiosis of the intestinal microbiota and the effects on immunity and disease. Nutrients 2012; 4: 1095–1119.

61. Clarke SF, Murphy EF, O'Sullivan O, et al. Exercise and associated dietary extremes impact on gut microbial diversity. Gut 2014; 63(12): 1913–1920.

62. Mach N, Fuster-Botella. Endurance exercise and gut microbiota: A review. J Sport Health Sci 2016. In press.

63. Rivière A, Selak M, Lantin D, Leroy F, De Vuyst L. Bifidobacteria and Butyrate-Producing Colon Bacteria: Importance and Strategies for Their Stimulation in the Human Gut. Front Microbiol 2016; 28(7): 979.

64. Costa RJS, Teixiera A, Rama L, et al. Water and sodium intake habits and status of ultra-endurance runners during a multi-stage ultra-marathon conducted in a hot ambient environment: An observational study. Nutri J 2013; 12(13): 1–16.

65. American College of Sports Medicine, Sawka MN, Burke LM, et al. American college of sports medicine position stand. Exercise and fluid replacement. Med Sci Sports Exerc 2007; 39: 377–390.

66. Wendt D, van Loon LJ, Lichtenbelt WD. Thermoregulation during exercise in the heat: Strategies for maintaining health and performance. Sports Med 2007; 37: 669–682.

67. Goulet EDB. Effect of exercise-induced dehydration on endurance performance: evaluating the impact of exercise protocols on outcomes using a meta-analytic procedure. Br J Sports Med 2012; 70(Suppl 2): S132-S136.

68. van Nieuwenhoven MA, Vriens BE, Brummer RJ, Brouns F. Effect of dehydration on gastrointestinal function at rest and during exercise in humans. Eur J Appl Physiol. 2000; 83(6): 578–584.

69. Snipe R, Dixon D, Gibson P, Costa RJS. The effects of exercise-induced dehydration on gastrointestinal integrity and symptoms. Sports Dietitians Australian 2015; abstract.

70. Lambert GP, Lang J, Bull A, Pfeifer PC, et al. Fluid restriction during running increases GI permeability. Int J Sports Med 2008; 29(3): 194–198.

71. Gill SK, Allerton DM, Ansley-Robson P, Hemming K, Cox M, Costa RJS. Does Acute High Dose Probiotic Supplementation Containing Lactobacillus casei Attenuate Exertional-Heat Stress Induced Endotoxaemia and Cytokinaemia? Int J Sports Nutr Exerc Metab 2016; 26: 268–275.

72. Zuhl M, Dokladny K, Mermier C, Schneider S, Salgado R, Moseley P. The effects of acute oral glutamine supplementation on exercise-induced gastrointestinal permeability and heat shock protein expression in peripheral blood mononuclear cells. Cell Stress Chaperones 2015; 20(1): 85–93.

73. Brock-Utne JG, Gaffin SL, Wells MT, et al. Endotoxemia in exhausted runners after a long-distance race. S Afr Med J 1988; 73: 533–536.

74. Buchman AL, Killip D, Ou CN, et al. Short-term vitamin E supplementation before marathon running: a placebo-controlled trial. Nutr 1999; 15(4): 278–283.

75. Ashton T, Young IS, Davison GW, et al. Exercise-induced endotoxemia: the effect of ascorbic acid supplementation. Free Radic Biol Med 2003; 35(3): 284–291.

76. Buchman AL, O'Brien W, Ou CN, et al. The effect of arginine or glycine supplementation on gastrointestinal function, muscle injury, serum amino acid concentrations and performance during a marathon run. Int J Sports Med 1999; 20(5): 315–321.

77. Zuhl MN, Lanphere KR, Kravitz L, et al. Effects of oral glutamine supplementation on exercise-induced gastrointestinal permeability and tight junction protein expression. J Appl Physiol 2014; 116(2): 183–191.

78. van Wijck K, Wijnands KA, Meesters DM, et al. L-citrulline improves splanchnic perfusion and reduces gut injury during exercise. Med Sci Sports Exerc 2014; 46(11): 2039–2046.

79. Buckley JD, Butler RN, Southcott E, Brinkworth GD. Bovine colostrum supplementation during running training increases intestinal permeability. Nutrients 2009; 1(2): 224–234.

80. Carol A, Witkamp RF, Wichers HJ, Mensink M. Bovine colostrum supplementation's lack of effect on immune variables during short-term intense exercise in well-trained athletes. Int J Sport Nutr Exerc Metab 2011; 21(2): 135–145.

81. Morrison SA, Cheung SS, Cotter JD. Bovine colostrum, training status, and gastrointestinal permeability during exercise in the heat: a placebo-controlled double-blind study. Appl Physiol Nutr Metab 2014; 39(9): 1070–1082.

82. Davison G, Marchbank T, March DS, Thatcher R, Playford RJ. Zinc carnosine works with bovine colostrum in truncating heavy exercise-induced increase in gut permeability in healthy volunteers. Am J Clin Nutr 2016; 104(2): 526–536.

83. Matherson PJ, Wilson MA, Garrison RN. Regulation of intestinal blood flow. J Surg Res 2000; 93(1): 182–196.

84. Rehrer NJ, Goes E, DuGardeyn C, Reynaert H, DeMeirleir K. Effect of carbohydrate on portal vein blood flow during exercise. Int J Sports Med 2005; 26: 171–176.

85. Lambert GP, Broussard LJ, Mason BL, Mauermann WJ, Gisolfi CV. Gastrointestinal permeability during exercise: effects of aspirin and energy-containing beverages. J Appl Physiol 2001; 90(6): 2075–2080.

86.  Snipe R, Kitic C, Gibson P, Costa RJS. Carbohydrate and protein intake during exertional-heat stress ameliorates intestinal epithelial damage. Nutri Diet 2016; 73(Suppl 1): 19 abstract.

87.  Burke LM, Hawley JA, Wong SH, Jeukendrup AE. Carbohydrates for training and competition. J Sports Sci 2011; 29(Suppl 1): S17-S27.

88.  Sator BR. Therapeutic manipulation of the enteric microflora in inflammatory bowel diseases: antibiotics, probiotics, and prebiotics. Gastroenterol 2004; 126: 1620–1633.

89.  Christensen HR, Larsen CN, Kaestel P, et al. Immunomodulating potential of supplementation with probiotics: a dose–response study in healthy young adults. FEMS Immunol Med Microbiol 2006; 47: 380–390.

90.  Lamprecht M, Bogner S, Schippinger G, et al. Probiotic supplementation affects markers of intestinal barrier, oxidation, and inflammation in trained men; a randomized, double-blinded, placebo-controlled trial. J Int Soc Sports Nutr 2012; 9(1): 45.

91.  Halmos EP, Christophersen CT, Bird AR, Shepherd SJ, Gibson PR, Muir JG. Diets that differ in their FODMAP content alter the colonic luminal microenvironment. Gut 2015; 64: 93–100.

92.  Enko D, Kriegshäuser G, Kimbacher C, Stolba R, Mangge H, Halwachs-Baumann G. Carbohydrate Malabsorption and Putative Carbohydrate-Specific Small Intestinal Bacterial Overgrowth: Prevalence and Diagnostic Overlap Observed in an Austrian Outpatient Center. Digestion 2015; 92(1): 32–38.

93.  Parodi A, Dulbecco P, Savarino E, et al. Positive glucose breath testing is more prevalent in patients with IBS-like symptoms compared with controls of similar age and gender distribution. J Clin Gastroenterol 2009; 43(10): 962–966.

94.  Lis DM, Stellingwerff T, Shing CM, Ahuja KD, Fell JW. Exploring the popularity, experiences, and beliefs surrounding gluten-free diets in nonceliac athletes. Int J Sport Nutr Exerc Metab 2015; 25(1): 37–45.

95.  Lis D, Stellingwerff T, Kitic CM, Ahuja KD, Fell J. No Effects of a Short-Term Gluten-free Diet on Performance in Nonceliac Athletes. Med Sci Sports Exerc 2015; 47(12): 2563–2570.

96.  Muir JG, Gibson PR. The Low FODMAP Diet for Treatment of Irritable Bowel Syndrome and Other Gastrointestinal Disorders. Gastroenterol Hepatol 2013; 9(7): 450–452.

97.  Halmos EP, Power VA, Shepherd SJ, Gibson PR, Muir JG. A diet low in FODMAPs reduces symptoms of irritable bowel syndrome. Gastroenterol 2014; 146(1): 67–75.

98.  Lis D, Ahuja KD, Stellingwerff T, Kitic CM, Fell J. Case Study: Utilizing a Low FODMAP Diet to Combat Exercise-Induced Gastrointestinal Symptoms. Int J Sport Nutr Exerc Metab 2016; 24: 1–17.

## Chapter 17

1.  National Weather Service website: http: //www.nws.noaa.gov/om/hazstats.shtml. Accessed August 29, 2016.

2.  National Weather Service website: http: //www.nws.noaa.gov/om/hazstats/light15.pdf. Accessed August 29, 2016.

3.  National Geographic Lightning Profile. Environment.nationalgeographic.com/environment/natural-disasters/lightning-profile. Accessed August 29, 2016.

4.  Diclose, PJ, Sanderson LM. An Epidemiological Description of Lightning-Related Deaths in the United States. Int J Epidemiology. 1990 Sep; 19(3): 673–9.

5.  Cherington, M, Walker, I, Boyson M, et al. Closing the gap on the actual numbers of lightning casualties and deaths. Preprints, 11th Conference on applied climatology, Dallas, January 10–15. Boston: American Meteorological Society; 1999.

6.  Elson, DM. Deaths and Injuries caused by lightning in the United Kingdom: analyses of two databases. Atm Res. 2001 Jan; 56(1–4): 325–334.

7.  Cooper, MA, Holle, RL, Andres, CJ, et al. Lightning Injuries. In: Auerbach, PS. Wilderness Medicine. 6th ed. Philadelphia, PA: Elsevier Mosby; 2012.

8.  Lengyel MM, Brooks HE, Rolle RL, et al. Lightning Casualties and their proximity to surrounding cloud-to-ground lightning. Proceedings of the 14th Symposium on education, American Meteorological Association, San Diego, January 2005.

9.  Davis C, Engeln A, Johnson E, McIntosh SE, Zafren K, Islas AA, McStay C, Smith W, Cushing T; Wilderness Medical Society. Wilderness medical society practice guidelines for the prevention and treatment of lightning injuries. Wilderness Environ Med. 2012 Sep; 23(3): 260–9. doi: 10.1016/j.wem.2012.05.016. Epub 2012 Jul 31.

10. Holle, RL, Lopez, RE, Zimmermann, C. Updated recommendations for lightning safety. Bull Am Meteorological Soc. 1998; 80: 2035. [1999].

11. Cooper, MA, Holle, R, Lopez, R. Recommendations for lightning safety. JAMA. 1999; 282: 1132.

12. Hodanish, SJ, Torgerson, K, Jensenius, JS et al. Leon the lightning safety lion says: "When Thunder roars go indoors!" NOAA's efforts regarding children's lightning safety. Third Conference on Meteorological Applications of Lightning Data. New Orleans: American Meteorological Society; 2008.

13. National Weather Service website. www.lightningsafety.noaa.gov. Accessed August 28, 2016.

14. The National Severe Storms Labaratory: Floods. http: //www.nssl.noaa.gov/education/svrwx101/floods/ Accessed August 16, 2016.

15. National Weather Service website. http: //www.floodsafety.noaa.gov/. Accessed August 28, 2016.

16. Flash flood and other canyoneering hazards. http: //www.canyoneeringusa.com/utah/introduction/hazards/. Accessed August 29, 2016.

17. Weiss, EA. Whitewater Medicine and Rescue. In: Auerbach, PS. Wilderness Medicine. 6th ed. Philadelphia, PA: Elsevier Mosby; 2012.

18. Giesbrecht, GG, Steinman, AM. Immersion Into Cold Water. In: Auerbach, PS. Wilderness Medicine. 6th ed. Philadelphia, PA: Elsevier Mosby; 2012.

19. Vanggaard, L. Physiological reactions to wet-cold. Aviat Space Environ Med. 1975; 46: 33.

20. Liu, J.C., Mickley, L.J., Sulprizio, M.P. et al. Climatic Change (2016). doi: 10.1007/s10584–016–1762–6.

21. Alexander, ME, Mutch, RW, Davis, KM, et al. Wildland Fires Dangers and Survival. In: Auerbach, PS. Wilderness Medicine. 6th ed. Philadelphia, PA: Elsevier Mosby; 2012.

22. Alexander, ME: Predicting fire behavior in wildland/urban environments. Proceedings of the international ymposium on fire and environment: Ecological and cultural perspectives. 1991.
23. Alexander, ME. Surviving a wildland fire entrapment or burnover. Can Silviculture. 2007; August: 23.

## Chapter 18

1. Adams BB. Dermatologic disorders of the athlete. Sports Med. 2002; 32(5): 309–321.
2. Adams BB. Sports dermatology. New York, NY: Springer; 2006.
3. Helm MF, T NH, W FB. Skin problems in the long-distance runner 2500 years after the Battle of Marathon. Int J Dermatol. 2012; 51(3): 263–270.
4. Mailler EA, Adams BB. The wear and tear of 26.2: dermatological injuries reported on marathon day. Br J Sports Med. 2004; 38(4): 498–501.
5. Mailler-Savage EA, Adams BB. Skin manifestations of running. J Am Acad Dermatol. 2006; 55(2): 290–301.
6. Conklin RJ. Common cutaneous disorders in athletes. Sports Med. 1990; 9(2): 100–119.
7. Auerbach PS, Constance BB, Freer L, Donner HJ, Weiss EA, Auerbach PS. Field guide to wilderness medicine. 4th ed. Philadelphia, PA: Elsevier/Mosby; 2013.
8. Stevens DL, Bryant AE. Impetigo, Erysipelas and Cellulitis. In: Ferretti JJ, Stevens DL, Fischetti VA, eds. Streptococcus pyogenes: Basic Biology to Clinical Manifestations. Oklahoma City (OK) 2016.
9. Cohen PR, Grossman ME. Management of cutaneous lesions associated with an emerging epidemic: community-acquired methicillin-resistant Staphylococcus aureus skin infections. J Am Acad Dermatol. 2004; 51(1): 132–135.
10. Cohen PR. The skin in the gym: a comprehensive review of the cutaneous manifestations of community-acquired methicillin-resistant Staphylococcus aureus infection in athletes. Clin Dermatol. 2008; 26(1): 16–26.
11. Holdiness MR. Management of cutaneous erythrasma. Drugs. 2002; 62(8): 1131–1141.
12. Pranteda G, Carlesimo M, Pranteda G, et al. Pitted keratolysis, erythromycin, and hyperhidrosis. Dermatol Ther. 2014; 27(2): 101–104.
13. Bristow IR, Lee YL. Pitted keratolysis: a clinical review. J Am Podiatr Med Assoc. 2014; 104(2): 177–182.
14. Greywal T, Cohen PR. Pitted keratolysis: successful management with mupirocin 2 percent ointment monotherapy. Dermatol Online J. 2015; 21(8).
15. Dreno B, Bettoli V, Perez M, Bouloc A, Ochsendorf F. Cutaneous lesions caused by mechanical injury. Eur J Dermatol. 2015; 25(2): 114–121.
16. Caputo R, De Boulle K, Del Rosso J, Nowicki R. Prevalence of superficial fungal infections among sports-active individuals: results from the Achilles survey, a review of the literature. J Eur Acad Dermatol Venereol. 2001; 15(4): 312–316.
17. Purim KS, Leite N. Sports-related dermatoses among road runners in Southern Brazil. An Bras Dermatol. 2014; 89(4): 587–592.
18. Pharis DB, Teller C, Wolf JE, Jr. Cutaneous manifestations of sports participation. J Am Acad Dermatol. 1997; 36(3 Pt 1): 448–459.

19. Goldstein AO, Goldstein BG. Dermatophyte (tinea) infections. In: Post TW, ed. UpToDate. Waltham, MA: UpToDate; 2016. www.uptodate.com Accessed July 26, 2016.

20. Kaushik N, Pujalte GG, Reese ST. Superficial Fungal Infections. Prim Care. 2015; 42(4): 501–516.

21. Sahoo AK, Mahajan R. Management of tinea corporis, tinea cruris, and tinea pedis: A comprehensive review. Indian Dermatol Online J. 2016; 7(2): 77–86.

22. Rotta I, Ziegelmann PK, Otuki MF, Riveros BS, Bernardo NL, Correr CJ. Efficacy of topical antifungals in the treatment of dermatophytosis: a mixed-treatment comparison meta-analysis involving 14 treatments. JAMA Dermatol. 2013; 149(3): 341–349.

23. Rashid RS, Shim TN. Contact dermatitis. BMJ. 2016; 353: i3299.

24. Madden CC. Netter's sports medicine. Philadelphia: Saunders/Elsevier; 2010.

25. Gladman AC. Toxicodendron dermatitis: poison ivy, oak, and sumac. Wilderness Environ Med. 2006; 17(2): 120–128.

26. Boelman DJ. Emergency: Treating poison ivy, oak, and sumac. Am J Nurs. 2010; 110(6): 49–52.

27. Grevelink SA, Murrell DF, Olsen EA. Effectiveness of various barrier preparations in preventing and/or ameliorating experimentally produced Toxicodendron dermatitis. J Am Acad Dermatol. 1992; 27(2 Pt 1): 182–188.

28. Montgomery SL. Cholinergic urticaria and exercise-induced anaphylaxis. Curr Sports Med Rep. 2015; 14(1): 61–63.

29. Siebenhaar F, Weller K, Mlynek A, et al. Acquired cold urticaria: clinical picture and update on diagnosis and treatment. Clin Exp Dermatol. 2007; 32(3): 241–245.

30. Altrichter S, Koch K, Church MK, Maurer M. Atopic predisposition in cholinergic urticaria patients and its implications. J Eur Acad Dermatol Venereol. 2016.

31. Beattie PE, Dawe RS, Ibbotson SH, Ferguson J. Characteristics and prognosis of idiopathic solar urticaria: a cohort of 87 cases. Arch Dermatol. 2003; 139(9): 1149–1154.

32. Maurer M. Cold urticaria. In: Saini S, Callen J, eds. UpToDate. Waltham, MA: UptoDate; 2016. www.uptodate.com. Accessed July 26, 2016.

33. Gozali MV, Zhou BR, Luo D. Update on treatment of photodermatosis. Dermatol Online J. 2016; 22(2).

34. Ramelet AA. Exercise-induced purpura. Dermatology. 2004; 208(4): 293–296.

35. Ambros-Rudolph CM, Hofmann-Wellenhof R, Richtig E, Muller-Furstner M, Soyer HP, Kerl H. Malignant melanoma in marathon runners. Arch Dermatol. 2006; 142(11): 1471–1474.

36. Richtig E, Ambros-Rudolph CM, Trapp M, et al. Melanoma markers in marathon runners: increase with sun exposure and physical strain. Dermatology. 2008; 217(1): 38–44.

37. Harrison SC, Bergfeld WF. Ultraviolet light and skin cancer in athletes. Sports Health. 2009; 1(4): 335–340.

38. Hussain MS, Cripwell L, Berkovsky S, Freyne J. Promoting UV Exposure Awareness with Persuasive, Wearable Technologies. Stud Health Technol Inform. 2016; 227: 48–54.

39. American Academy of Dermatology. Position Statement on VITAMIN D. https: // www.aad.org/forms/policies/uploads/ps/ps-vitamin percent20d percent20postition percent20statement.pdf. Published November 14, 2009. Approved November 1, 2008. Accessed July 26, 2016.

## Chapter 19

1. Hoffman MD, Pasternak A, Rogers IR, et al. Medical services at ultra-endurance foot races in remote environments: medical issues and consensus guidelines. Sports Med. 2014; 44(8): 1055–1069.

2. Cass SP. Ocular injuries in sports. Curr Sports Med Rep. 2012; 11(1): 11–15.

3. Leivo T, Haavisto AK, Sahraravand A. Sports-related eye injuries: the current picture. Acta Ophthalmol. 2015; 93(3): 224–231.

4. Olsen DE, Sikka RS, Pulling T, Broton M. Eye Injuries in Sports. Netter's Sports Medicine. Philadelphia, Pennsylvania, USA: Saunders, an imprint of Elsevier Inc.; 2010: 332–339.

5. Rodriguez JO, Lavina AM, Agarwal A. Prevention and treatment of common eye injuries in sports. Am Fam Physician. 2003; 67(7): 1481–1488.

6. Ellerton JA, Zuljan I, Agazzi G, Boyd JJ. Eye problems in mountain and remote areas: prevention and onsite treatment—official recommendations of the International Commission for Mountain Emergency Medicine ICAR MEDCOM. Wilderness Environ Med. 2009; 20(2): 169–175.

7. Hoffman MD, Fogard K. Factors related to successful completion of a 161-km ultra-marathon. Int J Sports Physiol Perform. 2011; 6(1): 25–37.

8. Hoeg TB, Corrigan GK, Hoffman MD. An investigation of ultramarathon-associated visual impairment. Wilderness Environ Med. 2015; 26(2): 200–204.

9. Khodaee M, Torres DR. Corneal Opacity in a Participant of a 161-km Mountain Bike Race at High Altitude. Wilderness Environ Med. 2016; 27(2): 274–276.

10. Cope TA, Kropelnicki A. Eye injuries in the extreme environment ultra-marathon runner. BMJ Case Rep. 2015; 2015.

11. Daly R. Frozen corneas - treatment in an ultra-cold climate. EyeWorld Online: EyeWorld News Service; 2004.

12. Jha KN. High Altitude and the Eye. Asia Pac J Ophthalmol (Phila). 2012; 1(3): 166–169.

13. Pescosolido N, Barbato A, Di Blasio D. Hypobaric hypoxia: effects on contrast sensitivity in high altitude environments. Aerosp Med Hum Perform. 2015; 86(2): 118–124.

14. Willmann G, Schatz A, Zhour A, et al. Impact of acute exposure to high altitude on anterior chamber geometry. Invest Ophthalmol Vis Sci. 2013; 54(6): 4241–4248.

15. Bosch MM, Barthelmes D, Merz TM, et al. New insights into changes in corneal thickness in healthy mountaineers during a very-high-altitude climb to Mount Muztagh Ata. Arch Ophthalmol. 2010; 128(2): 184–189.

16. Morris DS, Somner JE, Scott KM, McCormick IJ, Aspinall P, Dhillon B. Corneal thickness at high altitude. Cornea. 2007; 26(3): 308–311.

17. Ettl AR, Felber SR, Rainer J. Corneal edema induced by cold. Ophthalmologica. 1992; 204(3): 113–114.

18. Feiz V. Corneal Edema. In: Krachmer JH, Mannis MJ, Holland EJ, eds. Cornea. 3rd ed: Mosby is an imprint of Elsevier Inc.; 2011: 283–287.

19. McMonnies CW. Intraocular pressure and glaucoma: Is physical exercise beneficial or a risk? J Optom. 2016; 9(3): 139–147.

20. Williams PT. Relationship of incident glaucoma versus physical activity and fitness in male runners. Med Sci Sports Exerc. 2009; 41(8): 1566–1572.

21. Aerni GA. Blunt visual trauma. Clin Sports Med. 2013; 32(2): 289–301.
22. Labriola LT, Friberg TR, Hein A. Marathon runner's retinopathy. Semin Ophthalmol. 2009; 24(6): 247–250.

## Chapter 20

1.  Forrester JA, Holstege CP, Forrester JD. Fatalities from venomous and nonvenomous animals in the United States (1999–2007). Wilderness Environ Med 2012; 23: 146–152.
2.  Herrero S, Higgins A, Cardoza JE, et al. Fatal attacks by American black bear on people: 1900–2009. J Wildl Manage 2011; 75: 596–603.
3.  Smith TS, Herrero S, Debruyn TD, et al. Efficacy of Bear Deterrent Spray in Alaska. J Wildl Manage 2008; 72: 640–645.
4.  Beier P. Cougar attacks on humans in the United States and Canada. Wildernes Soc Bull 1991; 19: 403–412.
5.  Manning SE, Rupprecht CE, Fishbein D, et al.: Human rabies prevention—United States, 2008: recommendations of the Advisory Committee on Immunization Practices. MMWR Morb Mortal Wkly Rep 2008; 57(No. RR-3): 1–28.
6.  Fernandez R, Griffiths R. Water for wound cleansing. Cochrane Database of Syst Rev 2012; 2: 1–32.
7.  Dire DJ, Welsh AP. A comparison of wound irrigation solutions used in the emergency department. Ann Emerg Med 1990; 19(6): 704–8.
8.  Moscati, R, Mayrose J, Fincher L, et al. Comparison of normal saline with tap water for wound irrigation. Am J Emerg Med 1998; 16(4): 379–381.
9.  Jackson, CA. Update on Rabies Diagnosis and Treatment. Curr Infect Dis Rep 2009; 11: 296–301.
10. Goldstein EJ. Bite wounds and infection. Clin Infect Dis 1992; 14: 633–638.
11. Fleisher GR. The Management of Bite Wounds. N Engl J Med 1999; 340(2): 138–40.
12. Novotny V, Basset Y, Miller SE, et al. Low host specificity of herbivorous insects in a tropical forest. Nature 2002; 416: 841–4.
13. Lee H, Halverson S, Mackey R. Insect Allergy. Prim Care Clin Office Pract 2016; 43: 417–431.
14. Bilò MB, Bonifazi F. The natural history and epidemiology of insect venom allergy: clinical implications. Clin Exp Allergy 2009; 39(10): 1467–76.
15. Ribeiro JMC, Francischetti IMB. Role of arthropod saliva in blood feeding: Sialome and Post-Sialome Perspectives. Annu Rev Entomol 2003; 48: 73–88.
16. Braack L, Hunt R, Koekemoer LL, et al. Biting behaviour of African malaria vectors: 1. where do the main vector species bite on the human body? Parasit Vectors 2015; 4(8): 76.
17. Nasci RS, Wirtz RA, Brogdon WG. Chapter 2.The pre-travel consultation. Protection against mosquitoes, ticks, and other insects and arthropods. US Centers for Disease Control and Prevention. Available at: http://wwwnc.cdc.gov/travel/yellowbook/2016/the-pre-travel-consultation/protection-against-mosquitoes-ticks-other-arthropods.
18. Katz TM, Miller JH, Hebert AA. Insect repellents: historical perspectives and new developments. J Am Acad Dermatol 2008; 58: 865–871.
19. Brown M, Hebert AA. Insect repellents: An overview. J Am Acad Dermatol 1997; 36: 243–9.

20. Diaz JH. Chemical and Plant-Based Insect Repellents: Efficacy, Safety, and Toxicity. Wilderness Environ Med 2016; 27: 153–163.

21. Petrucci N, Sardini S. Severe neurotoxic reaction associated oral ingestion of low-dose diethyltoluamide containing insect repellent in a child. Pediatr Emerg Care 2000; 16: 341–342.

22. Rutledge LC, Wirtz PA, Buescher MD, et al. Mathematical models of the effectiveness and persistence of mosquito repellents. J Am Mosq Control Assoc 1985; 1: 56–61.

23. Frances SP, Waterston DGE, Beebe NW, et al. Field evaluation of repellent formulations containing DEET and picaridin against mosquitoes in Northern Territory, Australia. J Med Entomol 2004; 41: 414–417.

24. Goodyer LI, Croft AM, Frances SP. Expert review of the evidence base for arthropod bite avoidance. J Travel Med 2010; 17: 182–192.

25. Trigg JK, Hill N. Laboratory evaluation of a eucalyptus- based repellent against four biting arthropods. Phytother Res 1996: 10313–10316.

26. Fradin MS, Day JF. Comparative efficacy of insect repellents against mosquito bites. N Engl J Med 2002; 347: 13–8.

27. Burkhard PR, Burkhardt K, Haenggeli CA, et al. Plant-induced seizures: reappearance of an old problem. J Neurol 1999; 246(8): 667–670.

28. Rajan TV, Hein M, Porte P, et al. A double-blinded, placebo-controlled trial of garlic as a mosquito repellent; a preliminary study. Med Vet Entomol 2005; 19: 84–89.

29. Vetter RS, Visscher PK, Camazine S. Mass envenomations by honey bees and wasps. West J Med 1999; 170: 223–227.

30. Freeman TM. Hypersensitivity to hymenoptera stings. N Engl J Med 2004; 351: 1987–84.

31. Diaz-Sanchez, CL, Lifshitz-Guinzberg A, Ignacio-Ibarra G, et al. Survival after massive (>2000) Africanized Honeybee stings. Arch Intern Med 1998; 158: 925–927.

32. Hahn I, Lewin NA: Arthropods, in Goldfrank LR, Flomenbaum NE, Lewin NA, et al (eds). Goldfrank's Toxicologic Emergencies (ed 7). New York: McGraw-Hill, 2002.

33. Golden DBK, Kagey-Sobotka A, Norman PS, et al. Outcomes of allergy to insect stings in children, with and without venom immunotherapy. N Engl J Med 2004; 351: 668–74.

34. Ludman SW, Boyle RJ. Stinging insect allergy: current perspectives on venom immunotherapy. J Asthma Allergy 2015; 23(8): 75–86.

35. Ellis AK, Day JH. Incidence and characteristics of biphasic anaphylaxis: a prospective evaluation of 103 patients. An Allergy Asthma Immunol 2007; 98: 64–9.

36. Golden DB, Moffitt, JE, Nicklas RA, et al. Stinging insect hypersensitivity: a practice parameter update. J Allergy Clin Immunol 2011; 127(4): 852.e23–854.e23.

37. Fitzgerald KT, Flood AA. Hymenoptera Stings. Clin Tech Small Anim Pract 2006; 21: 194–204.

38. Truskinovsky AM, Dick JD, Hutchins GM. Fatal infection after a bee sting. Clin Infect Dis 2001; 32(2): E36–8.

39. Petricevich VL. Scorpion venom and the inflammatory response. Mediators Inflamm 2010; (Article ID# 903295).

40. Isbister GK, Bawaskar HS. Scorpion Envenomation. N Engl J Med 2014; 371: 457–463.

41. Uluğ M, Yaman Y, Yapıcı F, et al. Scorpion envenomation in children: an analysis of 99 cases. Turk J Pediatr 2012; 54: 119–127.
42. Özkan Ö, Adıgüzel S, Yakıştıran S, et al. Androctonus crassicauda (Oliver 1807) scorpionism in the Şanlıurfa provinces of Turkey. Turkiye Parazitol Derg 2006; 30: 239–245.
43. Berg RA, Tarantino MD. Envenomation by the scorpion Centruroides exilicuada (C. sculpturatus): severe and unusual manifestations. Pediatrics 1991; 87: 930–3.
44. LoVecchio F, McBride C. Scorpion envenomations in young children in central Arizona. J Toxicol Clin Toxicol 2003; 41: 937–40.
45. Quinter-Hernandez V, Jimenez-Vargas JM, Gurrola GB, et al. Scorpion venom components that affect ion-channels function. Toxicon 2012; 76: 328–42.
46. Boyer LJ, Theodorou AA, Berg RA, et al. Antivenom for Critically Ill Children with Neurotoxicity from Scorpion Stings. N Engl J Med 2009; 360: 2090–8.
47. Chippaux JP, Goyffon M. Epidemiology of scorpionism: a global appraisal. Acta Trop 2008; 107: 71–9.
48. Bawaskar HS, Bawaskar PH. Efficacy and safety of scorpion antivenom plus prazosin compared with prazosin alone for venomous scorpion (Mesobuthus tamulus) sting: randomised open label clinical trial. BMJ 2011; 342: c7136.
49. Boyer LV, Theodorou AA, Chase PB, et al. Effectiveness of Centruroides scorpion antivenom compared to historical controls. Toxicon 2013; 76: 377–85.
50. Boyer L, Degan J, Ruha AM, et al. Safety of intravenous equine F(ab')2: insights following clinical trials involving 1534 recipients of scorpion antivenom. Toxicon 2013; 76: 386–93.
51. Kanaan CN, Ray J, Stewart M, et al. Wilderness medical Society Practice Guidelines for the Treatment of Pitviper Envenomations in the United States and Canada. Wilderness Environ Med 2015; 26: 472–487.
52. O'Neil ME, Mack KA, Gilchrist J, et al. Snakebite injuries treated in United States emergency departments, 2001–2004. Wilderness Environ Med 2007; 18: 281–287.
53. Herbert SS, Hayes WK. Denim clothing reduces venom expenditure by rattlesnakes striking defensively at model human limbs. Anne Emerg Med 2009; 54: 830–836.
54. Young BA, Zahn K. Dry bites are real. Venom flow in rattlesnakes: mechanic and metering. J Exp Biol 2001; 204: 4345–4351.
55. Whitaker PB, Ellis K, Shine R. The defensive strike of the Eastern Brown snake, Pseudonaja textilis (Elapidae). Funct Ecol 2000; 14(1): 25–31.
56. Lavonas EJ, Ruha AM, Banner W, et al. Unified treatment algorithm for the management of cotaline snake bite in the United States: results of an evidence-informed consensus workshop. BMC Emerg Med. 2011; 11: 2.
57. Bucaretchi F, Capitani EM, Vieira RJ, et al. Coral snake bites (Micrurus spp.) in Brazil: a review of literature reports. Clin Toxicol (Phila) 2016; 54(3): 222–34.
58. Alberts MB, Shalit M, LoGalbo F. Suction for venomous snakebite: a study of "mock venom" extraction in a human model. Ann Emerg Med 2004; 43: 181–186.
59. Bush SP, Hegewald K, Green SM, et al. Effects of a negative-pressure venom extraction device [Extractor] on local tissue injury after artificial rattlesnake envenomation in a porcine model. Wilderness Environ Med 2000; 11: 180–188.

60. Hardy DL. A review of first aid measures for pit viper bite in North America with an appraisal of Extractor suction and stun gun electro shock. In: Campbell JA, Brodie ED, eds. Biology of the Pitvipers. Tyler, TX: Selva Publishing; 1992: 405–441.

61. Johnson E, Kardong K, Mackessy S. Electric shocks are ineffective in treatment of lethal effects of rattlesnake envenomation in mice. Toxicon 1987; 25: 1347–1349.

62. Amaral CF, Campolina D, Dias MB, et al. Tourniquet ineffectiveness to reduce the severity of envenoming after Crotalus durissus snakebite in Belo Horizonte, Minas Gerais, Brazil. Toxicon1998; 36: 805–808.

## Chapter 21

1. Centers for Disease Control and Prevention. National Center for Health Statistics: Heart Disease. Atlanta, GA: Centers for Disease Control and Prevention, US Dept of Health and Human Services; 2016.

2. Mozaffarian D, Benjamin EJ, Go AS, et al.; on behalf of the American Heart Association Statistics Committee and Stroke Statistics Subcommittee. Heart disease and stroke statistics—2015 update: a report from the American Heart Association. Circulation. 2015; 131(4): e29–322.

3. Shah R, Lima J. Association of Fitness in Young Adulthood With Survival and Cardiovascular Risk: The Coronary Artery Risk Development in Young Adults (CARDIA) Study. Jama Intern Med. 2016; 176(1): 87–95.

4. Anderson L, Taylor R. Exercise-based cardiac rehabilitation for coronary heart disease. Cochrane Database syst rev. 2016; 5: CD001800.

5. Anderson K, Kannel W. Cardiovascular Disease Risk Profiles. Am Heart Jour. 1991; 121(1): 293–98.

6. Thompson P, Wenger N. Exercise and Physical Activity in the Prevention and Treatment of Atherosclerotic Cardiovascular Disease. Circulation. 2003; 107: 2989.

7. Lee D, Blair S. Leisure-time running reduces all-cause and cardiovascular mortality risk. J Am Coll Cardiol. 2014; 64(5): 472–81.

8. O'Keefe J, McCullough P. Potential adverse cardiovascular effects from excessive endurance exercise. Mayo Clin Proc. 2012; 87: 587–595.

9. Lavie C, Sallis R. Exercise and the heart—the harm of too little and too much. Curr Sports Med Rep. 2015; 14: 104–9.

10. Neidfeldt M. Managing Hypertension in Athletes and Physically Active Patients. Am Fam Physician. 2002; 66(3): 445–453.

11. Reibe D, Pescatello L. Updating ACSM's Guidelines for Exercise Preparticipation Health Screening. Med and Sci in Sports & Exer. 2015; 47(11): 2473–2479.

12. Shipe M. Exercising with Coronary Heart Disease. Amer Coll of Sports Med. 2012.

13. Faris R, Coats A. Diuretics for Heart Failure. Cochrane Database Syst Rev. 2012; 15(2): CD003838.

14. Sagar V, Taylor R. Exercise-based Rehabilitation for Heart Failure: systematic review and meta-analysis. Open Heart. 2015; 2(1): e000163.

15. Elosua R, Molina L. Sport practice and the risk of lone atrial fibrillation: a case-control study. Int J Cardiol. 2006; 108: 332–7.

16. Mont L, Sambola A, Brugada J, Vacca M, Marrugat J, Elosua R, et al. Long-lasting sport practice and lone atrial fibrillation. Eur Heart J. 2002; 23: 477–82.

17. Williams T, Franklin B. Reduced incidence of cardiac arrhythmias in walkers and runners. Plos One. 2013; 8(6): e65302.

18. Heidbuchel H, Biffi A. Recommendations for participation in leisure-time physical activity and competitive sports in patients with arrhythmias and potentially arrhythmogenic conditions. Eur J Cardiovasc. 2006; 13: 475–84.

19. Walker J, Nazarian S. Evaluation of cardiac arrhythmia among athletes. Am J Med. 2010; 123: 1075–81.

20. Helenius I, Sarna S. Asthma and increased bronchial responsiveness in elite athletes: atopy and sport event as risk factors. Jour of Allergy and Immunol. 1998; 101: 646–52.

21. Krafczyk M. Exercise-Induced Bronchoconstriction: Diagnosis and Management. Am Fam Physician. 2011; 84(4): 427–34.

22. Schwartz L, Weiler J. Exercise-induced hypersensitivity syndromes in recreational and competitive athletes: a PRACTALL consensus report. Allergy. 2008; 63(8): 953–61.

23. Koch S, Koehle M. Inhaled salbutamol does not affect athletic performance in asthmatic and non-asthmatic cyclists. Br J Sports Med. 2015; 49: 51–5.

24. Elkins M, Brannan J. Warm-up exercise can reduce exercise-induced bronchoconstriction. Br J Sports Med. 2013; 47: 657–8.

25. Molis M, Molis W. Exercise-Induced Bronchospasm. Sports Health. 2010; 2(4): 311–317.

26. Plishka C, Marciniuk D. Effects of clinical pathways for chronic obstructive pulmonary disease (COPD) on patient, professional and systems outcomes: protocol for a systematic review. Syst Rev. 2016; 5: 135.

27. Maldonado D, Casas A. Effects of clinical pathways for chronic obstructive pulmonary disease patients at an altitude of 2640 meters breathing air and oxygen (FiO2 28 percent and 35 percent): a randomized crossover trial. COPD. 2014; 11(4): 401–6.

28. Rizk A, Pepin V. Acute responses to exercise training and relationship with exercise adherence in moderate chronic obstructive pulmonary disease. Chronic Respir Dis. 2015; 12(4): 329–39.

29. Winwood R. Asthma, COPD and me. COPDathlete.com.

30. Nici L, Troosters T. American Thoracic Society/European Respiratory Society statement on pulmonary rehabilitation. Am J Respir Crit Care Med. 2006; 173(12): 1390.

31. Capovilla G, Arida R. Epilepsy, seizures, physical exercise, and sports: A report from the ILAE Task Force on Sports and Epilepsy. Epilepsia. 2016; 57(1): 6–12.

32. Arida R, Scorza F. Physical Activity and Epilepsy. Sports Med 2008; 38: 607–615.

33. Arida R, Scorza F. Physical exercise in epilepsy: what kind of stressor is it? Epilepsy Behav. 2009; 16: 381–7.

34. Pimentel J, Morgado J. Seizure. 2015; 25: 87–94.

35. Arida R, Scorza F. Physical activity and epilepsy: proven and predicted benefits. Sports Med. 2008; 38(7): 607–15.

36. Carter A, Saxton J. Participant recruitment into a randomized controlled trial of exercise therapy for people with multiple sclerosis. Trial. 2015; 16: 468.

37. Motl R, Sandroff B. Benefits of Exercise Training in Multiple Sclerosis. Curr Neurol Neurosci Rep. 2015; 9: 62.

38. Heine M, Kwakkel G. Exercise Therapy for Fatigue in Multiple Sclerosis. Cochrane Database Syst Rev. 2015; 9.

39. Pleis J, Lucas J. Summary health statistics for U.S. adults: National Health Interview Survey, 2009. Vital Health Stat. 2010; 10(249).

40. Robbins L. Precipitating Factors in Migraine: A Retrospective Review of 494 Patients. Headache. 1994; 34(4): 214–216.

41. Ahn A. Why does increased exercise decrease migraine? Curr Pain Headache Rep. 2013; 12: 379.

42. Gil-Martinez A, La Touche R. Therapeutic exercise as treatment for migraine and tension-type headaches: a systematic review of randomized clinical trials. Rev Neurol. 2013; 57(10): 433–43.

43. Irby M, Penzien D. Aerobic Exercise for Reducing Migraine Burden: Mechanisms, Markers, and Models of Change Processes. Headache. 2016; 56: 357–69.

44. Koseoglu E, Bilgen M. The role of exercise in migraine treatment. J Sports Med Phys Fitness. 2015; 55: 1029–36.

45. Centers for Disease Control and Prevention. National Diabetes Statistics Report: Estimates of Diabetes and its Burdens in the United States. US Department of Health and Human Services, 2014.

46. Bally L, Stettler C. Exercise-associated glucose metabolism in individuals with type I diabetes mellitus. Curr Opin Clin Nutr Metab Care. 2015; 18: 428–33.

47. Clarke SF, Foster JR. A history of blood glucose meters and their role in self-monitoring of diabetes mellitus. Br J Biomed Sci. 2012; (3)2: 83–93.

48. Ratjen I, Weber K. Type I diabetes mellitus and exercise in competitive athletes. Exp Clin Endocrinol Diabetes. 2015; 123: 419–22.

49. Shetty V, Jones T. Effects of Exercise Intensity on Glucose Requirements to Maintain Euglycemia During Exercise in Type I Diabetes. J Clin Endocrinol Metab. 2016; 101(3): 972–80.

50. Toni S, Festini F. Managing insulin therapy during exercise in Type I diabetes mellitus. Acta Biomed. 2006; 77(1): 34–40.

51. American Thyroid Association. Prevalence and Impact of Thyroid Disease. Thyroid. org. 2016. Accessed Aug 10, 2016.

52. Ciloglu F, Ozmerdivenli R. Exercise intensity and its effects on thyroid hormones. Neuro Endocrinol Lett. 2005; 26(6): 830–4.

53. Hackney A, Battaglini C. Thyroid hormonal responses to intensive interval versus steady-state endurance exercises sessions. Hormones. 2012; 11: 54–60.

54. Lankhaar J, Backx F. Impact of overt and subclinical hypothyroidism on exercise tolerance, a systematic review. Res Q Exerc Sport. 2014; 85(3): 365–89.

55. Mainenti M, Vaisman M. Effect of levothyroxine replacement on exercise performance in subclinical hypothyroidism. J Endocrinol Invest. 2009; 32(5): 470–3.

56. Loftus EV, Jr. Clinical epidemiology of inflammatory bowel disease: Incidence, prevalence, and environmental influences. Gastroenterology. 2004; 126: 1504–17.

57. Klare P, Huber W. The impact of a ten-week physical exercise program on health-related quality of life in patients with inflammatory bowel disease: a prospective randomized controlled trial. Digestion 2015; 91: 239–47.

58. Packer N, Ward G. Does physical activity affect quality of life, disease symptoms and immune measures in patients with inflammatory bowel disease? A systematic review. J Sports Med Phys Fitness. 2010; 50: 1–18.
59. Narula N, Fedorak R. Exercise and inflammatory bowel disease. Can J Gastroenterol. 2008; 22: 497–504.
60. Stuempfle K, Hoffman M. Gastrointestinal distress is common during a 161km ultra-marathon. J Sports Sci. 2015; 33(17): 1814–21.
61. Simons S, Kennedy R. Gastrointestinal problems in runners. Curr Sports Med Rep. 2004; 3(2): 112–6.
62. Cohen D, Skipworth J. Marathon-induced ischemic colitis: why running is not always good for you. Am J Emerg Med. 2009; 27: 255–7.
63. Williams P. Effects of running and walking on osteoarthritis and hip replacement risk. Med Sci Sports Exerc. 2013; 45: 1292–7.
64. French S, Hinman R. What do people with hip or knee osteoarthritis need to know? An international consensus list of essential statements for osteoarthritis. Arthritis Care Res. 2015; 67: 809–16.
65. Klein GR, Levine BR, Hozack WJ, et al. Return to athletic activity after total hip arthroplasty. J Arthroplasty. 2007; 22: 171–175.
66. Nance J, Mammen A. Diagnostic Evaluation of Rhabdomyolysis. Muscle Nerve. 2015; 51(6): 793–810.
67. Clarkson P. Exertional Rhabdomyolysis and acute renal failure in marathon runners. Sports Med. 2007; 37: 361–3.
68. Tietze D, Borchers J. Exertional rhabdomyolysis in the athlete: a clinical review. Sports Health. 2014; 6(4)336–9.
69. Landau M, Campbell W. Rhabdomyolysis: A clinical review with a focus on genetic influences. J Clin Neuromuscul Dis. 2012; 13: 122–36.
70. Sczcepanik M, O'Connor F. Exertional Rhabdomyolysis: Identification and evaluation of the athlete at risk of recurrence. Curr Sports Med Rep. 2014; 13: 119–9.
71. Witchardt E, Henrikssen-Larsen K. Rhabdomyolysis/myoglobinemia and NSAID use during 48 hr ultra-endurance exercise. Eur J Appl Phys. 2011; 111: 1541–4.

## Chapter 22

1. P. von Rosen, A. Frohm, A. Kottorp, C. Fridén, A. Heijne Too little sleep and an unhealthy diet could increase the risk of sustaining a new injury in adolescent elite athletes. Scandinavian Journal of Medicine & Science in Sports. 19 August 2016.
2. Burke L, Deakin V. Clinical Sports Nutrition. 5th Edition. 2015.
3. Beelen M, Burke L, Gibala M, van Loon L. Nutritional Strategies to Promote Postexercise Recovery. J of Phys Activity and Health, 2010.
4. Sousa M, Teixeira V, Soares J. Dietary Strategies to recover from exercise-induced muscle damage. Int J Food Sci Nutr, 2014; 65(2): 151–163.
5. ACSM Position of the Academy of Nutrition and Dietetics of Canada and the American College of Sport Medicine: Nutrition and Athletic Performance. 2016.
6. Peternelj TT, Coombes JS. Antioxidant supplementation during exercise training: Beneficial or detrimental? Sports Med. 2011; 41 (12): 1043–1069.

7. Roberts, CK, Barnard RJ. Effects of exercise and diet on chronic disease. J Appl Physiol 2005; 98 (1): 3–30.
8. Herrera E, Jimenez R. Aruoma OI, et al. Aspects of antioxidant foods and supplements in health and disease. Nutr Rev 2009; 67: S140–4.
9. Levers, K, et al. Effects of powdered Montmorency tart cherry supplementation on acute endurance exercise performance in aerobically trained individuals. J of Int Society of Sport Nutrition. 2016; 13: 22.
10. Connolly DA1, McHugh MP, Padilla-Zakour OI, Carlson L, Sayers SP. Efficacy of a tart cherry juice blend in preventing the symptoms of muscle damage. Br J Sports Med. 2006 Aug; 40(8): 679–83; .
11. Shirreffs, S., Sawka, M. Fluid and electrolyte needs for training, competition and recovery. Journal of Sports Sciences, 2011; 29 (S!): S39-S49.
12. Dietary Guidelines 2015.
13. Bartlett JD Hawley, JA, Morton JP. Carbohydrate availability and exercise training adaptation: too much of a good thing? Eur J Sport Sci 2015; 15: 3–12.
14. Phillips, S. Dietary Protein Requirements and Adaptive Advantages in athletes. British Journal of Nutrition (2012). 108, S158–167.
15. Louis, J, et al. The impact of sleeping with reduced glycogen stores on immunity and sleep in triathletes. Eur J Appl Physiol (2016) 116: 1941–1954.
16. von Rosen, P, et al. Too little sleep and an unhealthy diet could increase the risk of sustaining a new injury in adolescent elite athletes. Scand J Med Sci Sports 2016: Aug. 1–8.
17. Burke, L., et al. Carbohydrates for training and competition. Journal of Sports Sciences, 2011; 29 (S1): S17–S27.

## Chapter 23

1. van Gent RN, Siem D, van Middelkoop M, van Os AG, Bierma-Zeinstra SM, Koes BW. Incidence and determinants of lower extremity running injuries in long distance runners: a systematic review. British journal of sports medicine. 2007; 41(8): 469–480; discussion 480.
2. Tenforde AS, Sayres LC, McCurdy ML, Collado H, Sainani KL, Fredericson M. Overuse injuries in high school runners: lifetime prevalence and prevention strategies. PM & R : the journal of injury, function, and rehabilitation. 2011; 3(2): 125–131; quiz 131.
3. Lopes AD, Hespanhol Junior LC, Yeung SS, Costa LO. What are the main running-related musculoskeletal injuries? A Systematic Review. Sports Med. 2012; 42(10): 891–905.
4. Tenforde AS, Sayres LC, Liz McCurdy M, Sainani KL, Fredericson M. Identifying Sex-Specific Risk Factors for Stress Fractures in Adolescent Runners. Medicine and science in sports and exercise. 2013.
5. Kelsey JL, Bachrach LK, Procter-Gray E, et al. Risk factors for stress fracture among young female cross-country runners. Medicine and science in sports and exercise. 2007; 39(9): 1457–1463.
6. Nattiv A, Loucks AB, Manore MM, Sanborn CF, Sundgot-Borgen J, Warren MP. American College of Sports Medicine position stand. The female athlete triad. Medicine and science in sports and exercise. 2007; 39(10): 1867–1882.

7.  Barrack MT, Gibbs JC, De Souza MJ, et al. Higher incidence of bone stress injuries with increasing female athlete triad-related risk factors: a prospective multisite study of exercising girls and women. The American journal of sports medicine. 2014; 42(4): 949–958.

8.  Tenforde AS, Barrack M, Nattiv A, Fredericson M. Parallels with the Female Athlete Triad in Male Athletes. Sports Med. 2015.

9.  Mountjoy M, Sundgot-Borgen J, Burke L, et al. The IOC consensus statement: beyond the Female Athlete Triad—Relative Energy Deficiency in Sport (RED-S). British journal of sports medicine. 2014; 48(7): 491–497.

10. Nieves JW, Melsop K, Curtis M, et al. Nutritional factors that influence change in bone density and stress fracture risk among young female cross-country runners. PM & R : the journal of injury, function, and rehabilitation. 2010; 2(8): 740–750; quiz 794.

11. Institute of Medicine Dietary reference intakes for calcium and vitamin D. National Academy of Sciences; November 2010, Report Brief. 2010. http: //wwwiomedu/~/media/ Files/Report Files/2010/Dietary-Reference-Intakes-for-Calcium-and-Vitamin-D /Vitamin D and Calcium 2010 Report Brief.pdf.

12. McKeon PO, Hertel J, Bramble D, Davis I. The foot core system: a new paradigm for understanding intrinsic foot muscle function. British journal of sports medicine. 2015; 49(5): 290.

13. Davis IS, Bowser BJ, Mullineaux DR. Greater vertical impact loading in female runners with medically diagnosed injuries: a prospective investigation. British journal of sports medicine. 2016; 50(14): 887–892.

14. Ben-Sasson SA, Finestone A, Moskowitz M, et al. Extended duration of vertical position might impair bone metabolism. Eur J Clin Invest. 1994; 24(6): 421–425.

15. Cook JL, Purdam CR. Is tendon pathology a continuum? A pathology model to explain the clinical presentation of load-induced tendinopathy. British journal of sports medicine. 2009; 43(6): 409–416.

16. Tenforde AS, Sainani KL, Carter Sayres L, Milgrom C, Fredericson M. Participation in ball sports may represent a prehabilitation strategy to prevent future stress fractures and promote bone health in young athletes. PM & R : the journal of injury, function, and rehabilitation. 2015; 7(2): 222–225.

17. Davis IS, Futrell E. Gait Retraining: Altering the Fingerprint of Gait. Phys Med Rehabil Clin N Am. 2016; 27(1): 339–355.

# INDEX

Page numbers in **bold** indicate a picture or graph. When one or more page numbers are bolded in a run of pages such as 3–**6**, there are pictures or graphs within the page run.

# Contributing Authors

William M. Adams, PhD, LAT, ATC
Assistant Professor
Director, Athletic Training Program
Department of Kinesiology School of Health & Human Sciences
University of North Carolina Greensboro

Kevin N. Alschuler, PhD
Department of Rehabilitation Medicine
University of Washington
Seattle, Washington

Natalie Badowski Wu, MD
Department of Emergency Medicine
Kaiser Permanente – San Jose Medical Center
San Jose, California

Aaron L. Baggish, MD, FACC, FACSM
Division of Cardiology
Harvard University and Massachusetts General Hospital
Boston, Massachusetts

Leslie Bonci, MPH, RDN, CSSD
Active Eating Advice
Pittsburgh, Pennsylvania

Ricardo José Soares da Costa, PhD, MSc, BSc (Hon), PGCE, PGCHE, RD,
    RSEN, APD
Department of Nutrition & Dietetics
Monash University
Melbourne, Australia

Tracy A. Cushing, MD, MPH
Department of Emergency Medicine
University of Colorado School of Medicine
Aurora, Colorado

Irene S. Davis, PhD, PT, FAPTA, FACSM, FASB
Department of Physical Medicine and Rehabilitation
Harvard Medical School, Spaulding Rehabilitation Hospital
Harvard Medical School
Cambridge, Massachusetts

Erin Drasler, MD
Department of Emergency Medicine
St. Joseph's Hospital
Denver, Colorado

Jonathan Dugas, PhD
The Science of Sports
Chicago, Illinois

Michael Fredericson, MD
Division of Physical Medicine and Rehabilitation
Department of Orthopedic Surgery
Stanford University School of Medicine
Stanford, California

Jessie R. Fudge, MD
Department of Activity, Sports, and Exercise Medicine
Group Health Conservative
Everett, Washington

N. Stuart Harris, MD
Department of Emergency Medicine
Harvard Medical School
Cambridge, Massachusetts

Tamara Hew-Butler, DPM, PhD, FACSM
Department of Exercise Science
Oakland University
Rochester, Michigan

Yuri Hosokawa, MAT, ATC
Korey Stringer Institute
Department of Kinesiology

University of Connecticut
Storrs, Connecticut

Alicia Kendig, MS, RD, CSSD
Department of Sport Science
United States Olympic Committee
Colorado Springs, Colorado

Morteza Khodaee, MD
Department of Family Medicine
University of Colorado School of Medicine
Denver, Colorado

Brian J. Krabak, MD, MBA, FACSM
Department of Rehabilitation, Orthopedics and Sports Medicine
University of Washington and Seattle Children's Sports Medicine
Seattle, Washington

Emily Krauss, MD
Division of Physical Medicine and Rehabilitation
Department of Orthopedic Surgery
Stanford University School of Medicine
Stanford, California

Erek Latzka, MD
Department of Rehabilitation, Orthopedics and Sports Medicine
University of Washington
Seattle, Washington

Daniel E. Lieberman, PhD
Department of Human Evolutionary Biology
Harvard University
Boston, Massachusetts

Grant S. Lipman, MD, FACEP, FAWM
Department of Emergency Medicine
Stanford University School of Medicine
Stanford, California

Andrew M. Luks, MD
Division of Pulmonary and Critical Care Medicine
Department of Medicine
University of Washington
Seattle, Washington

Sarah Terez Malka, MD
Department of Emergency Medicine
Harvard Medical School
Cambridge, Massachusetts

Eric K. O'Neal, CSCS, PhD
Department of Health, Physical Education and Recreation
University of North Alabama
Florence, Alabama

Jeremiah W. Ray, MD
Department of Orthopedic Surgery
Stanford University School of Medicine
Stanford, California

Rebecca L. Stearns, PhD
Korey Stringer Institute
Department of Kinesiology
University of Connecticut
Storrs, Connecticut

Trevor C. Steinbach, MD
Department of Medicine
University of Washington
Seattle, Washington

Adam S. Tenforde, MD
Department of Physical Medicine and Rehabilitation
Spaulding Rehabilitation Hospital, Spaulding National Running Center
Harvard Medical School
Cambridge, Massachusetts

Kate M. Tenforde
Cambridge, Massachusetts

Brian Toedebusch, MD
Department of Physical Medicine and Rehabilitation
University of California Davis School of Medicine
Sacramento, California

Karin VanBaak, MD
Department of Family Medicine
University of Colorado School of Medicine
Aurora, Colorado

Brandee L. Waite, MD, FAAPMR
Department of Physical Medicine and Rehabilitation
University of California Davis School of Medicine
Sacramento, California

Kendall Wu, PhD
San Jose, California